TENDINOPATHY IN ATHLETES

TENDINOPATHY IN ATHLETES

VOLUME XII OF THE ENCYCLOPAEDIA OF SPORTS MEDICINE

AN IOC MEDICAL COMMISSION PUBLICATION

IN COLLABORATION WITH

THE INTERNATIONAL FEDERATION OF SPORTS MEDICINE

EDITED BY

SAVIO L-Y. WOO, PhD, DSc

PER A.F.H. RENSTRÖM, MD, PhD

and

STEVEN P. ARNOCZKY, DVM

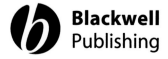

© 2007 International Olympic Committee
Published by Blackwell Publishing Ltd
Blackwell Publishing, Inc., 350 Main Street, Malden, Massachusetts 02148-5020, USA
Blackwell Publishing Ltd, 9600 Garsington Road, Oxford OX4 2DQ, UK
Blackwell Publishing Asia Pty Ltd, 550 Swanston Street, Carlton, Victoria 3053, Australia

First published 2007

2   2008

Library of Congress Cataloging-in-Publication Data
Tendinopathy in athletes / edited By Savio L-Y. Woo, Per A.F.H. Renström, and Steven P.
Arnoczky.
        p. ; cm. — (Encyclopaedia of sports medicine ; v. 12)
   "An IOC Medical Commission publication in collaboration with the International Federation
of Sports Medicine."
   Includes bibliographical references and index.
   ISBN-13: 978-1-4051-5670-7 (alk. paper)
   1. Tendons—Wounds and injuries.   2. Sports injuries.   I. Woo, Savio L-Y.
II. Renström, Per.   III. Arnoczky, Steven P.   IV. IOC Medical Commission.
V. International Federation of Sports Medicine.   VI. Series.
   [DNLM: 1. Tendinopathy.   2. Athletic Injuries.   WE 600 T2095 2007]

   RD688.T45 2007
   617.4'74044—dc22

                                                                              2006019906

ISBN-13: 978-1-4051-5670-7

A catalogue record for this title is available from the British Library

Set in 9/12pt Palatino by Graphicraft Limited, Hong Kong
Printed and bound in Singapore by Markono Print Media Pte Ltd

Commissioning Editor: Gina Almond
Editorial Assistant: Victoria Pittman
Development Editor: Nick Morgan, Adam Gilbert
Project Manager: Helen Harvey
Production Controller: Debbie Wyer

For further information on Blackwell Publishing, visit our website:
http://www.blackwellpublishing.com

Contents

List of Contributors

PAUL W. ACKERMANN MD, PhD, *Orthopedic Laboratory, Research Center, Karolinska Institutet, S-171 76 Stockholm, Sweden*

HÅKAN ALFREDSON MD, PhD, *Sports Medicine Unit, Department of Surgical and Perioperative Science, University of Umeå, 901 87 Umeå, Sweden*

LOUIS C. ALMEKINDERS MD, *North Carolina Orthopedic Clinic, Duke University Health System, 3609 Watkins Road, Durham, NC 27707, USA*

STEVEN P. ARNOCZKY DVM, *Laboratory for Comparative Orthopedic Research, College of Veterinary Medicine, Michigan State University, East Lansing, MI 48824, USA*

ALBERT J. BANES PhD, *Orthopedics Department, Biomolecular Research Building, University of North Carolina at Chapel Hill, Chapel Hill, NC 27599-7052, USA*

FRANCESCO BENAZZO MD, *Clinica Ortopedica e Traumatologica dell'Università di Pavia, Fondazione IRCCS Policlinico San Matteo, Piazzale Golgi 2, 27100 Pavia, Italy*

ROBERT BOUSHEL PhD, DMSci, *Sports Medicine Research Unit and Copenhagen Muscle Research Centre, Bispebjerg Hospital, Bispebjerg Bakke 23, DK-2400 Copenhagen NV, Denmark*

DANIEL K-I. BRING MD, *Department of Molecular Medicine and Surgery, Section for Orthopedics and Sports Medicine, Karolinska Institutet, S-171 76 Stockholm, Sweden*

DONALD BYNUM MD, *Orthopedics Department, University of North Carolina at Chapel Hill, Chapel Hill, NC 27599-7052, USA*

KAI-MING CHAN MB BS, MCh (Orth), *Department of Orthopaedics and Traumatology, The Chinese University of Hong Kong, and Department of Orthopaedics and Traumatology, Clinical Science Building, Prince of Wales Hospital, Shatin, New Territories, Hong Kong*

FRANCO COMBI MD, *F.C. Internazionale, Via Durini 24, Milano, Italy*

JILL L. COOK PhD, *Musculoskeletal Research Centre, La Trobe University, Bundoora, Victoria 3086, Australia*

JOHAN DAHL MD, *Department of Molecular Medicine and Surgery, Section for Orthopedics and Sports Medicine, Karolinska Institutet, S-171 76 Stockholm, Sweden*

VINCENT DURONIO PhD, *University of British Columbia, 2660 Oak Street, Vancouver BC, V6H 3Z6, Canada*

MONICA EGERBACHER DVM, PhD, *Laboratory for Comparative Orthopedic Research, College of Veterinary Medicine, Michigan State University, East Lansing, MI 48824, USA*

ANN MARIE FOX PhD, *Biomedical Engineering, University of North Carolina at Chapel Hill, Chapel Hill, NC 27599-7052, USA*

METTE HANSEN MSci, *Institute of Sports Medicine, Bispebjerg Hospital, Bispebjerg Bakke 23, DK 2400 Copenhagen NV, Denmark*

PHILIP HANSEN MD, *Institute of Sports Medicine, Bispebjerg Hospital, Bispebjerg Bakke 23, DK 2400 Copenhagen NV, Denmark*

DAVID A. HART PhD, *Departments of Surgery, Microbiology and Infectious Diseases and Medicine, University of Calgary, 3330 Hospital Drive NW, Calgary, AB T2N 4N1, Canada*

KATJA HEINEMEIER MSci, *Institute of Sports Medicine, Bispebjerg Hospital, Bispebjerg Bakke 23, DK 2400 Copenhagen NV, Denmark*

WEI-HSIU HSU MD, *Musculoskeletal Research Center, Department of Bioengineering, Center for Bioengineering, 300 Technology Drive, University of Pittsburgh, Pittsburgh, PA 15219, USA*

MASAKI ISHIKAWA PhD, *Neuromuscular Research Center, Department of the Biology of Physical Activity, University of Jyväskylä, FIN-40014 Jyväskylä, Finland*

DEIARY KADER MD, *Department of Orthopaedic Surgery, Queen Elizabeth Hospital, Sheriff Hill, Gateshead NE9 6SX, UK*

SPERO KARAS MD, *Orthopedics Department, University of North Carolina at Chapel Hill, Chapel Hill, NC 27599-7052, USA*

KARIM M. KHAN MD, PhD, *Department of Family Practice, University of British Columbia, 320–5950 University Boulevard, Vancouver BC, V6T 1Z3, Canada*

MICHAEL KJÆR MD, DMSci, *Sports Medicine Research Unit and Copenhagen Muscle Research Centre, Bispebjerg Hospital, Bispebjerg Bakke 23, DK-2400 Copenhagen NV, Denmark*

PAAVO V. KOMI PhD, *Neuromuscular Research Center, Department of the Biology of Physical Activity, University of Jyväskylä, FIN-40014 Jyväskylä, Finland*

SATU KOSKINEN PhD, *Institute of Sports Medicine, Bispebjerg Hospital, Bispebjerg Bakke 23, DK 2400 Copenhagen NV, Denmark*

HENNING LANGBERG PhD, *Institute of Sports Medicine, Bispebjerg Hospital, Bispebjerg Bakke 23, DK 2400 Copenhagen NV, Denmark*

MICHAEL LAVAGNINO MS, MSE, *Laboratory for Comparative Orthopedic Research, College of Veterinary Medicine, Michigan State University, East Lansing, MI 48824, USA*

NICOLA MAFFULLI MD, MS, PhD, *Department of Trauma and Orthopaedic Surgery, Keele University School of Medicine, North Staffordshire Hospital, Thornburrow Drive, Hartshill, Stoke on Trent, Staffordshire ST4 7QB, UK*

S. PETER MAGNUSSON DMSci, *Institute of Sports Medicine, Bispebjerg Hospital, Bispebjerg Bakke 23, DK 2400 Copenhagen NV, Denmark*

BENJAMIN MILLER PhD, *Department of Sport and Exercise Science, University of Auckland, 1142-NZ, New Zealand*

MARIO MOSCONI MD, *Clinica Ortopedica e Traumatologica dell'Università di Pavia, Fondazione IRCCS Policlinico San Matteo, Piazzale Golgi, 27100 Pavia, Italy*

ALLISON NATION MS, *Biomedical Engineering, University of North Carolina at Chapel Hill, Chapel Hill, NC 27599-7052, USA*

JENS L. OLESEN MD, PhD, *Institute of Sports Medicine Copenhagen, University of Copenhagen, Copenhagen, Denmark*

ALBERTO PIO MD, PhD, *Clinica Ortopedica e Traumatologica dell'Università di Pavia, Fondazione IRCCS Policlinico San Matteo, Piazzale Golgi 2, 27100 Pavia, Italy*

JIE QI PhD, *Flexcell International Corporation, 437 Dimmocks Mill Road, Hillsborough, NC 27278, USA*

PER A.F.H. RENSTRÖM MD, PhD, *Stockholm Sports Trauma Research Center, Section of Orthopedics and Sports Medicine, Department of Molecular Medicine and Surgery, Karolinska Institutet, S-171 76 Stockholm, Sweden*

ALEXANDER SCOTT MSc, BSc(PT), PhD, *University of British Columbia, Vancouver Coastal Health & Research Institute, CIHR and Michael Smith Foundation for Health Research Fellow, 2660 Oak Street, Vancouver BC, V6H 3Z6, Canada*

DAVID A. STONE MD, *MechanoBiology Laboratory and Musculoskeletal Research Center, Department of Orthopaedic Surgery, University of Pittsburgh, Pittsburgh, PA 15213, USA*

MARI TSUZAKI DDS, PhD, *Biomedical Engineering, University of North Carolina at Chapel Hill, Chapel Hill, NC 27599-7052, USA*

MICHELLE WALL PhD, *Orthopedics Department and Biomedical Engineering, University of North Carolina at Chapel Hill, Chapel Hill, NC 27599-7052, USA*

JAMES H-C. WANG PhD, *MechanoBiology Laboratory, Departments of Orthopaedic Surgery, Bioengineering, and Mechanical Engineering, Biomedical Science Tower, 210 Lothrop Street, Pittsburgh, PA 15213, USA*

NICK WEBBORN MB, MSc, *The Sussex Centre for Sport and Exercise Medicine, University of Brighton, The Welkin, Carlisle Road, Eastbourne BN20 7SN, UK*

SAVIO L-Y. WOO PhD, DSc (Hon), *Musculoskeletal Research Center, Department of Bioengineering, 405 Center for Bioengineering, 300 Technology Drive, Pittsburgh, PA 15219, USA*

XI YANG RN, *Orthopedics Department, University of North Carolina at Chapel Hill, Chapel Hill, NC 27599-7052, USA*

Forewords

The IOC Medical Commission workshop, held in October 2003 in Athens, on the understanding and prevention of tendinopathy in the athlete was a major event in the study of this debilitating condition for participants in a wide variety of sports activities. The participants in this workshop represented the most knowledgeable and experienced clinicians and scientists in the world. An outcome of this important meeting is this volume, which becomes an integral and important addition to the IOC Medical Commission's *Encyclopaedia of Sports Medicine*.

The manuscripts received from the workshop participants represent the highest quality of science. The diligent interaction of the three co-editors with the contributing authors has resulted in a highly readable text that should serve in excellent fashion as a resource for thousands of clinicians and scientists around the world. The health and welfare of athletes, not only in Olympic events, but also at all levels of international, regional, and national competition, are important objectives for the IOC.

Tendinopathy in Athletes will help the medico-scientific community to better understand this problem and constitutes the most valuable reference for this medical condition for many years to come.

I express my sincere appreciation for the excellent work of the co-editors and contributing authors who participated in this project.

Dr Jacques Rogge
President of the International Olympic Committee

The publication of *The Encyclopaedia of Sports Medicine* began in 1988 and, through the years, the eleven volumes have included a wide variety of topics as applied to sports. This has involved such areas as clinical medicine, physiology, biochemistry, and biomechanics including such special considerations as endurance, strength and power, children and adolescents, nutrition, and women in sport. This volume, *Tendinopathy in Athletes*, is unique in that it brings focus to a medical condition that prevents athletes from preparing for competition and from the competition, itself, in a wide variety of sports.

The information presented by the contributing authors consists of a blend of basic science, clinical science, and the practical application of this science to the treatment of patients. The successful dissemination of state-of-the-art information about tendinopathy for the edification of medical doctors and sports scientists around the world should provide an excellent basis for the improved medical treatment of athletes.

The IOC Medical Commission is immensely pleased that this valuable contribution is being made to the international literature of sports medicine and sports science.

Arne Ljungqvist, MD
Chairman, IOC Medical Commission

Preface

Tendinopathy remains one of the most common injuries encountered in sports or at the workplace. It encompasses various tendon injuries including tendinosis, tendonitis, paratenonitis, as well as paratenonitis with tendinosis (Khan *et al*. 1999). In effect, tendinopathies are the inability of the tendon to return to its homeostatic balance. It accounts for 30–50% of all sports injuries (Renstrom *et al*. 1991), while being involved in more than 48% of reported occupational maladies (NIOSH 1996). However, despite its high incidence, the precise etiopathogenesis and effective treatment(s) of tendinopathy remain elusive. The often insidious progression and potentially catastrophic sequelae of this problem have made the study of tendinopathy a priority topic by the International Olympic Academy of Sports Science.

The IOC Olympic Academy of Sports Science is an honor society founded in 1999 by the late Prince Alexander De Merode within the IOC Medical Commission and sponsored by Parke-Davis/Werner-Lambert/Pfizer. In October 2003, the Academy convened a workshop on "Understanding and Prevention of Tendinopathy in the Athlete" in Athens, Greece. The workshop brought together clinicians and scientists from all over the world to discuss the latest information available on tendinopathy. The topics covered were epidemiology, tendon biology and biomechanics, training and physical therapy, and clinical management including alternative approaches to the treatment of these ailments. We have taken the information presented at this workshop and have asked the authors to update and expand their discussions for this book.

The result is a comprehensive reference which covers all aspects of tendinopathy. We have organized our chapters logically for the reader, starting with defining the problem of tendinopathy to etiology and epidemiology, followed by the molecular, metabolic, cellular, tissue and nerve pathologies, as well as particular molecular and cellular mechanisms. These chapters are followed by a biomechanical study of *in vivo* tendon function, as well as new information on the innervation of tendons and its potential role in tendinopathy. Finally, treatment modalities including new molecular and biological approaches, plus surgical and alternative approaches for tendinopathies are discussed. For the ease of the reader, the text in each chapter has a uniform format consisting of an abstract, introduction, what we know and its' clinical significance; the authors conclude their chapters with suggestions for future research directions. By doing this, we hope the text will not only serve as a comprehensive reference for scientists, clinicians and students, but also provide a stimulus and "roadmap" for continued basic science and clinical investigations into the prevention and treatment of tendinopathy.

We are extremely pleased that *Tendinopathy in Athletes* is included in the prestigious series of the *IOC Encyclopedia of Sports Medicine*. We are indebted to many who have helped so much in the publication of this book. We are especially grateful to Dr. Arne Ljungqvist for his distinguished leadership of the IOC medical commission and his enthusiastic and continued support of the workshop and the publication of this book. We are also greatly appreciative of Professor Howard "Skip" Knuttgen for his guidance and support, and Dr. Patrick Schamasch and the IOC Medical Commission for their cooperation in this effort. In addition, we wish to recognize Gina Almond and Nick Morgan at Blackwell Publishing for their assistance with the commissioning and production of the book, and Mrs Serena Saw for her tireless efforts in helping the editors and authors throughout this entire process.

Savio L-Y. Woo, PhD, DSc (Hon)
Per Renström, MD, PhD
Steven P. Arnoczky, DVM

References

Khan KM, Cook JL, Bonar F, Harcourt P, Åström M. (1999) Histopathology of common tendinopathies. Update and implications for clinical management. *Sports Medicine* **27**(6), 393–408.

Renström P. (1991) Sports traumatology today. A review of common current sports injury problems. *Annales Chirurgiae et Gynaecologiae* (Helsinki) **80**(2), 81–93.

Chapter 1

Tendinopathy: A Major Medical Problem in Sport

PER A.H.F. RENSTRÖM AND SAVIO L-Y. WOO

Tendinopathy is a major medical problem associated with sports and physical activity in active people over 25 years of age. It can be defined as a syndrome of tendon pain, localized tenderness, and swelling that impairs performance. The clinical diagnosis is determined mainly through the history, although the exact relationship between symptoms and pathology remains unknown. In chronic tendinopathy, there is an increasing degree of degeneration with little or no inflammation present. Increasing age results in decline of the ultimate load of the muscle–tendon–bone complex, ultimate strain, as well as modulus of elasticity and tensile strength of the tendon.

The management of tendinopathy is often based on a trial and error basis. Controlled motion and exercise are the cornerstone of treatment, as human tendon tissue responds to mechanical loading both with a rise in metabolic and circulatory activity as well as with an increase in extracellular matrix synthesis. These changes contribute to the training-induced adaptation in biomechanical properties whereby resistance to loading is altered, tolerance towards strenuous exercise can be improved, and further injury avoided. Using eccentric exercise has been shown to be effective. Extracorporal shock wave therapy and sclerosing therapy are fairly recent and promising techniques but more research is needed. Surgery is also an option but return to sports after surgery is reported in only 60–85% of cases. It should be noted that those reports with higher success rates following surgery are associated with a poor overall methodologic scoring system.

The treatment of tendinopathy is difficult and can be frustrating. Recovery takes time as there is no quick fix. The patient's return to sports after surgery may take a long time to avoid re-injury. Thus, tendinopathy remains one of the most challenging areas in orthopedic sports medicine. In this chapter, we review topics in tendinopathy including the incidence of injury in sports, factors associated with its development, pathology, diagnosis, and clinical management.

Introduction

Tendinopathy, a major medical problem associated with sports and physical activity, is a generic descriptor of the clinical conditions in and around tendons resulting from overload and overuse. As it is difficult to determine the pathologic changes for most patients, investigators today use a classification system based on pain and function. Tendinopathy can be defined as a syndrome of tendon pain, localized tenderness, and swelling that impair performance. This condition is aggravated by additional physical and sports activity.

The physiology of tendinopathy remains largely unknown. The condition may be called tendinosis, which is defined as intratendinous degeneration (i.e. hypoxic, mucoid or myxoid, hyaline, fatty, fibrinod, calcific, or some combination of these) resulting from a variety of causes such as ageing, microtrauma, and vascular compromise (Jósza & Kannus 1997). It is often detected when the clinical examination is supplemented with magnetic resonance imaging (MRI) and/or ultrasonography which shows changes in the tendon tissue. The syndrome can include inflammatory changes in the tendon sheath and terms such as tenosynovitis, paratenonitis, and peritendinitis have been used. Others further suggest that the terms tendinosis and paratendinitis should not be used until after histologic examination (Maffulli *et al.* 1998).

Diagnosis is mostly determined through the history, although the exact relationship between symptoms and pathology remains unknown (Curwin & Stanish 1984). Pain during activity is the cardinal symptom in tendinopathy and swelling is often present. Tenderness on palpation will support the diagnosis. MRI and ultrasonography can be used to verify the diagnosis.

The most well-known problems are Achilles tendinopathy, patellar tendinopathy, quadriceps and hamstrings tendinopathy, rotator cuff tendinopathy, tennis and golf elbow epicondylitis, as well as paratendinopathy in the wrist and hand (de Quervain disease). These issues are discussed in this book. The findings can, to a large extent, be applied to most chronic tendon problems around the ankle, knee, hip, wrist, elbow, and shoulder joints.

Tendon has a unique structure. Its parallel collagen fibers are suitable for the tendon to resist high tensile load without excessive elongation. The muscle–tendon–bone complex is involved in almost every human motion. Some of the strongest tissues in the body are the Achilles and the patellar tendons. Nevertheless, these tendons can still be frequently injured and the unanswered question is why are they so prone to injury.

Biomechanically, tendons are subjected to very high loads—thus causing tendons to be injured and result in pain that could lead to chronic pathology. Repair and remodeling are unusually slow and are not evident in great amounts. In addition, the injury takes a long time to heal. In acute tendon injury, however, repair tissues are present in the healing process. Biomechanical changes include a decrease in ultimate load and strain, decrease in tensile strength, and changes in collagen cross-links (Józsa & Kannus 1997).

Tendinopathy is to a large extent a work and sports-induced problem. In the initial phase of tendon injury, there is often inflammation present. However, in a more chronic setting, there is an increasing degree of degeneration, especially with increasing age, with little or no inflammation. Most inflammatory changes take place in the paratenon and are accompanied by areas of focal degeneration within the tendon (Backman *et al.* 1990). It would be uncommon for tendon degeneration to occur without some inflammatory changes around the tendon.

The etiology and pathology are still not well known and therefore the management of tendinopathy is often based on a trial and error basis. The treatment can vary from country to country, from clinic to clinic, and from clinician to clinician (Kannus & Jósza 1997).

Tendon and sport

Tendinopathy is thought to follow frequent actions involving quick accelerations and decelerations, eccentric activities, and quick cutting actions. Thus, the location of such injuries is sports specific.

Achilles tendinopathy can occur in sports activities such as running, jumping, or in team sports, such as football and team handball, as well as in racquet sports, such as tennis and badminton. The incidence in tennis players is 2–4% and 9% in dancers (Winge *et al.* 1989). The incidence in nonathletes is 25–30% (Åström 1997). However, for a long time, Achilles tendinopathy had been considered to be a running injury, with a high incidence, 6–18% of all injuries, especially during the running boom during the 1980s (Clement *et al.* 1984). The incidence seems to have decreased during the last 15 years, partly because of increasing awareness and prevention, but also perhaps a result of the improved quality and design of footwear. Still, there is a yearly incidence of 24–64% in runners (Hoeberigs 1992; van Mechelen 1995) while the prevalence in middle and long-distance runners is 7–11% (James *et al.* 1978; Lysholm & Wiklande 1987; Winge *et al.* 1989; Teitz 1997). The rate of Achilles tendinopathy among orienteering runners was 29% compared with 4% in the control group (Kujala *et al.* 1999).

Thirty percent of patients with Achilles tendinopathy have bilateral problems (Paavola *et al.* 2002b). In most cases, the problems are located to the medial side of the Achilles tendon while the lateral side is involved in every fifth case (Gibbon 2000).

Patellar tendinopathies are often associated with jumping sports such as basketball, volleyball, tennis, and high jump, as well as ice-hockey, football, downhill running, and weight lifting. Tennis players, baseball players, and golfers may develop lateral and medial elbow epicondylitis. Hamstring syndromes involving the proximal tendons are common in athletics. Rotator cuff tendinopathy occurs in throwing sports such as baseball, javelin, and team handball, as well as in volleyball, tennis, and gymnastics.

Known factors associated with tendinopathy

Many factors contribute to the development of tendinopathy: extrinsic factors, such as training errors and environmental conditions, as well as intrinsic factors, such as malalignment. In addition, increasing age as well as gender are also overall factors that can influence the development of tendinopathy.

Extrinsic factors

Tendinopathy can be caused by an interaction of extrinsic factors including training errors, such as excessive distance, intensity, hill work, technique, and fatigue, as well as playing surface, which seems to be predominant in acute injuries. Clinically, it is known that a change in load, training errors (linked to a change in load), changes in the environment, and changes or faults with equipment such as racquets can result in an onset of tendon symptoms (Jósza & Kannus 1997). Environmental conditions such as cold weather during outdoor training can also be a risk factor (Milgrom 2003). Footwear and equipment may also play a part. However, there is little evidence to support other extrinsic factors and further research is required.

Intrinsic factors

Intrinsic factors related to Achilles tendinopathy include the malalignment of the lower extremity, which occurs in 60% of Achilles disorders. There is an increased forefoot pronation (Nigg 2001), limited mobility of the subtalar joint, decrease of range of motion of the ankle (Kvist 1991), varus deformity of the forefoot, increased hind foot inversion, and decreased dorsiflexion with the knee in extension (Kaufmann et al. 1999). Other factors that have been discussed include decreased flexibility, leg length discrepancy, muscle weakness, or imbalance. Åström (1997) concluded in his PhD thesis that malalignments may not be of clinical importance. Biomechanical abnormalities may still be corrected but the clinical outcome has yet to be validated. We should remember that there is a lack of high-quality prospective studies, which limit the conclusions that can be drawn regarding these factors.

Age

Even though the rate of tendon degeneration with age can be reduced by regular activity (Józsa & Kannus 1997), age is indeed a factor with respect to tendon injury. In patients less than 18 years of age, the problems are usually located in the muscle tendon junction or tendon insertion to bone. Younger tendons are smaller and can withstand more stress than older tendons (Ker 2002). Between 18 and 55 years of age there is an increasing incidence of tendinopathy in Achilles and patellar tendinopathy with clinical problems especially after 30–35 years of age. Patellar tendinopathy seems to have a similar prevalence in adolescents as adult athletes (Cook et al. 2000a). Shoulder injuries, especially rotator cuff problems, are increasingly frequent with increasing age especially in patients over 55 years of age. They account for 18% of cases.

Increasing age also results in changes in the structure and function of human tendons as the collagen fibers increase in diameter and decrease in tensile strength. The ultimate strain, ultimate load, modulus of elasticity, and tensile strength of the tendon also declines (Kannus & Józsa 1991). The most characterized age-related changes are degeneration of the tenocytes and collagen fibers and accumulation of lipids and calcium deposits (Kannus & Józsa 1991). Well-structured, long-term exercise appears to have a beneficial effect and minimize the negative effects on aging tendons (Tuite et al. 1997).

Gender

Achilles tendinopathy seems equally common in men and women (Mafi et al. 2001; Mafulli et al. 2005). However, larger cohort studies have found that there may be a decreased risk for females to develop patellar tendinopathy (Cook et al. 2000a).

In running, 60% of injuries occur in men. Many of these injuries involve tendinopathy and related issues. Women under 30 years are at the highest risk (Järvinen 1992). However, some studies have found no decreased risk of tendinopathy in females compared to males.

Work-induced tendinopathy, especially involving repetitive overloading of the muscle–tendon unit, is also common. This is characterized by being present in over 60% of women with a mean age of 41 years. The upper limb is involved in 93% of the cases of which 63% occur in the forearm and 24% is elbow epicondylitis. The remaining problems come from the neck, back, and lower limbs (Kivi 1984).

Pathology

In chronic tendinopathy, science has shown minimal or no inflammation (Arner et al. 1959; Puddu et al. 1976). This was verified by Alfredson et al. (1999), who found no physiologic increase in prostataglandin E_2 in the injured human Achilles tendon. Animal models also suggest that inflammation does not occur in the overused tendinopathy process. However, it is important to know that the absence of inflammatory mediators in end-stage disease does not mean that they were not present in early-stage disease. These mediators may still be a factor in the cause of tendinopathy. Mechanical load can increase the tendinosus and peritendinous levels of prostataglandins (Almekinders et al. 1993). Thus, inflammation could be associated with tendinopathy at some point in time.

Tendon impingement could also be a contributing factor to tendon pathology. For example, between the Achilles tendon and the calcaneal bone there is a retrocalcaneal bursa, which can be impinged between the Achilles tendon and the bony posterior aspect of the calcaneus. In some cases with bony prominence, impingement is likely, with resulting bursitis and tendinopathy. Another example of impingement may involve patellar tendinopathy (Johnson et al. 1996). However, others have found that the superficial attachment of the proximal patellar tendon is far stronger than its depth would indicate. There is pain in the early phases of landing with the knee in an extended position. Pain increases on palpation with the knee in full extension, making it less likely that such impingement could be a major contributing factor.

Where is the pain coming from in tendinopathy?

What causes tendon pain? Tendon degeneration with mechanical breakdown of collagen could theoretically explain the pain mechanism but clinical and surgical observations challenge this view (Khan et al. 2003). Structural changes are unlikely to be the main cause. Recently, the combination of biomechanical and biochemical changes has become a more plausible explanation for the cause of pain. Preliminary evidence shows that unidentified biochemical noxious compounds such as glutamate, substance P, or calcitonin gene-related peptide (CGRP) may be involved (Ackermann 2003; Alfredson 1999; Danielson et al. 2006).

Neural factors such as sensory neuropeptides show that tendinous tissues are supplied with a complex network of neuronal mediators involved in the regulation of nociception vasoactivity and inflammation (Ackermann et al. 2003). In response to injury, the expression of neuropeptides is significantly altered, suggesting a synchronized mechanism in nociception and tissue repair. Further studies must be performed to determine if the neuronal pathways of tendon healing can be stimulated by specific rehabilitation programs or by external delivery of mediators and/or nerve growth factors.

Diagnosis of tendinopathy

In most cases, the patient's history should secure a correct diagnosis. Pain with activity, often combined with impaired performance, is the key component. The catchwords "Too much, too soon, too often" are often heard in the patient's history. Careful clinical examination will verify the diagnosis as the pain is often associated with localized tenderness and swelling.

Robinson *et al.* (2001) has developed a questionnaire, the Victorian Institute of Sports Assessment—Achilles questionnaire (VISA-A score), which can be used to evaluate the clinical severity of Achilles tendinopathy. This has also been used to evaluate the outcome of treatment (Peers *et al.* 2003) and can provide a guideline for treatment as well as for monitoring the effect of treatment (Silbernagel *et al.* 2005). This score is also useful for patellar tendinopathy (Frohm *et al.* 2004).

Ultrasonography is a valuable but not perfect tool for the diagnosis and evaluation of tendinopathy, particularly for patellar tendinopathy (Cook *et al.* 2000a). Ultrasonography is a very helpful guiding tool when minor biopsies are to be taken from the tendon tissue. MRI detects abnormal tissue with greater sensitivity than ultrasound (Movin 1998). In a recent observation, both ultrasound and MRI showed a moderate correlation with clinical abnormality at baseline (Peers *et al.* 2003). In Achilles tendinopathy, MRI was associated with clinical findings. However, it should be mentioned that tendon imaging findings can still be asymptomatic. Therefore, MRI must always be correlated to the clinical symptoms.

Management of tendinopathy—what do we know?

As the exact etiology, pathophysiology, and healing mechanisms of tendinopathy are not well known, it is difficult to prescribe a proper treatment regimen. So far, the given treatments are frequently based on empirical evidence and so recommended treatment strategies by different clinicians can vary greatly (Paavola *et al.* 2002b). Nevertheless, the first course would be to identify and remove those external factors and forces, especially excessive training regimens. Also, intrinsic factors, such as lack of flexibility, increased foot pronation, and impingement, should also be corrected.

Exercise—key to success in prevention and management

Exercise is an important factor in the prevention of tendinopathy but it has emerged also as a successful factor in the management of tendinopathy. Exercise combined with specified loading conditions will make the tendon more resistant to injury. Human tendon tissue responds to mechanical loading both with a rise in metabolic and circulatory activity as well as with an increase in extracellular matrix synthesis. These changes contribute to the training-induced adaptation in mechanical properties whereby resistance to loading is altered and tolerance towards strenuous exercise can be improved and injury avoided (Kjaer 2004). In other words, exercise during healing of an injury stimulates faster healing (Jósza *et al.* 1992).

The concept of using eccentric exercise in tendinopathy was introduced by Stanish and Curwin in 1984 and has been shown to function well in a number of studies (Curwin & Stanish 1984; Stanish *et al.* 1986; Fyfe & Stanish 1992; Alfredson & Lorentzon 2003). It has been shown to be superior to concentric training (Niesen-Vertommen *et al.* 1992) and effective in prospective randomized studies (Alfredson *et al.* 1998; Mafi *et al.* 2001; Alfredson & Lorentzon 2003). More than 80% of patients were satisfied with the treatment and could return to previous activity levels. However, the results for insertional injuries were not satisfactory. Curwin and Stanish (1984) stressed careful attention to the level of pain as a high level of pain or pain too early in the exercise program could cause worsening of the symptoms.

There was increased collagen synthesis and cross-sectional area after a session with eccentric exercise (Magnusson & Kjaer 2003; Crameri *et al.* 2004). An ongoing study indicated that weekly overload eccentric exercises, using weights up to 300 kg in a specifically constructed machine called Bromsman, might be effective in the management of tendinopathy (Frohm, personal communication). These studies support the results from previous studies by Woo *et al.* (1982) which showed prolonged exercise is effective and results in an increase in the cross-sectional area of extensor tendons as well as its mechanical properties.

A well-defined exercise regimen should be the cornerstone of treatment of tendinopathy. Knowledge of the tendon in response to tensile loading can be used successfully to manage most tendon overuse injuries (Stanish *et al.* 1986; Magnusson & Kjaer 2003). However, it should be pointed out that exercise alone does not solve all cases of tendinopathy.

Patients with long-standing Achilles tendinopathy may be instructed to continue Achilles tendon loading activity with the use of a pain monitoring model during the treatment (Silbernagel 2006). This model may help the patient as well as the clinician to handle the pain and determine how the exercises should progress.

Physical therapy

Physical therapy is important. Regular attention to the problem in combination with hands-on techniques enables the patient to feel more relaxed and better as a whole. Some rehabilitation techniques such as eccentric training can be very difficult for the patient to perform properly without supervision. Although the scientific evidence is limited and in some cases controversial, modalities such as heat, ultrasound, electrical stimulation, laser stimulation, and acupuncture may be effective. Systematic reviews of the effect of ultrasound to treat soft tissues in general showed little efficacy except in the treatment of calcific tendinopathy and lateral epicondylitis (van der Windt et al. 1999).

Recently, some newer treatment techniques have been introduced. Extracorporal shock wave therapy has been reported effective (Rompe et al. 1996) and shows a comparable outcome to surgery of patellar tendinopathy (Peers et al. 2003). Sclerosing therapy focusing on destroying the new vessels and accompanying nerves showed very promising short-term clinical results (Alfredson & Öhberg 2004). As a whole, much more research is needed before these new procedures can be recommended routinely.

Corticosteroid injections

Corticosteroid injections are designed to suppress inflammation. As tendinopathy is not an inflammatory condition, the value of injection may be to reduce adhesions between the tendon and sheath as well as to medicate pain in the short term. However, the adverse effects of corticosteroids may be recognized and caution is needed. A corticosteroid injection may inhibit collagen synthesis and delay tendon healing. Partial ruptures are also common (Åström 1998). In addition, peritendinous injections may also have deleterious effects (Paavola et al. 2002). In conclusion, it is fair to say that the biologic basis of the effect of corticoid injections and benefits are largely lacking. Above all, one should avoid injections into the tendon substance.

Surgical management

It should be remembered that a surgical incision, in itself, results in a strong healing response. Clinicians have suggested needling, coblation, percutateous tenotomy, arthroscopic debridement, percutaneous paratenon stripping, open tenotomy, paratenon stripping, and tendon grafting (Maffulli et al. 2005). However, the surgical technique as such in open surgery is probably not very important in the management of tendinopathies. Furthermore, endoscopic arthroscopic techniques have seemed to gradually take over.

As the physiologic, biomechanical, and biologic base of the effect of surgery are not clearly understood, it is not possible to establish the relationship between operative treatment and the healing and reparative process. In general, a return to sports after surgery has been reported in 60–85% of cases. Again, we caution that the higher the reported success rates of surgery, the worse the overall methodologic score in published paper (Tallon et al. 2001).

Healing and return to sport take time

Patients' return to sports following surgical management of tendinopathy may take a long time. The rule of thumb for their return has been no increase of symptoms. First time ailments may require 2–3 months to recover but chronic cases may take 4–6 months in the case of Achilles tendinopathy, 6–8 months for patellar tendinopathy, and 8–12 months for rotator cuff tendinopathy.

So, why does it take such a long time? As tendons have limited vascularity and a slow metabolic rate, the tenocytes that produce collagen have a very slow turnover rate of 50–100 days (Peacock 1959). Healing and remodeling of the Achilles tendon of the rabbit requires 4 months (Williams 1986) and complete regeneration of the tendon is never achieved. If a tendon is given inadequate time to repair, tenocytes may undergo apotosis because of excessive strain. So, the message here is that even though the athlete would like to return to their sport quickly, the clinician must advocate that time for healing be allowed in order to avoid re-injury. Recovery from tendinopathy often takes time and there is no quick fix. Such treatment regimens often lead to frustration and re-injury. The use of controlled exercise programs can be effective but a clear understanding of the mechanisms is largely lacking.

Future directions

Aging and exercise influence the degenerative process, which has an important role in the development of tendinopathy. However, regular exercise appears to have a beneficial effect on aging tendons and may delay the degenerative changes. Therefore, more studies need to be performed in order to define a quantitative relationship: what would be the appropriate amount of usage and at what stress levels for the maintenance of homeostasis. Meanwhile, it is also important to recognize the large differences in the development of tendinopathies between normal and diseased tendons. Because these tendinopathies come from different origins, they do not have the same cell phenotypes and will respond to the mechanical and biologic milieu differently (Fig. 1.1). Therefore, different strategies are needed for the appropriate management of these tendinopathies. As such, appropriate strategies for management and maintenance of tendon homeostasis and tendon remodeling must be developed to avoid tendinopathy.

Many athletes are at risk for developing tendinopathy. Activities such as basketball, triple jump, tennis, badminton, and running continue to be the main sports that increase risk. Downhill eccentric activities can also be a problem. With increasing demands, intensified training, and more frequent athletic contests, it is vital to analyze these sports and activity schedules in order to design preventive programs.

Exercise and load are the key parameters for an ideal and effective treatment. Too much load and activity too early may generate pain and more severe injury as well as significantly delay the healing process. During passive static stretching, the mechanical properties of the muscle–tendon unit are affected during the actual stretch maneuver and stress relaxation occurs. However, this mechanical effect appears to disappear rapidly within minutes. Stretching produces gains in maximal joint range of motion and habitual stretching may improve maximal muscle strength and the height of a jump. The currently available evidence does not support the notion that stretching prior to exercise can effectively reduce risk of injury. However, stretching includes exercise and load, and may favorably affect the homeostatis of tendons. As such, the effect of stretching on tendons needs to be further studied.

Tendon healing after injury will not result in a normal tendon. The results may be often functionally

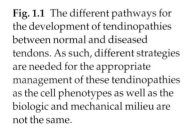

Fig. 1.1 The different pathways for the development of tendinopathies between normal and diseased tendons. As such, different strategies are needed for the appropriate management of these tendinopathies as the cell phenotypes as well as the biologic and mechanical milieu are not the same.

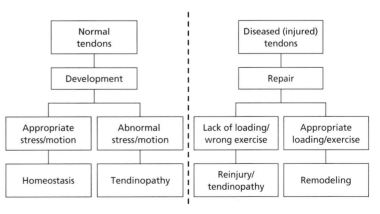

satisfactory despite its biomechanical weakness and morphologic inferiority. The effect of growth factors and gene therapy with the aim to "normalize" the healing tendon are intriguing and seem promising but are far from being ready for clinical use. However, there are exciting possibilities on prevention of tendon degeneration as well as promoting tendon regeneration after injury.

Tendinopathy is without doubt one of the most difficult areas in orthopedic sports medicine. The research on this common problem needs to be intensified in the coming years. This IOC workshop was therefore an important catalyst as it allowed many front line researchers to get together, share their knowledge, and discuss future directions that can lead to solving the enigma of tendinopathy.

References

Ackermann, P.W., Ahmed, M. & Kreicsbergs, A. (2003) Early nerve regeneration after Achilles tendon rupture: a prerequisite for healing? *Journal of Orthopedic Research* **20**, 849–856.

Alfredson, H., Pietilä, T. & Jonsson, P., *et al.* (1998) Heavy-load eccentric calf muscle training for the treatment of chronic Achilles tendinosis. *American Journal of Sports Medicine* **26**, 360–366.

Alfredson, H., Thorsen, K. & Lorentzon, R. (1999) *In situ* microdialysis in tendon tissue high levels of glutamate but not of prostaglandin E$_2$ in chronic Achilles tendon pain. *Knee Surgery, Sports Traumatology, Arthroscopy* **7**, 378–381.

Alfredson, H. & Lorentzon, R. (2003) Intratendinous glutamate levels and eccentric training in chronic Achilles tendinosis: a prospective study using microdialysis technique. *Knee Surgery, Sports Traumatolology, Arthroscopy* **11**, 196–199.

Alfredson, H. & Öhberg, L. (2004) Sclerosing injections to areas of neovascularisation reduce pain in chronic Achilles tendinopathy: a double-blind randomized controlled trial. *Knee Surgery, Sports Traumatology, Arthroscopy* **13**, 74–80.

Almekinders, L.C., Banes, A.J. & Ballenger, C.A. (1993) Effects of repetitive motion on human fibroblasts. *Medicine and Science in Sports and Exercise* **25**, 603–607.

Arner, O., Lindholm, A. & Orell, S.R. (1959) Histologic changes in subcutaneous rupture of the Achilles tendon; a study of 74 cases. *Acta Chirurgica Scandinavica* **116**, 484–490.

Åström, M. (1997) *On the nature and etiology of chronic Achilles tendinopathy* [dissertation]. University of Lund, Sweden.

Åström, M. (1998) Partial rupture in chronic Achilles tendinopathy: a retrospective analysis of 342 cases. *Acta Orthopaedica Scandinavica* **69**, 404–407.

Åström, M. & Westlin, N. (1992) No effect of piroxicam on Achilles tendinopathy: a randomized study of 70 patients. *Acta Orthopaedica Scandinavica* **63**, 631–634.

Backman, C., Boquist, L., Friden, J., Lorentzon, R. & Toolanen, G. (1990) Chronic achilles paratenonitis with tendinosis: an experimental model in the rabbit. *Journal of Orthopaedic Research* **8**, 541–547.

Clement, D.B., Taunton, J.E. & Smart, G.W. (1984) Achilles tendonitis and peritendinitis: etiology and treatment. *American Journal of Sports Medicine* **12**, 179–184.

Cook, J.L., Kiss, Z.S., Khan, K.M., Purdam, C. & Griffiths, L. (2000a) Prospective imaging study of asymptomatic patellar tendinopathy in elite junior basketball players. *Journal of Ultrasound in Medicine* **19**, 473–479.

Cook, J.L., Khan, K.M., Kiss, Z.S., Coleman, B. & Griffiths, L. (2000b) Asymptomatic hypoechoic regions on patellar tendon US do not foreshadow symptoms of jumper's knee: a 4 year followup of 46 tendons. *Scandinavian Journal of Science and Medicine in Sports* **11**, 321–327.

Crameri, R.M., Langberg, H., Teisner, B., *et al.* (2004) Enhanced procollagen processing in skeletal muscle after a single bout of eccentric loading in humans. *Matrix Biology* **23**, 259–264.

Curwin, S. & Stanish, W.D. (1984) *Tendinitis: Its Etiology and Treatment.* Collamore Press, Lexington.

Danielson, P., Alfredson, H. & Forsgren, S. (2006) Distribution of general (PGP 9.5) and sensory (substance P/CGRP) innervations in the human patellar tendon. *Knee Surgery, Sports Traumatology, Arthroscopy* **14**, 125–132.

Frohm, A., Saartok, T., Edman, G. & Renstrom, P. (2004) Swedish translation of the VISA-P outcome score for patellar tendinopathy. *BMC Musculoskeletal Disorders* **18**, 49.

Fyfe, I. & Stanish, W.D. (1992) The use of eccentric training and stretching in the treatment and prevention of tendon injuries. *Clinical Sports Medicine* **11**, 601–624.

Gibbon, W.W. (2000) Musculoskeletal ultrasound. *Baillieres Clinical Rheumatology* **10**, 561–588.

Frohm A., Saartok T., Edman G. & Renstrom P. (2004) Swedish translation of the VISA-P outcome score for patellar tendinopathy. *BMC Musculoskeletal Disorders* **18**, 4.

Fyfe, I. & Stanish, W.D. (1992) The use of eccentric training and stretching in the treatment and prevention of tendon injuries. *Clinical Sports Medicine* **11**, 601–624.

Gibbon, W.W. (2000) Musculoskeletal ultrasound. *Baillieres Clinical Rheumatology* **10**, 561–588.

Hoeberigs, J.H. (1992) Factors related to the incidence of running injuries: a review. *Sports Medicine* **13**, 408–422.

James, S.L., Bates, B.T. & Osternig, L.R. (1978) Injuries to runners. *American Journal of Sports Medicine* **6**, 40–50.

Järvinen, M. (1992) Epidemiology of tendon injuries in sports. *Clinical Sports Medicine* **11**, 493–504.

Johnson, D.P., Wakeley, C.J. & Watt, I. (1996) Magnetic resonance imaging of patellar tendonitis. *Journal of Bone and Joint Surgery. British volume* **78**, 452–457.

Józsa, L., Renström, P., Järvinen, M., *et al.* (1992) The effects of training, immobilization and remobilization on musculoskeletal tissue. *Scandinavian Journal of Medicine and Science in Sports* **2**, 100–118.

Józsa, L.G. & Kannus, P. (1997) *Human Tendons: Anatomy, Physiology, and Pathology.* Human Kinetics, Champaign, IL: 164–253.

Kannus, P. & Józsa, L.G. (1991) Histopathological changes preceding spontaneous rupture of a tendon: a controlled study of 891 patients. *Journal of Bone and Joint Surgery. American volume* **73**, 1507–1525.

Kaufmann, K.R., Brodine, S., Schaffer R.A., Johnson, C.W. & Cullison T.R. (1999) The effect of foot structure and range of motion on musculoskeletal overuse injuries. *American Journal of Sports Medicine* **27**, 585–593.

Ker, R.F. (2002) The implications of the adaptable fatigue quality of tendons for their construction, repair, and function. *Comparative Biochemistry and Physiology and Molecular and Integrative Physiology* **133**, 987–1000.

Khan, K.M., Forster, B.B., Robinson, J., *et al.* (2003) Are ultrasound and magnetic resonance imaging of value in assessment of Achilles tendon disorders? A two year prospective study. *British Journal of Sports Medicine* **37**, 149–153.

Kivi, P. (1984) Rheumatic disorders of the upper limbs associated with repetitive occupational tasks in Finland in 1975–1979. *Scandinavian Journal of Rheumatology* **13**, 101–107.

Kjaer, M. (2004) Role of extracellular matrix in adaptation of tendon and skeletal muscle in response to physical activity. *Physiology Review* **84**, 64998.

Kujala, U.M., Sarna, S., Kaprio, J., Konskenvuo, M. & Karjalainen, J. (1999) Heart attacks and lower limb function in master endurance athletes. *Medicine and Science in Sports and Exercise* **31**, 1041–1046.

Kvist, M. (1991) Achilles tendon injuries in athletes. *Annals Chirurgie Gynecologie* **80**, 88–201.

Lysholm, J. & Wiklande, J. (1987) Injuries in runners. *American Journal of Sports Medicine* **15**, 168–171.

Maffulli, N., Kahn, K. & Puddu, G. (1998) Overuse tendon conditions: time to change a confusing terminology. *Arthroscopy* **14**, 840–843.

Maffulli, N., Renström, P., Leadbetter, W.B. (2005) *Tendon Injuries: Basic Science and Clinical Medicine.* Springer, London.

Mafi, N., Lorentzon, R. & Alfredson, H. (2001) Superior results with eccentric calf-muscle training compared to concentric training in a randomized prospective multi-center study of patients with chronic Achilles tendinosis. *Knee Surgery, Sports Traumatology, Arthroscopy* **9**, 42–47.

Magnusson, S.P. & Kjaer, M. (2003) Region-specific differences in Achilles tendon cross-sectional area in runners and non-runners. *European Journal of Applied Physiology* **90**, 549–553.

Milgrom, C. (2003) Cold weather training: a risk factor for Achilles paratendinitis among recruits. *Foot & Ankle International* **24**, 398–401.

Movin, T. (1998) *Aspects of aetiology, pathoanatomy and diagnostic methods in chronic mid-portion Achillodynia* [dissertation]. Karolinska Institutet, Stockholm, Sweden.

Niesen-Vertommen, S., Taunton, J., Clement, D. & Mosher, R. (1992) The effect of eccentric exercise in the management in the management of Achilles tendinitis. *Clinical Journal of Sports Medicine* **2**, 109–113.

Nigg, B. (2001) The role of impact forces and foot pronation: a new paradigm. *Clinical Journal of Sport Medicine* **11**, 2–9.

Paavola, M., Kannus, P., Jarvinen, T.A., Jarvinen, T.L., Józsa, L. & Jarvinen, M. (2002a) Treatment of tendon disorders: is there a role for corticosteroid injection? *Foot & Ankle Clinics* **7**, 501–513.

Paavola, M., Kannus, P., Jarvinen, T.A., Khan, K., Józsa, L., Jarvinen, M. (2002b) Achilles tendinopathy. *Journal Bone and Joint Surgery. American volume*, **84**, 2062–2076.

Peacock, E.E. (1959) A study of the circulation in normal tendons and healing grafts. *Annals of Surgery.* **149**, 415–28.

Peers, K., Brys, P.P. & Lysens, R. (2003) Correlation between power Doppler ultrasonography and clinical severity in Achilles tendinopathy. *International Orthopaedics* **27**, 180–183.

Puddu, G., Ippolito, E. & Postacchini, F. (1976) A classification of Achilles tendon disease. *American Journal of Sports Medicine* **4**, 146–150.

Robinson, J.M., Cook, J.L., Purdam, C., *et al.* (2001) Victorian Institute Of Sport Tendon Study Group. The VISA-A questionnaire: a valid and reliable index of the clinical severity of Achilles tendinopathy. *British Journal of Sports Medicine* **35**, 335–341.

Rompe, J.D., Hopf, C., Nafe, B. & Burger, R. (1996) Low-energy extracorporeal shock wave therapy for painful heel: a prospective controlled single-blind study. *Archives of Orthopedic Trauma and Surgery* **115**, 75–79.

Silbernagel, K.G. (2006) *Achilles tendinopathy: evaluation and treatment* [PhD thesis]. Sahlgrenska Academy of Göteborg University, Sweden.

Silbernagel, K.G., Thomee, R. & Karlsson, J. (2005) Cross-cultural adaptation of the VISA-A questionnaire, an index of clinical severity for patients with Achilles tendinopathy, with reliability, validity and structure evaluations. *BMC Musculoskeletal Disorder* **6**, 12.

Stanish, W.D., Rubinovich, R.M. & Curwin, S. (1986) Eccentric exercise in chronic tendonitis. *Clinical Orthopaedics* **208**, 65–68.

Tallon, C., Maffulli, N. & Ewen, S.W. (2001) Ruptured Achilles tendons are significantly more degenerated than tendinopathic tendons. *Medicine and Science in Sports and Exercise* **33**, 1983–1990.

Teitz, C.C., Garrett, W.E. Jr, Miniaci, A., Lee, M.H. & Mann, R.A. (1997) Tendon problems in athletic individuals. *Journal of Bone and Joint Surgery. American volume* **79**, 138–152.

Tuite, D.J., Renström, P.A. & O'Brien, M. (1997) The aging tendon. *Scandinavian Journal of Medicine and Science in Sports* **7**, 72–77.

van der Windt, D.A., van der Heijden, G.J., van der Berg, S.G., ter Riet, G., de Winter, A.F., Bouter, L.M. (1999) Ultrasound therapy for musculoskeletal disorders; a systematic review. *Pain* **81**, 257–281.

van Mechelen, W. (1995) Can running injuries be effectively prevented? *Sports Medicine* **19**, 161–165.

Williams, J.G.P. (1986). Achilles tendon lesions in sport. *Sports Medicine* **3**, 114–135.

Winge, S., Jorgensen, U. & Lassen Nielsen, A. (1989) Epidemiology of injuries in Danish championship tennis. *International Journal of Sports Medicine* **10**, 368–371.

Woo, S.L-Y., Gomez, M.A., Woo, Y.K. & Akeson, W.H. (1982) Mechanical properties of tendons and ligaments. I. Quasistatic and nonlinear viscoelastic properties. *Biorheology* **19**, 385–396.

Chapter 2

Etiology of Tendinopathy

JILL L. COOK AND KARIM M. KHAN

Understanding the etiology of tendinopathy is a critical aspect of improving knowledge in this area, as it would allow active intervention in athletes prior to the onset of debilitating symptoms or tendon rupture. The investigation of tendinopathy is hindered by experimental and ethical factors, such as the lack of a suitable animal model, the onset of pathology in humans before pain and the limitations of investigating cellular processes without an intact matrix. Currently, very little is understood about the cause of tendinopathy, mechanical load is implicated in the etiology of both pain and pathology; however, the type and magnitude of load is not known. As the tensile model of overload does not explain many aspects of tendinopathy, a primary shift is occurring from a tensile cause to the addition of compression and stress-shielding as a load factor in tendon disease.

The processes of tendinopathy at a cellular level is also under review. Cellular process including inflammation, apoptosis, vascular, and neural changes have been proposed as the initiating event in tendinopathy, although one single instigating process is not likely. In addition, factors that are unique to each individual must be considered; gender, disease, age, flexibility, previous injury, and genetic profile will all impact on the development of tendinopathy. Each athlete may have a preset load tolerance, over which they develop tendinopathy. Understanding this individual variation will allow better management of athletes in the future. The load required, the cellular responses, and the athlete profile that underpin the development of tendino-

pathy all require more investigation and integration before the etiology of tendinopathy can be fully understood.

Introduction

Tendinopathy primarily affects active people; the more active they are, the greater chance of developing tendon pathology and pain. The recreational athlete has some risk of developing tendinopathy, but the elite athlete has the greatest prospect of tendon pain and pathology. Tendinopathy can curtail or even end an athletic career and, as treatment options are limited, understanding the etiology of tendinopathy and identifying risk factors for tendinopathy may allow for the implementation of preventative strategies.

Currently, the cause of tendinopathy is unknown. Experimental and clinical research is clarifying aspects of the etiology of pain and pathology but the relationship between them is unclear. Elucidating reasons for the onset of pain has clinical utility; however, acute tendon pain may not equal acute tendon pathology. Pathology is likely to have temporally preceded symptoms and symptoms may be the consequence of the combination of pathology and load. Thus, defining the etiology of pain does not necessarily also define the etiology of pathology.

The etiology of pain in tendinopathy is often examined at an organism level; in humans the athlete is the ideal subject. Tendon pain is correlated with performance, capacity, or function of the athlete. The etiology of pathology is examined by necessity *in vitro* or in animal models. Understanding the relationship and interaction between factors examined microscopically and those examined in the athlete is problematic, and this remains one of the key challenges in tendon research.

Some factors, such as tendon load and vascular changes, are implicated in the etiology of both pathology and pain and, as such, these must be a priority to investigate. However, both tendon load and vascularity may be factors that are responsible for, and affected by, a cascade of smaller changes. Only investigation of factors on both a small and large scale will allow the etiology of tendinopathy to be fully understood. Consequently, a chapter on the etiology must examine both the etiology of tendon pathology and the etiology of tendon pain. This chapter also examines the risk factors associated with tendon pathology and pain. Risk factors have clinical relevance and may help the clinician treat athletes, but may also aid researchers understand the etiology of tendinopathy.

Does pathology precede pain?

Kannus and Józsa's seminal study on tendon rupture clearly defines the relationship between pain and pathology (Kannus & Józsa 1991). In their series of 891 tendon ruptures, they demonstrated that although virtually all tendons were pathologic prior to rupture, only 34% were symptomatic. This study demonstrated that tendon pathology is not always painful.

This has been further examined in several longitudinal imaging studies of tendon pathology in athletes. These studies have demonstrated that pathology not only preceded symptoms in both the Achilles and patellar tendons, but abnormal tendons could remain pain free for years despite continued athletic activity (Khan *et al.* 1997; Cook *et al.* 2000b,c; Fredberg & Bolvig 2002). In this series of imaging studies a consistent pattern of outcomes was demonstrated; approximately one-third of pathologic tendons resolved on imaging, of the remaining two-thirds, only one-third of these became symptomatic. The remaining pathologic tendons stayed both abnormal and asymptomatic.

If the presence of abnormal imaging is taken *sine qua non* for tendon pathology (Khan *et al.* 1996; Green *et al.* 1997), this demonstrates that the etiology of tendon pathology may be very different to tendon pain.

Where does tendon pathology occur in athletes?

Although tendon pathology is considered primarily to occur in the tendon, most problematic tendon injuries occur at the bone–tendon junction (enthesis). The Achilles tendon is clearly predisposed to develop midtendon pathology more often than enthesis pathology, but tendinopathies in athletes primarily occur at the bone tendon junction, or at sites of functional entheses (where tendons abut but do not attach to bone; Benjamin & McGonagle 2001).

While most tendon disease in athletes occurs at the enthesis, the majority of research has been directed at the tendon. It is unclear if results from research directed at a pure tendinopathy are applicable to pathology and processes at the bone–tendon junction. The presence of unmineralized and mineralized fibrocartilage and the vascular and neural morphology of the enthesis must vary the enthesis' response to injury from pure tendinopathy.

The enthesis is clearly structurally and histologically different from the tendon proper. The enthesis has four transitional layers from bone to tendon (through mineralized and unmineralized fibrocartilage) with several changes in collagen type (I, II, V, IX, and X) and proteoglycans. The fibrocartilages of the enthesis are primarily avascular as vessels from the bone can reach, but not breach, the tidemark. Neurally, the enthesis is richly endowed with type C and A delta pain fibers and substance P nerve fibers (Benjamin & McGonagle 2001).

Entheseal layering increases the capacity of the enthesis to bear all types of load, and the stress levels at the enthesis may be four times that of the tendon midsubstance (Woo *et al.* 1988; McGonagle *et al.* 2003). However, the enthesis is strong enough to withstand high forces, and disruption occurs most commonly in the underlying bone. The bone of the enthesis may become reactive to high load, and osteitis and positive bone imaging have been demonstrated in disease (Woo *et al.* 1988; McGonagle *et al.* 2003) and athletically induced enthesis injury (Green *et al.* 1996).

Enthesis fibrocartilage response to mechanical load may vary with activity levels and type of load (Benjamin & McGonagle 2001). Fibrocartilage is reactive to the addition or removal of compressive and shear loads (Benjamin & McGonagle 2001) and reaction may result in pathologic changes in thickness, as in patellar tendinopathy (Ferretti *et al.* 1983).

Other reported pathology at the enthesis includes bony spurs, fissures, and cracks, and pathology similar to that seen in tendons—fatty, hyaline, cystic, calcific or mucoid degeneration. Fibrocartilage and its associated proteoglycans (aggrecan and possibly versican; Thomopoulos *et al.* 2003) have been implicated in the breakdown process of the enthesis (McGonagle *et al.* 2003). It is unclear if inflammation is part of the enthesis pathology, as very few studies have investigated inflammation in the pathologic enthesis.

Why does the Achilles tendon suffer midtendon pathology more often than bone–tendon pathology? The Achilles tendon in humans and the superficial digital flexor tendon in horses have been called energy storage tendons, called upon to store and release energy to make athletic activity more efficient (Komi & Bosco 1978). Smith *et al.* (2002) consider these tendons to be more at risk of developing tendinopathy than tendons that are stabilizers or segment positioners. As many tendons other than the Achilles store and release energy in athletic activity (patellar tendon, medial elbow tendons, shoulder internal rotators), breakdown is not only influenced by its capacity to store energy, but also by the dimensions of the tendon. Long tendons appear more at risk of midtendon tendinopathy and fatigue rupture than shorter, broader tendons (Ker 2002). Ker (2002) hypothesizes that tendons have a structural unit of a designated length, and fatigue (and consequent pathology) may occur if the tendon is longer than the structural unit.

Although the enthesis is affected by pathology more commonly than the tendon itself, by necessity we will examine the etiology of tendon pathology, and assume that factors that affect the tendon also impact on the enthesis.

Etiology of tendon pathology

Mechanical load

Overloading at the organism level and at the tendon level are often hypothesized to be the reason for the onset of pain and pathology, respectively. However, the nature and the timing of the stimuli needed to cause tendon pathology are unknown. As a number of tendon pathologies have been described (hypoxic, hyaline, mucoid, fibrinoid, lipoid) it is possible that there is an equal number of etiologies. Alternately, the type of tendon pathology may be determined by factors that occur subsequent to the onset of a primary pathologic state.

Although the literature suggests that tendon overload is critical, what constitutes overload is undefined. Overload must vary from tendon to tendon and between athletes. In addition, overload can not be the sole reason for tendon pathology, and tendon pathology may be caused by many factors that are either working alone, in cooperation or as a cascade. The relationship between the factors reported in this section is complex and remains undefined.

Traditionally, pathology is reported to be caused by repeated strain that is less than the force necessary to rupture. The strain is reported to disrupt collagen cross-links and fibrils and may damage blood vessels, resulting in impaired metabolic and oxygen delivery (Kannus 1997). Collagen tearing caused by tensile load has long been considered to be the primary event in tendinopathy. Ker (2002) suggests that the failure of tendon is primarily in the region between collagen fibrils, with the separated fibrils then breaking independently. Although logical, this hypothesis lacks evidence, and the response of tendon cells to load must be considered.

Mechanical load at physiologic levels has been shown to deform tendon cells *in situ* (Arnoczky *et al.* 2002) and cells respond to load with an increase in nitrous oxide levels (van Griensven *et al.* 2003) and cytosolic calcium (Shirakura *et al.* 1995). The presence of load is then communicated to adjacent cells through gap junctions (Banes *et al.* 1995). This normal cellular response to mechanical load may be supplemented when larger or repetitive loads are applied. Repetitive motion has been shown to increase an inflammatory mediator, prostoglandin E_2 (PGE_2) produced by tendon fibroblasts (Almekinders et al. 1993). Similarly, exercise has been demonstrated to increase levels of PGE_2 in the Achilles peritendinous space (Langberg et al. 1999).

A reaction to excessive tendon strain may result in tendon pathology, as a response to low level tendon strain may implement tendon repair. The capacity of the tendon to recover after load centers on the ability of the tendon cells to manufacture extracellular components of the tendon, and to organize these proteins into a structured extracellular matrix. It is the matrix that bears load, and deficiencies in the matrix structure determine decreased load capacity and tolerance.

In tendon pathology, the amount of strain is hypothesized to exceed the tendon's capacity to repair (Leadbetter 1992). Smith et al. (2002) suggest an incapacity for matrix adaptation after maturity is paramount in energy storage tendons and that overload after maturity only serves to accelerate degeneration. They hypothesize that this incapacity for adaptation is brought about by a lack of cellular communication and the loss of growth factors to stimulate the cells to manufacture matrix components. Growth factors are critical in determining a tendon's response to load. Growth factors with load stimulated mitogenesis in tendon cells (Banes et al. 1995). However, continued load without growth factors may induce cell death and matrix degradation.

Conversely, Ker (2002) suggests that tendon load during life must create tendon damage and tendon repair must be occurring constantly. Decorin and collagen VI (links type I collagen and may transmit force between fibrils) show the greatest turnover in tendons suggesting that these proteins are affected by everyday load and replaced during maintenance (Ker 2002). Similarly, collagen showed continued remodeling when collagen cross-links were investigated in human rotator cuff tendon, indicating regular, and continued matrix replacement (Banks et al. 1999).

In addition to remodeling, repair must also encompass adaptation to repeated overload. The response of tendons to exercise is ambiguous because of the range of tendon tissue examined (age, species, and tendon) and variation in exercise loads. Energy storage tendons, those that develop tendinopathy in athletes, are reported to be incapable of adapting to repeated load with tendon hypertrophy (Woo et al. 1982). Buchanan and Marsh (2002) report increase in tensile strength and stiffness apparently resultant from collagen cross-link changes. This minimal response to exercise in experimental studies supports the concept of minimal tendon adaptation to load proposed by Smith et al. (2002).

Impingement

Impingement is a form of mechanical load, and adds compressive or shearing load to the tendon's normal tensile load. Combinations of load types have been shown to create changes in tissue response (Forslund & Aspenberg 2002) and tendon reaction to impingement may result in cartilaginous and bony pathology in tendon. Compressive loads also upregulate endostatin (an antiangiogeneis factor), which in normal tendon may create and maintain the avascular nature of fibrocartilage. However, in pathologic tissue, it may perpetuate the tendinopathy cycle (Pufe et al. 2003).

Impingement in the Achilles tendon, rotator cuff, and the patellar tendon have been reported to cause tendinopathy. The shape of the calcaneus appears to affect the morphology of the Achilles insertion (Rufai et al. 1995) and may be the result of anatomical impingement. Tendons with a prominent, square, superior calcaneus have greater amounts of fibrocartilage in both the bone and tendon and have a more distinct retrocalcaneal bursa as compared to those with rounded and lower calcaneal shape.

Johnson et al. (1996) hypothesized that the inferior pole of the patella impinges on the tendon during knee flexion. A dynamic magnetic resonance study that investigated this hypothesis (Schmid et al. 2002) indicated that there was no difference in patellar movement between symptomatic tendons and those tendons without pain and pathology. The angle of the tendon to the patella either with or without quadriceps contraction was similar in both these groups. Clinical testing of patellar tendinopathy suggests that pain can occur at or near full extension in both the loaded and unloaded knee. In combination, clinical and research findings suggest that impingement from the patella may not be a factor in patellar tendinopathy.

In the rotator cuff tendons, arguments to counter impingement come from Uhthoff and Matsumoto (2000) who suggest that if impingement was the cause of rotator cuff disease, then the pathology should be consistently on the bursal side of the tendon. Yet, rotator cuff pathology is in fact nearly always on the articular side of the tendon.

Compressive or stress-shielding as an etiological cause of tendon pain have recently been proposed by several authors (Almekinders et al. 2003; Hamilton & Purdam 2003). The compression hypothesized is not mechanical (impingement) in nature, but more intrinsic to the tendon. Stress shielding may also induce compression on the tendon, commonly seen on the "interior" or joint surface of tendon attachments in the patellar, supraspinatus, elbow, and adductor tendons. These theories need investigation as it is clear that critical etiologic questions such as the nature of tendon load must be answered quickly, as it is the essence of adequate management.

Tendon load can take many forms, tensile, compressive or shearing. Tendon load may be directly responsible for tendon pathology, and induce many changes in the tendon. However, tendon load may also provoke other reactions in the tendon as a response to load. These tendon reactions may initiate or accelerate tendon pathology, alone or in conjunction with other tendon reponses, and are considered in the following sections.

Thermal

The storage and release of elastic energy in tendons discharge intratendinous heat. Equine studies suggest that the resultant increase in tendon temperature after exercise may induce cell death (Wilson & Goodship 1994). Cell loss affects the tendons ability to respond to stress and remodel the matrix. This particular model of etiology of tendon pathology explains central core tendinopathies very well. Hyperthermia also induces production of reactive oxygen species (see next section), and this in turn

may affect tendon tissue (Bestwick & Maffulli 2000). Good vascularity may allow for adequate cooling of the tendon. However, the relationship between the increase in vascularity seen in tendinopathy and thermal model of pathology has not been established.

Chemical

Reactive oxygen species are oxygen molecules with an unpaired electron (Bestwick & Maffulli 2000). There is a similar species of nitrogen based molecules, and a combined nitrogen and oxygen species may also be formed. These molecules are important in normal tissue function but are also capable of inducing cellular and matrix damage (Bestwick & Maffulli 2000) and can inflict damage at sites distant to their production.

Although these species are formed during normal cell function, strong stimuli such as exercise may enhance their formation. During exercise, bouts of ischemia and reperfusion may stimulate formation of reactive oxygen species (Kannus 1997). This mechanism for pathology is possible, as blood flow in normal tendons (Åström & Westlin 1994b) and neovascularization associated with pathology (Öhberg et al. 2001) are both affected by stretch and contraction.

Cell death may be a consequence of reactive species, and has been shown to be increased by greater amounts and longer exposure to hydrogen peroxide (Yuan et al. 2003). Peroxiredoxin eliminates hydrogen peroxide, and this has been shown to have its expression upregulated by fibroblasts and endothelial cells in torn supraspinatus tendons when compared to normal subscapularis tendons (Wang et al. 2001).

Similarly, nitrous oxide has been extensively investigated as a messenger molecule that responds to shear stress in cells (van Griensven et al. 2003). Measured nitrous oxide levels were increased with cyclic strain and these increased levels were hypothesized to positively modulate cellular function (Murrell et al. 1997). Recent research indicates that the treatment of tendinopathy may be enhanced by the addition of nitrous oxide (Paoloni et al. 2003).

Tendons may adapt to the presence of reactive species when exposed continually to them, as in regular and similar exercise routines, by increasing antioxidant defense mechanisms. When exercise is suddenly undertaken or changed, this adaptation may not have occurred and the tendon may be exposed to higher levels of reactive species and the potential for damage that follows (Bestwick & Maffulli 2000).

Inflammation

Although inflammation has not been demonstrated in tendon pathology in humans, tissue from end-stage disease has been commonly examined. End-stage disease in humans have shown no physiologic increase in PGE_2 in tendinopathic tissue at several different sites when compared with normal tendon tissue (Alfredson et al. 1999; Alfredson et al. 2001). Animal models where tendon sampling can be made early in the tendinopathy process also suggest that inflammation does not occur in the overuse tendinopathy process (Zamora & Marini 1988).

It is important to note that the absence of inflammatory modulators at end-stage disease does not mean that they are absent in early-stage disease and are not a factor in the cause of tendinopathy. PGE_2 has been shown to increase in the peri-tendinous space after exercise (Langberg et al. 1999). Long-term peritendinous increases in PGE_1 have been shown to lead to degenerative as well as inflammatory changes in the tendon (Sullo et al. 2001). As mechanical load can increase the tendinous (Almekinders et al. 1993) and peritendinous levels of PG, it is possible that inflammation is associated with the etiology of tendinopathy at some point in time.

Autocrine and paracrine substances

Cells in or near to the tendon produce many substances (cytokines and enzymes) that act on tendon tissue. The cytokines produced by the tendon and peritendon cells act in many different ways including as growth factors (Molloy et al. 2003), differentiation factors, and chemotactic factors as well as affecting enzyme production in any of these domains. The peritenon cells appear to be more active than, and respond differently to, the tendon cells themselves (Banes et al. 1995; Hart et al. 1998).

Very small amounts of cytokines are needed to affect tissue changes, and more of these substance does not necessarily increase its effectiveness (Evans 1999). Cytokines interact with other cytokines and substances, so investigation of single cytokines may not be relevant to in vivo tendon pathophysiology. Consideration of all substances is beyond the scope of this chapter. The role of matrix metallopro-teinases (MMP) and other substances that have been investigated including stress-activated protein kinases can be found in other chapters in this book.

Hypoxia and vascularity

Hypoxia has been hypothesized as a cause of tendinopathy (Kannus 1997), although the exact mechanism is not defined. Theoretically, cell disablement or death should be the main effect of hypoxia, with a consequent decrease or abolition of the capacity of the tendon to produce tendon matrix components and repair. Hypoxic changes have been reported in tendon cells (Józsa et al. 1982), with swollen mitochondria, pyknotic nuclei, and dilatation and degranulation of the endoplasmic reticulum. Importantly, these changes were seen in cells from samples taken after tendon rupture, which does not delineate cause and effect. The hypoxic changes may have occurred during the process of tendon pathology, during tendon rupture or after rupture prior to sampling.

The presence of hypoxia in tendon pathology prior to rupture is supported by reports of increased lactate levels in Achilles tendinopathy (Alfredson et al. 2002) compared with normal tendons. Increased lactate suggests anaerobic metabolism, used by tendon cells with a limited supply of oxygen. This study did not report if the pathologic tendons demonstrated increased vascularity on imaging, a common occurrence in tendon pathology that should preclude hypoxia.

Although there is some evidence of hypoxia in tendon pathology affecting tendon cells, other studies suggest that fibroblasts are somewhat resistant to hypoxia. Cells exposed to decreased oxygen tension still exhibited cell proliferation but demonstrated decreases in collagen production (Mehm *et al.* 1988). Tendon cells specifically also appear resistant to low oxygen levels, with cellular proliferation unchanged by low oxygen tissue levels (Rempel & Abrahamsson 2001). Similar to Mehm *et al.* (1988), this study demonstrated a decrease in collagen synthesis in hypoxia.

These two studies suggest that hypoxia may affect the extracellular structure of tendon, rather than the cellular components. This is consistent with what is seen histopathologically in tendon pathology, where cellular presence is maintained in most situations, but the extracellular structure is disrupted. Interestingly, the presence of myofibroblasts, another common feature of tendon pathology, is reported to diminish the tendon capacity to repair, resulting in more immature collagen in tendons with myofibroblasts than those without (Moyer *et al.* 2003).

The link between hypoxia and changes in vascularity in tendon pathology is unclear. Hypoxia is a powerful stimulant to angiogenesis. Alternatively, impaired vascularity may lead to hypoxia. Increased vascularity is the cornerstone of tendinopathy and has been demonstrated histopathologically (Kraushaar & Nirschl 1999), with imaging on Doppler ultrasound (Öhberg *et al.* 2001; Terslev *et al.* 2001), and with laser flowmetry (Åström & Westlin 1994a,b).

Angiogenesis is controlled by a variety of mitogenic, chemotactic, or inhibitory peptide and lipid factors (Pufe *et al.* 2003). Vascular endothelial growth factor is absent in adult tissue (Pufe *et al.* 2003), this suggests that neovascularization may be a reaction to a hypoxic state.

Some pathologic tendons do not demonstrate increased vascularity on imaging (Zanetti *et al.* 2003), but few studies have examined both histopathology and vascularity demonstrated on imaging. It is unknown why some tendons react by markedly increasing vascularity (visible on imaging) and others do not.

In vivo, Biberthaler *et al.* (2003) have shown that areas of tendon degeneration or rupture of the supraspinatus tendon in humans have a decreased microcirculation density and vessel number compared to areas of normal tendon insertion (1–2 mm from the insertion). Lower vascularity may be associated with areas of decreased oxygen levels. Other authors do not support this, Uhthoff and Matsumoto (2000) consider that the area of hypovascularity is not related to the etiology of tendinopathy, and that the pathology process starts at the insertion.

Neural

The body of a tendon is poorly innervated. The myotendinous and osseotendinous junctions and the peritendon are well innervated, but the tendon proper does not have a good neural supply. Nerve fibres in the tendon are associated with the vascular, lymphatic, and connective tissue channels, some of these nerve fibres have been reported to have direct contact with tendon collagen (Andres *et al.* 1985).

Although sparse in sections, the nerve supply of the tendon may have important roles in the onset of pathology, pain production, and tendon repair. Neurogenic inflammation, inflammation initiated by neuropeptides may also be implicated in tendon pathology. Neuropeptides substance P and calcitonin gene-related peptide (CGRP) increase nociception (Ackermann *et al.* 2003), affect angiogenesis, vascular permeability, and cell proliferation. Substance P can induce mast cells to release other substances that affect tendon tissue (Hart *et al.* 1999). However, histopathologic examination of tendon pathology at the elbow did not demonstrate a close proximity between mast cells and nerve fibres with substance P and CGRP (Ljung *et al.* 1999).

Substance P and CGRP seem to exert more influence on the peritendon than the tendon itself (Hart *et al.* 1998). Substance P upregulates cyclooxygenase 2 (COX 2) and interleukin β (IL-β) in the peritendon but not the tendon (Hart *et al.* 1998). Neurogenic inflammation could initiate peritendinopathy, with substance P and CGRP both implicated in this pathway (Hart *et al.* 1998). As it has been shown that long-term peritendon inflammation can lead to degenerative changes in the tendon (Sullo *et al.* 2001), this could initiate the tendinopathy cycle.

The role of neural substances in tendon repair has also been reported. After experimental rupture in the rat Achilles tendon, there was significant neural ingrowth to week 6 (Ackermann *et al.* 2003). Increases in heat and mechanical sensitivity were associated with these changes.

Apoptosis

Cell death (apoptosis) is a physiologic event that maintains, protects, and develops the body, and may be programmed or occur in response to trauma. Pathologically, apoptosis is associated with neural and joint disease, with impaired apoptosis being associated with cancer (Yuan *et al.* 2002). Apoptosis is completed with an intact cell membrane whereas trauma induces cell death with membrane destruction and leakage of cellular substrates which provokes a consequent inflammatory reaction (Bestwick & Maffulli 2000). Apoptosis is closely associated with the levels and actions of reactive nitrogen and oxygen species.

Investigations of apoptosis in tendinopathy have increased dramatically in the last few years. Although apoptosis has been demonstrated in pathologic tissue, it is not yet been shown if apoptosis is a cause or a consequence of tendon pathology. Apoptosis has been reported in the following circumstances; secondary to areas of partial rupture and repair, as myofibroblasts typically regress from scar tissue, accompanying vascular remodelling, secondary to hypoxia and secondary to mechanical load. Only mechanically induced apoptosis is likely to be a direct cause of tendinopathy, whereas in the remaining circumstances other events must precede apoptosis (Scott *et al.* 2005). Although demonstrated *in vitro*, mechanical loads sufficient to cause apoptosis *in vivo* have not yet been demonstrated.

Pathologic tissue has been examined in the ruptured rotator cuff, and the amount of apoptosis in the tendon cells was greater than normal tendon (Yuan *et al.* 2002). It is unclear from this data whether apoptosis is a cause or effect of the tendon rupture; if a ruptured tendon is not under tension, it may well change its nature and content. The authors suggest that the apoptosis could be secondary to ischaemia, hypoxia, free radical generation, and nutritional imbalances. This same study also demonstrated that increasing age and pathology in associated tendons might increase the amount of apoptosis in normal tissue.

Ground substance

Tendon remodeling and response to load may be implicated in tendon pathology. An investigation of the patellar tendons in a cohort of young active individuals suggests that there may be a sequence of pathologic changes in tendon (Cook *et al.* 2004a). In this study, activation of tenocytes occurred in isolation in some tendons while increased ground substance only existed in conjunction with activated tenocytes. Tendons with collagen separation were associated with both increased ground substance and tenocyte activation. Neovascularization was not evident in this cohort of asymtomatic tendons that were mostly normal on imaging, suggesting that changes in vascularity may be associated with both pain and imaging changes.

Although the study was cross-sectional in nature, it is tempting to speculate that a temporal sequence of events occurs in tendon exposed to load. Ground substance increases underpin many of the changes seen in tendinopathy, and may be responsible for some or all of the collagen changes seen. This study suggests that activated tenocytes preferentially manufacture ground substance, rather than collagen. Alternatively, increased ground substance as a result of compression has been suggested to be a source of pain either directly or as a result of the compression in the patellar tendon (Hamilton & Purdam 2003).

Pharmacology

There are medications that are known to directly and adversely affect tendon tissue. These substances induce tendon damage and can affect symptoms negatively (fluroquionolones) or positively (corticosteroids). Many studies indicate an association between fluroquionolones and tendon pathology, with a reported incidence among the general population of 0.4%. The Achilles tendon is most affected and rupture occurs in approximately one-third of affected patients (Movin *et al.* 1997b). Symptoms in those that do not rupture settle in several months.

The histopathology is identical to that seen in overuse tendinopathy (Movin *et al.* 1997b).

Corticosteroids are unique in that they are used to treat tendon pain, but at the same time are reported to potentially have adverse effects on tendon tissue. As defined in this chapter, painful tendons that are treated with corticosteroids must already be pathologic, hence corticosteroids do not necessarily induce pathology in athletes with tendon pain.

Intratendinous injection has demonstrated catabolic and negative mechanical effects on tendon tissue by causing collagen necrosis and decreasing force to failure (Kennedy & Willis 1976). Because of this, corticosteroid is usually infiltrated into the area around the tendon, and the effect of this on tendon tissue is debatable. Although clinically and anecdotally it has been associated with rupture, and most clinicians are hesitant to use corticosteroids to treat tendon pain, there is little evidence to suggest that it has any impact on tendon tissue. Some studies report an increase in tendon pathology after corticosteroid injection (placement not reported) (Åström & Rausing 1995), others have reported no greater pathology in ruptured tendons that had received corticosteroid injection compared with those that had not (Kannus & Józsa 1991). Painless tendons rupture more commonly than painful ones (Kannus and Józsa 1991), hence rupture occurs regardless of corticosteroid treatment. It could be hypothesized that rupture after corticosteroid injection occurs because the pain is removed, and the athlete places increased load on the tendon. Until there is a clearer understanding of the role of corticosteroids in tendon pathology and repair, their clinical use should be minimal.

Prolonged oral use of corticosteroids has been associated with tendon rupture (Aydingoz & Aydingoz 2002; Khurana *et al.* 2002) although in patients with significant and/or systemic disease, the use of corticosteroids may only be one factor in the cause of tendon pathology and subsequent rupture. Animal studies indicate that systemic use of corticosteroids may be beneficial to tendons, although high doses may be deleterious (Fredberg 1997).

In vitro, corticosteroids have been shown to affect tendon cell migration. The authors hypothesize that this may be a factor in the relationship between corticosteroid and tendon pathology (Tsai *et al.* 2003). Corticosteroids have also been shown to inhibit the upregulation of MMP-2 and MMP-9, something that should benefit the tendon matrix (Ritty & Herzog 2003).

Etiology of tendon pain

Clinically, tendon pain is considered to be the onset of tendinopathy. Athletes who present with first time tendon pain are commonly treated with the principles that underpin acute injury: rest, ice, and anti-inflammatory medications. Acknowledging that there is likely to be a pre-existing pathology challenges both clinical acumen and treatment options.

The source of pain in tendinopathy is obscure. Although biochemical substances have been proposed (Ljung *et al.* 1999; Alfredson *et al.* 2001), none have yet been shown conclusively to be the sole agent (Alfredson & Lorentzon 2003). Vascular and neural mechanisms have also been investigated (Ohberg *et al.* 2001; Öhberg & Alfredson 2002); however, it is clear that research is still yet to resolve this clinically essential question (Khan *et al.* 2003; Zanetti *et al.* 2003). An unknown pain pathway compromises our understanding of the etiology of symptoms, as both the stimulus for pain and its perpetuation are unknown. It is then certain that the treatment for tendon pain must also be obscure.

Although this chapter suggests that the presence of pathology is a prerequisite for tendon pain, there are imaging based studies that indicate symptoms are possible in normal tendons (Shalaby & Almekinders 1999). Although the imaging is normal, the tendon may not be. Tendon imaging is a wonderful clinical tool, but it does not show low levels of tendon disease. Several studies have shown pathology in imaging normal areas of tendon (Movin *et al.* 1997b; Cook 2003; Cook *et al.* 2004a). Tendon pain may exist in imaging normal tendons, but low levels of pathology may still exist for tendon pain. Most importantly, the clinician must be an accurate diagnostician as many tendons are surrounded by complex anatomic areas, and non tendinous structures may be the source of pain.

Tendon load

Clinically, an increase in tendon load is often linked to the onset of tendon symptoms. The load reported by the athlete is nearly always associated with a change in training type, volume, intensity, or frequency. The quantity and quality of overload needed to exacerbate symptoms may vary between individuals and depend on physical capacity, tendon capacity, tendon pathology, or individual characteristics such as biomechanical alignment.

The type of muscle contraction, the frequency, speed, and amount of tendon load may have independent or cumulative effects on tendon pain. However, clinically it is clear that eccentric load is implicated in the onset of tendon pain. Sports that do not have a large eccentric component or eccentric/concentric contraction turn around such as cycling and rowing do not have intratendinous pathology and pain in their profile of common injuries. Rotator cuff pathology and pain is common in swimmers; however, this tendon condition is complicated by the anatomic, biomechanical, and functional complexity of the shoulder in swimming.

If eccentric exercise is associated with the onset of either pain and/or tendon pathology, it is paradoxical that eccentric exercise offers the best treatment to date for tendinopathy (Alfredson et al. 1998), as a disease trigger does not often masquerade as the cure as well. It must be remembered that eccentric exercise, although it reduces pain, may act on the musculotendinous unit, and not specifically on the tendon, although an effect on tendon tissue has been reported (Alfredson & Lorentzon 2003). Eccentric exercise offers its best outcomes in tendon pain in the midtendon, and is less effective in insertional tendinopathy (Fahlstrom 2001).

An increase or sudden change in load has been associated with an onset of pain in several tendons. Increasing training times has been linked to the onset of pain in the patellar tendon (Ferretti 1986), Achilles tendon (Clement et al. 1984) and the rotator cuff (Hagberg & Wegman 1987). Recent research has reported that female athletes with patellar tendon pathology (not necessarily pain) trained on average 2.14 hours/week (± 1.4 hours; $P < 0.05$) more than those athletes without pathology (Gaida et al. 2004). More weight training has been linked to symptoms in the patellar tendon (Lian et al. 2003), and in the same study linked to greater jumping ability.

Vacularity

Normal tendons have a low vascularity, but have sufficient supply for their metabolic needs. In the pathologic tendon, increases in vascularity (neovascularization) have been demonstrated using Doppler ultrasound (Öhberg et al. 2001) and laser flowmetry (Åstróm & Westlin 1994a). Further investigations have demonstrated that neovascularization has been associated with pain and furthermore, sclerosing the neovascularization decreases pain (Ohberg & Alfredson 2002).

Neovascularization may be associated with nerve fibers (Alfredson et al. 2001), including those immunoreactive to substance P and CGRP (Ljung et al. 1999). The association between pain and neovascularization is not absolute, as some studies demonstrate that tendons with neovascularization may not be painful (Khan et al. 2003; Zanetti et al. 2003). Conversely, pathologic tendons without neovascularization may also be painful. However, there is evidence that there is more pain in pathologic tendons with neovascularization compared with pathologic tendons without neovascularization (Cook et al. 2004c). Longitudinal studies demonstrate that neovascularization may come and go, and the stimulus for this and the relation to pain is currently undefined.

Biochemical sources

Inflammatory mediators (PGE_2) have been demonstrated to be similar in pathologic, symptomatic tendons compared with normal tendons (Alfredson et al. 2000, 2001). This suggests that inflammation is not implicated in chronic tendon pain, but does not exclude a possible role in the onset of tendon pathology and/or pain.

Glutamate has been demonstrated in several tendons of the body at significantly higher levels in pathologic tendons than in normal tendons (Alfredson et al. 1999, 2000, 2001). Glutamate as a neurotransmitter may have a role in tendon pain, although recent studies have reported the levels of glutamate do not decrease in those tendons that become asymptomatic after eccentric exercise treatment (Alfredson & Lorentzon 2003).

Neuropeptides

Neuropeptides transmit nociceptive information to the central nervous system, as well as have a local effect on tendon tissue. Their effect on regional tissue and the possible role in tendon pathology has been considered in this chapter, and their nociceptive role may be implicated in tendon pain. Neuropeptide substance P and the associated sensory nerves have been demonstrated in elbow tendinopathy (Ljung et al. 1999) and in the subacromial space in the shoulder (Gotoh et al. 1998). As these peptides increase with chronic pain they may be implicated in tendon pain.

Risk factors for tendinopathy

Many characteristics have been hypothesized to be risk factors for the development of tendon pathology and pain. These include biomechanical variations, leg length discrepancy, muscle weakness and imbalance, decreased flexibility, joint laxity, gender, youth, age, weight, and disease (Kannus 1997). These factors must be considered by clinicians when assessing an athlete with tendinopathy; however, little evidence underpins their role in tendon pain and pathology.

Demonstrated risk factors for tendinopathy are sparse in the literature as most studies of risk factors investigate all injuries. In addition, most risk factors have been investigated for the onset of symptoms as this has clinical importance. Few studies have reported risk factors for pathology, and as many pathologic tendons do not go on to cause symptoms or rupture, identifying risk factors for both symptoms and pathology has value.

Risk factors such as tendon load and pharmacology considered in other sections are not reviewed here. The majority of evidence has been found for intrinsic risk factors such as strength, flexibility, and biomechanical factors.

Intrinsic risk factors

GENETIC PROFILE

A link between tendinopathy and genetic profile is emerging. Mokone et al. (2005b) have reported an association between two genes, the COL5A1 and the tenscin-C gene (Mokone et al. 2005a). Both these genes are found near to the locus for the ABO blood group.

Wide variation in tendon strength and size between individual horses has been reported (Smith et al. 2002). If humans have various tendon sizes, and these tendons have limited capacity to adapt their matrix when under increased load (Smith et al. 2002), then some athletes may be more susceptible to tendinopathy. Individual susceptibility is supported by reports of individuals who have ruptured multiple tendons (Ho & Lee 2003). Also, an association between tissue type (HLA B-27) and Achilles tendinopathy has been reported (Olivieri et al. 1987). Psoriasis is also associated with this tissue type and tendon rupture (Aydingoz & Aydingoz 2002).

Although in this section we consider only gender and blood group, factors considered in their own entity as risk factors such as flexibility and disease may have a genetic contribution.

Blood group

Blood group has been reported to be associated with tendon rupture (Józsa et al. 1989). The ABO antigens of blood groups are found in other tissues including tendon, and may affect tendon tissue directly or through its genetic location on chromosome 9 (Maffulli et al. 2000b). In the Achilles tendon, studies have shown both a positive association (Kujala et al. 1992) and no association (Maffulli et al. 2000b). Ethnic group differences in the subjects of these studies may have impacted on the results.

Gender

Female gender is reported to increase the risk of tendinopathy (Kannus 1997) due to strength, body composition, and biomechanical differences in women compared with men. Despite these reports, women are much less likely than men to present for either conservative or surgical treatment for tendon injury. This suggests that women suffer less tendinopathy than men. However, reporting prevalence of a disease based only on those presenting with symptoms may not give a clear picture of the true gender distribution of tendinopathy.

Large cohort studies of patellar tendinopathy support a decreased risk for females to develop lower limb tendinopathy. In a large series of adolescent and adult patellar tendons, there was a greater ratio of tendon pathology (not symptoms) in males compared to females (2 : 1) (Cook et al. 1998; Cook et al. 2000a). Similar ratios are demonstrated in the Achilles tendon (Maffulli et al. 1999a).

Several studies report that the risk of tendinopathy for females compared with males increases with age. Biomechanically it has been reported that older female tendons were stiffer than male tendon, which may predispose to tendon pathology (Hart et al. 1998). Other studies report that Achilles tendons are thinner in older females compare with males and this was not found in younger subjects (Koivunen-Niemela & Parkkola 1995). Both these factors may increase the risk of tendon disease in older females (Maffulli et al. 1999a).

Females are also reported to have a greater inflammatory response to injury and also exhibit differences in neurogenic inflammation (Hart et al. 1998). This may explain the greater prevalence of repetitive motion disorders (often peritendon pathology) in females. Peritendon disorders are reported to be more common in women than men and hand and wrist disorders have a ratio of at least 4 : 1 women to men (Ta et al. 1999).

A proposed subset of sufferers of repetitive motion disorders has multiple sites of tendon disorders (mesenchymal syndrome). This is commonly seen in women over 30 years and is reported to be associated with diminished estrogen levels and premature menopause (Nirschl 1992). The syndrome has been reported in men.

Ligament injury has been linked to the phases of the menstrual cycle (Karageanes et al. 2000), although a relationship has not been fully established (Hewett 2000). Ligament tissue and tendon tissue are similar and it could be suggested that a similar situation existed in tendons. Both ligaments

and tendons have estrogen receptors (Hart et al. 1998) and it is possible that estrogen acts directly on tendon. It has also been shown that estrogen affects tissue repair (Liu et al. 1997) and both these factors may affect the gender distribution of tendon injury.

UNILATERAL/BILATERAL PATHOLOGY

Only one study of patellar tendinopathy with small subject numbers has suggested that athletes with unilateral tendinopathy may have unique risk factors compared with those with bilateral tendinopathy (Gaida et al. 2004). In this study, athletes with unilateral tendinopathy could be discriminated from normal subjects by a greater tibial length, a smaller waist : hip ratio and eccentric strength of the affected leg. Subjects with bilateral tendinopathy did not vary from normal subjects.

This is consistent with research that suggested that the prevalence of bilateral tendinopathy may be different from that of unilateral tendinopathy (Cook et al. 1998). In this study, women had 1 : 1 ratio of bilateral tendinopathy with men. Unilateral tendinopathy has a 2 : 1 ratio. Both these studies suggest that the cause of bilateral tendinopathy may be different than unilateral tendinopathy. Hypothetically, those athletes without a genetic predisposition to tendinopathy would sustain pathology in the tendon subject to a causative factor, such as load. Those predisposed to tendinopathy when exposed to a causative factor develop pathology in both knees. This further supports a link between tendinopathy and genetic profile.

PREVIOUS INJURY

Tendons can become repeatedly symptomatic (Cook et al. 1997), but it is unlikely pathology changes greatly when moving from symptomatic to asymptomatic. Therefore, redevelopment of symptoms in tendons may not be associated with injury to scar tissue from previous injury as seen in other types of injury such as musculotendinous sprain (Orchard 2001). Clinically, previous injury appears to affect muscle strength, which appears to place the tendon under increased potential to develop symptoms. Although quadriceps strength has been shown to be lower in affected patellar tendons (Gaida *et al.* 2004), cause and effect are not known.

DISEASE

Collagen disease such as Ehlers–Danlos syndrome, Marfan syndrome and Menke kinky hair syndrome can directly affect tendons; however, individuals with these diseases are predisposed to both musculoskeletal and vascular injury and they are often discouraged from undertaking athletic endeavors.

Several other systemic and genetic diseases predispose the tendon to symptoms. Systemic lupus erythematosus (Prasad *et al.* 2003) and rheumatoid arthritis (Fredberg 1997) can be associated with tendon rupture, and glycogen storage disease has been associated with Achilles tendinopathy (Carves *et al.* 2003). Psoriasis has also been associated with tendon rupture (Aydingoz and Aydingoz 2002). Vitamin C deficiency causes an excess of hydroxyproline in the urine and is reported to have an effect on collagen (O'Brien 1997).

Lipid metabolism

Increased levels of blood lipids may directly affect the tendon or tendon vascularity, both of which may lead to pathology and pain. Increased serum lipids levels have been associated with Achilles tendon rupture in several studies. Only one study has compared results with a control group and they reported serum cholesterol levels to be higher in subjects with tendinopathy than the control group (Ozgurtas *et al.* 2003). However, the control group in this study was not matched for activity levels, body mass, and time of blood collection, which renders the results difficult to interpret. Other studies of subjects with (Zehntner *et al.* 1984) and without (Mathiak *et al.* 1999b) frank lipid disorders suggest that further investigations are warranted.

AGE

Older age

Aging has been associated with an increase in prevalence of tendinopathy, to a point where the thirtieth birthday has been described as a risk factor for tendinopathy. Exactly what constitutes old age for a tendon is not defined; however, the incidence of ruptures increases in middle age. This suggests that old age for tendon pathology may in fact be earlier than middle age, as pathology precedes rupture.

In isolation, ageing does not mean that a tendon must be degenerate or have pathology. Maffulli *et al.* (2000a) demonstrated that the Achilles tendons of patients with peripheral vascular disease who underwent limb amputation had significantly less pathologic change than tendons of patients with symptomatic tendons.

Although most tendon ruptures occur later in life (Åström 1997), painful tendinopathy remains the domain of both the young, active athlete with large tendon loads and the older person, active or not. It seems that young people do not get symptomatic tendinopathy unless there is significant load, whereas older individuals can become symptomatic regardless of activity levels.

Major changes associated with aging include a decrease in ultimate strain and load, tensile strength, and an increase in stiffness. It is clear that these many changes must compromise the capacity of the tendon to absorb and respond to load. These changes in function are a result in structural change. For example, a decrease in cartilage oligomeric matrix protein whose function is to align collagen molecules (Smith *et al.* 2002) and transmit forces between collagen fibrils (Ker 2002) is correlated with a decrease in tensile stress and stiffness. Changes in collagen cross-links in aging tendon are also important in changing the mechanical properties of tendon (Banks *et al.* 1999).

Changes in vascularity with age are evident as a decrease in blood supply is reported (Kannus & Józsa 1991; Tuite *et al.* 1997). However, as increased peritendinous flow (and the tendon they supply) has been reported under conditions of exercise up to middle age (Langberg *et al.* 1998), vascular changes appear to occur later in life than middle age.

It seems self-evident in the face of changes in tendon structure and mechanical properties that when older people do get tendinopathy, the histopatholgy appears to be more severe than that seen in younger athletes (Åström & Rausing 1995). This may be because of the capacity of the original tissue as well as a decline in the ability of older tendons to repair.

Young age

Tendons of younger athletes may be structurally and functionally adaptable, but this does not protect them from tendon pathology and symptoms. As young tendons are smaller and can take less stress than mature tendons (Ker 2002), overload at this age may easily stimulate tendinopathy (Smith *et al.* 2002). Young partially disrupted ligament tissue repairs more quickly than older tissue and this may be analogous to tendon (Provenzano *et al.* 2002).

Tendinopathy has been shown to exist and to change in the patellar tendons of young athletes. Patellar tendinopathy seems to have a similar prevalence in adolescents as adult athletes, 23% of 268 tendons were abnormal on imaging in 14–18-year-old basketball players compared with 29% in a similar adult population (Cook *et al.* 1998, 2000a). More importantly, when followed over time, these young athletes were at a greater risk of developing symptoms than the adult athletes (Cook *et al.* 2000c).

RANGE OF MOTION

Both joint and muscle flexibility are assessed by clinicians when managing tendinopathy. There is evidence to support the importance of flexibility in the onset of pathology and onset of symptoms in several tendons. Witvrouw *et al.* (2001) assessed a cohort of subjects entering a physical education course and then examined which factors were found in those that developed tendon pain. They showed that hamstring and quadriceps inflexibility were associated with onset of patellar tendon pain. This finding is supported by Cook *et al.* (2004b) who examined hamstring flexibility (sit and reach) and patellar tendon pathology. They found a clear relationship between inflexibility and the presence of pathology in men and women with unilateral pathology.

Joint stiffness and joint hyperflexibility have also been suggested as risk factors for tendinopathy pain and pathology. Kaufmann *et al.* (1999) found that decreased ankle dorsiflexion and increased subtalar inversion increased the risk of Achilles tendon pain. Åström (1997) also reported that females with Achilles tendinopathy had decreased ankle and subtalar joint motion.

Foot posture remains very difficult to reliably measure and consequently, foot posture as a risk factor for tendinopathy is inherently difficult to investigate (Elveru *et al.* 1988). Åström (1997) found that foot posture was no different between subjects with Achilles tendon pain/pathology and matched controls. Clinically, assessing and treating foot mechanics remains an important part of a management plan.

STRENGTH

Strength has been reported as a risk factor for patellar tendinopathy, but both increased strength in athletes with symptoms and decreased strength have been reported. Gaida *et al.* (2004) reported a decrease in eccentric strength (measured isokinetically) in the quadriceps associated with patellar tendinopathy on imaging. Lian *et al.* (1996, 2003) reported an increase in work capacity and force produced (measured temporally with a contact mat) in athletes with symptoms. The difference in athlete gender, experimental method, and diagnostic criteria may explain the difference in the outcomes of these studies.

Very little research has been conducted that investigates strength in other tendons, except when the athlete presents for treatment of symptoms with conservative or surgical management. Recent success with heavy load eccentric exercise in the treatment of tendinopathy (Alfredson *et al.* 1998) suggest that musculotendinous strength may be important in ameliorating pain; however, it is not known if these subjects had muscle weakness before treatment or if the treatment takes them to "super" strength.

Extrinsic risk factors

It is clinically accepted that a change in load, training errors (linked to a change in load), changes in the environment, and change or faults with equipment such as racquets can result in an onset in tendon symptoms (Kannus 1997). Other extrinsic factors have little evidence to support them and further research is required.

Conclusions

This chapter has highlighted the challenges that face researchers and clinicians in understanding and treating tendinopathy. As pathology and pain may have different etiologies, and clinicians and researchers have different priorities, amalgamating knowledge in a form that will deliver better outcomes for athletes will be a long-term prospect.

Clinical relevance

The role of load in the etiology of both tendon pathology and tendon pain has great ramifications for athletes and coaches; however, load prescription that will prevent tendinopathy has not yet been determined. Eccentric load that occurs in many athletic activities is associated with the onset of tendinopathy, as those sports without large eccentric loads (cycling, rowing) do not have athletes with tendinopathy. However, reducing eccentric load in an athletic training program remains almost impossible. Tendon matrix response to load seems to be slow (several days) (see Chapter 5), and this suggests that high tendon load activity should not be undertaken daily.

Contrary to this, each individual may have the potential to respond differently to tendon load, and simple load management may not be applicable to every athlete. However, similar to load, it is not yet been completely defined which athletes will tolerate large amounts of tendon load. Gender, age, and disease are all known to directly affect tendons;

however, these are not under the control of either the coach or the athlete. Conversely, flexibility, strength, and extrinsic factors such as surface and equipment are controlled by the coach and athlete. The evidence that these are implicated in tendinopathy is incomplete; however, sufficient evidence is available to indicate that these factors must be managed in an athletic population.

Future directions

The direction of future research must focus on factors both within the tendon and within the athlete as well as extrinsic factors and preventative strategies. Tendon factors that require investigation include the stimulants to repair, understanding the source of pain, the relationship between pain and pathology, and the stimuli that set an athlete on the pathways to pathology and to pain. These simple pieces of knowledge may take many years to study, as human tendinopathy is difficult to study and animal models are poor substitutes. *In vitro* models of tendinopathy are improving but remain independent of so many factors intrinsic to an athlete. *In vivo* examination of tendon response is the future for this research.

Identifying athletes at risk may allow the athlete strategies to avoid tendon pain and pathology. This research must focus on research that allows modification of intrinsic factors such as flexibility, strength, and body composition.

In addition, quantification of a tendon's response to load is necessary for the development of appropriate training loads for athletes and correct prescription of training loads for athletes with painful tendinopathy. A step by step research program with multicenter collaborations will be the best approach to future tendinopathy research in all these areas.

References

Ackermann, P.W., Li, J., Lundeberg, T. & Kreicbergs, A. (2003) Neuronal plasticity in relation to nociception and healing of rat achilles tendon. *Journal of Orthopaedic Research* **21**, 432–441.
Alfredson, H. & Lorentzon, R. (2003) Intratendinous glutamate levels and eccentric training on chronic Achilles

tendinosis: a prospective study using microdialysis technique. *Knee Surgery Sports Traumatology Arthroscopy* **11**, 196–199.
Alfredson, H., Bjur, D., Thorsen, K., Lorentzon, R. & Sandstrom, P. (2002) High intratendinous lactate levels in painful chronic Achilles tendinosis.

An investigation using microdialysis technique. *Journal of Orthopaedic Research* **20**, 934–938.
Alfredson, H., Forsgren, S., Thorsen, K. & Lorentzon, R. (2001) *In vivo* microdialysis and immunohistochemical analyses of tendon tissue demonstrated high

amounts of free glutamate and glutamate receptors, but no signs of inflammation, in Jumper's knee. *Journal of Orthopaedic Research* **19**, 881–886.

Alfredson, H., Ljung, B.-O., Thorsen, K. & Lorentzon, R. (2000) *In vivo* investigation of ECRB tendons with microdialysis technique: no signs of inflammation but high amounts of glutamate in tennis elbow. *Acta Orthopaedica Scandinavica* **71**, 475–479.

Alfredson, H., Pietila, T., Jonsson, P. & Lorentzon, R. (1998) Heavy-load eccentric calf muscle training for the treatment of chronic Achilles tendinosis. *American Journal of Sports Medicine* **26**, 360–366.

Alfredson, H., Thorsen, K. & Lorentzon, R. (1999) *In situ* microdialysis in tendon tissue: high levels of glutamate, but not protoglandin E$_2$ in chronic Achilles tendon pain. *Knee Surgery, Sports Traumatology, Arthroscopy* **7**, 378–381.

Almekinders, L.C., Banes, A.J. & Ballenger, C.A. (1993) Effects of repetitive motion on human fibroblasts. *Medicine and Science in Sport and Exercise* **25**, 603–607.

Almekinders, L.C., Weinhold, P.S. & Maffulli, N. (2003) Compression etiology in tendinopathy. *Clinics in Sports Medicine* **22**, 703–710.

Andres, K.H., von During, M. & Schmidt, R.F. (1985) Sensory innervation of the Achilles tendon by group III and IV afferent fibres. *Anatomy and Embryology* **172**, 145–156.

Arnoczky, S., Lavagnino, M., Whallon, J.H. & Hoonjan, A. (2002) *In situ* cell nucleus deformation in tendons under tensile load: a morphological analysis using confocal laser microscopy. *Journal of Orthopaedic Research* **20**, 29–35.

Åström, M. (1997) *On the nature and etiology of chronic Achilles tendinopathy*. Lund University, Sweden.

Åström, M. & Rausing, A. (1995) Chronic Achilles tendinopathy: a survey of surgical and histopathological findings. *Clinical Orthopaedics* **316**, 151–164.

Åström, M. & Westlin, N. (1994a) Blood flow in chronic Achilles tendinopathy. *Clinical Orthopaedics* **308**, 166–172.

Åström, M. & Westlin, N. (1994b) Blood flow in the normal Achilles tendon assessed by laser Doppler flowmetry. *Journal of Orthopaedic Research* **12**, 246–252.

Aydingoz, U. & Aydingoz, O. (2002) Spontaneous rupture of the tibialis anterior tendon in a patient with psoriasis. *Clinical Imaging* **26**, 209–211.

Banes, A.J. & Hu, P., *et al.* (1995) Tendon cells of the epitenon and internal tendon compartment communicate mechanical signals through gap junctions and respond differentially to mechanical load and growth factors. In: *Repetitive Motion Disorders of the Upper Extremity* (Gordon, S.L., Blair, S.J. & Fine L.J., eds.) American Academy of Orthopaedic Surgeons, Park Ridge: 231–245.

Banks, R.A., TeKoppele, J.M., Oostingh, G., Hazleman, B.L. & Riley G.P. (1999) Lysylhydroxylation and non-reducible crosslinking of human supraspinatus tendon collagen: changes with age and in chronic rotator cuff tendinitis. *Annals of Rheumatic Diseases* **58**, 35–41.

Benjamin, M. & McGonagle, D. (2001) The anatomical basis for disease localisation in seronegative spondyloarthropathy at entheses and related sites. *Journal of Anatomy* **199**, 503–526.

Bestwick, C.S. & Maffulli, N. (2000) Reactive oxygen species and tendon problems: review and hypothesis. *Sports Medicine and Arthroscopy Review* **6**, 6–16.

Biberthaler, P., Weidemann, E., Nerlich, A., *et al.* (2003) Microcirculation associated with degenerative rotator cuff lesions. *Journal of Bone and Joint Surgery* **85-A**, 475–480.

Buchanan, C.I. & Marsh, R.L. (2002) Effects of exercsie on the biomechanical, biochemical and structural properties of tendons. *Comparative Biochemistry and Physiology Part A* **133**, 1101–1107.

Carves, C., Duquenoy, A., Toutain, F., *et al.* (2003) Gouty tendinitis revealing glycogen storage disease Type Ia in two adolescents. *Joint Bone Spine* **70**, 149–153.

Clement, D.B., Taunton, J.E. & Smart, G.W. (1984) Achilles tendinitis and peritendinitis: etiology and treatment. *American Journal of Sports Medicine* **12**, 179–184.

Cook, J. (2003) Tendon. In: *Physical Therapies in Sport and Exercise* (Kolt, G. & Snyder-Mackler, L., eds.) Harcourt Health Sciences.

Cook, J.L., Feller, J.A., Bonar, S.F. & Khan, K.M. (2004a) Abnormal tenocyte morphology is more prevalent than collagen disruption in asymptomatic athletes' patellar tendons: Is this the first step in the tendinosis cascade? *Journal of Orthopaedic Research* **24**, 34–38.

Cook, J.L., Khan, K.M., Kiss, Z.S. & Griffiths, L. (2000a) Patellar tendinopathy in junior basketball players: a controlled clinical and ultrasonographic study of 268 tendons in players aged 14–18 years.

Scandinavian Journal of Medicine and Science in Sports **10**, 216–220.

Cook, J.L., Khan, K.M., Harcourt, P.R., Grant, M., Younf, D.A. & Bonar, S.F. (1997) A cross-sectional study of 100 cases of jumper's knee managed conservatively and surgically. *British Journal of Sports Medicine* **31**, 332–336.

Cook, J.L., Khan, K.M., Harcourt, P.R., *et al.* (1998) Patellar tendon ultrasonography in asymptomatic active athletes reveals hypoechoic regions: a study of 320 tendons. *Clinical Journal of Sports Medicine* **8**, 73–77.

Cook, J.L., Khan, K.M., Kiss, Z.S., Coleman, B.D. & Griffiths, L. (2000b) Asymptomatic hypoechoic regions on patellar tendon US do not foreshadow symptoms of jumper's knee: a 4 year followup of 46 tendons. *Scandinavian Journal of Science and Medicine in Sports* **11**, 321–327.

Cook, J.L., Khan, K.M., Kiss, Z.S., *et al.* (2004b) Posterior leg tightness and vertical jump are associated with US patellar tendon abnormality in 14–18-year old basketball players: a cross-sectional anthropometric and physical performance study. *British Journal of Sports Medicine* **38**, 206–209.

Cook, J.L., Kiss, Z.S., Khan, K.M., *et al.* (2000c) Prospective imaging study of asymptomatic patellar tendinopathy in elite junior basketball players. *Journal of Ultrasound in Medicine* **19**, 473–479.

Cook, J.L., Malliaras, P., De Luca, J., *et al.* (2004c) Neovascularisation and pain in abnormal patellar tendons of active jumping athletes. *Clinical Journal of Sports Medicine* **14**, 296–299.

Elveru, R.A., Rothsein, J.M., Lamb, R.L. (1988) Goniometric reliability in a clinical setting. Subtalar and ankle joint measurements. *Physical Therapy* **68**, 672–677.

Evans, C. (1999) Cytokines and the role they play in the healing of ligaments and tendons. *Sports Medicine* **28**, 71–76.

Fahlstrom, M. (2001) *Badminton and the Achilles tendon*. Department of Surgical and Perioperative Sciences. Umea, Umea University: 126.

Ferretti, A. (1986) Epidemiology of jumper's knee. *Sports Medicine* **3**, 289–295.

Ferretti, A., Ippolito, E., Mariani, P. & Puddu, G. (1983) Jumper's knee. *American Journal of Sports Medicine* **11**, 58–62.

Forslund, C. & Aspenberg, P. (2002) CDMP-2 induces bone or tendon-like tissue depending on mechanical stimulation. *Journal of Orthopaedic Research* **20**, 1170–1174.

Fredberg, U. (1997) Local corticosteroid injection in sport: review of literature and guidelines for treatment. *Scandinavian Journal of Medicine and Science in Sports* **7**, 131–139.

Fredberg, U. & Bolvig, L. (2002) Significance of ultrasonographically detected asymptomatic tendinosis in the patellar and Achilles tendons of elite soccer players. *American Journal of Sports Medicine* **30**, 488–491.

Gaida, J., Cook, J., Bass, S.L., Austen, S. & Kiss, Z.S. (2004) Are unilateral and bilateral patellar tendinopathy distinguished by differences in anthropometry, body composition or muscle strength in elite female basketball players? *British Journal of Sports Medicine* **38**, 581–585.

Gotoh, M., Hamada, K., Yamakawa, H., Inoue, A. & Fukuda, H. (1998) Increased substance P in subacromial bursa and shoulder pain in rotator cuff disease. *Journal of Orthopaedic Research* **16**, 618–621.

Green, J.S., Morgan, B., Lauder, I., Finlay, D.B., Allen, M. & Belton, I. (1996) The correlation of bone scintigraphy and histological finding in patellar tendinitis. *Nuclear Medicine Communications* **17**, 231–234.

Green, J.S., Morgan, B., Lauder, I., Finlay, D.B. & Allen, M. (1997) Correlation of magnetic resonance imaging and histology in patellar tendinitis. *Sports Exercise and Injury* **3**, 80–84.

Hagberg, M. & Wegman, D.H. (1987) Prevalence rates and odds ratios of shoulder-neck diseases in different occupational groups. *British Journal of Industrial Medicine* **44**, 602–610.

Hamilton, B. & Purdam, C. (2003) Patellar tendinosis as an adaptive response: A new hypothesis. *British Journal of Sports Medicine* **38**, 758–761.

Hart, D., Archambault, J., Kydd, A., Reno, C., Frank, C.B. & Herzog, W. (1998) Gender and neurogenic variables in tendon biology and repetitive motion disorders. *Clinical Orthopaedics and Related Research* **351**, 44–56.

Hart, D., Kydd, A. & Reno, C. (1999) Gender and pregnancy affect neuropeptide responses of the rabbit Achilles tendon. *Clinical Orthopaedics and Related Research* **365**, 237–246.

Hewett, T. (2000) Neuromuscular and hormonal factors associated with knee injuries in female athletes. *Sports Medicine* **29**, 313–327.

Ho, H.-M. & Lee W.-K.E. (2003) Traumatic bilateral concurrent patellar tendon rupture: and alternative fixation method. *Knee Surgery, Sports Traumatology, Arthroscopy* **11**, 105–111.

Johnson, D.P., Wakeley, C.J. & Watt, I. (1996) Magnetic resonance imaging of patellar tendonitis. *Journal of Bone and Joint Surgery* **78-B**, 452–457.

Józsa, L., Bálint, J.B., Reffy A., *et al.* (1982) Hypoxic alterations of tenocytes in degenerative tendonopathy. *Archives of Orthopaedic and Traumatic Surgery* **99**, 243–246.

Józsa, L., Balint, J., Kannus, P., Reffy, A. & Barzo, M. (1989) Distribution of blood groups in patients with tendon injury. *Journal of Bone and Joint Surgery* **71**, 272–274.

Kannus, P. (1997) Etiology and pathophysiology of chronic tendon disorders in sport. *Scandinavian Journal of Medicine and Science in Sports* **7**, 78–85.

Kannus, P. & Józsa, L. (1991) Histopathological changes preceding spontaneous rupture of a tendon. *Journal of Bone and Joint Surgery* **73A**, 1507–1525.

Karageanes, S., Blackburn, K., Vangelos, Z.A. (2000) The association of the menstrual cycle with the laxity of the anterior cruciate ligament in adolescent female athletes. *Clinical Journal of Sport Medicine* **10**, 162–168.

Kaufman, K., Brodine, S., Shaffer, R.A., Johnson, C.W. & Cullison, T.R. (1999) The effect of foot structure and range of motion on musculoskeletal overuse injuries. *American Journal of Sports Medicine* **27**, 585–593.

Kennedy, J.C. & Willis, R.B. (1976) The effects of local steroid injections on tendons: a biomechanical and microscopic correlative study. *American Journal of Sports Medicine* **4**, 11–21.

Ker, R.F. (2002) The implications of the adaptable fatigue quality of tendons for their construction, repair and function. *Comparative Biochemistry and Physiology Part A* **133**, 987–1000.

Khan, K.M., Bonar, F., Desmond, P.M., *et al.* (1996) Patellar tendinosis (jumper's knee): findings at histopathologic examination, US and MR imaging. *Radiology* **200**, 821–827.

Khan, K.M., Cook, J.L., Kiss, Z.S., *et al.* (1997) Patellar tendon ultrasonography and jumper's knee in elite female basketball players: a longitudinal study. *Clinical Journal of Sports Medicine* **7**, 199–206.

Khan, K.M., Forster, B.B., Robinson, J., *et al.* (2003) Are ultrasound and magnetic resonance imaging of value in assessment of Achilles tendon disorders? A two year prospective study. *British Journal of Sports Medicine* **37**, 149–154.

Khurana, R., Torzillo, P., Horsley, M. & Mahoney, J. (2002) Spontaneous bilateral rupture of the Achilles tendon in a patient with chronic obstructive airways disease. *Respirology* **7**, 161–163.

Koivunen-Niemela, T. & Parkkola, K. (1995) Anatomy of the Achilles tendon (tendo calcaneus) with respect to tendon thickness measurements. *Surgical and Radiologic Anatomy* **17**, 263–268.

Komi, P.V. & Bosco, C. (1978) Utilization of stored elastic energy in leg extensor muscle by men and women. *Medicine and Science in Sports and Exercise* **10**, 261–265.

Kraushaar, B. & Nirschl, R. (1999) Tendinosis of the elbow (tennis elbow). Clinical features and findings of histological, immunohistochemical, and electron microscopy studies. *Journal of Bone and Joint Surgery America* **81**, 259–278.

Kujala, U.M., Jarvinen, M., Natri A., *et al.* (1992) ABO blood groups and musculoskeletal injuries. *Injury* **23**, 131–133.

Langberg, H., Bulow, J. & Kjaer, M. (1998) Blood flow in the peritendinous space of the human Achilles tendon during exercise. *Acta Physiologica Scandinavia* **163**, 149–153.

Langberg, H., Skovgaard, D., Karamouzis, M., Bulow, J. & Kjaer, M. (1999) Metabolism and inflammatory mediators in the peritendinous space measured by microdialysis during intermittent isometric exercise in humans. *Journal of Physiology* **515**, 919–927.

Leadbetter, W. (1992) Cell matrix response in tendon injury. *Clinics in Sports Medicine* **11**, 533–578.

Lian, O., Engebretsen, L., Ovrebo, R.V. & Bahr, R. (1996) Characteristics of the leg extensors in male volleyball players with jumper's knee. *American Journal of Sports Medicine* **24**, 380–385.

Lian, O., Refsnes, P.E., Engebretsen, L. & Bahr, R. (2003) Performance characteristics of volleyball players with patellar tendinopathy. *American Journal of Sports Medicine* **31**, 408–413.

Liu, S.H., Al-Shaikh, R.A., Panossian, V., Fineman, G.A. & Lane, J.M. (1997) Estrogen affects the cellular metabolism of the anterior cruciate ligament. A potential explanation for female athletic injury. *American Journal of Sports Medicine* **25**, 704–709.

Ljung, B., Forsgren, S. & Friden, J. (1999) Substance P and calcitonin gene-related peptide expression at the extensor carpi radialis brevis muscle origin: implications for the etiology of tennis elbow. *Journal of Orthopaedic Research* **17**, 554–559.

Maffulli, N., Barrass, V. & Ewen, S.W. (2000a) Light microscopic histology of Achilles tendon ruptures. *American Journal of Sports Medicine* **28**, 857–863.

Maffulli, N., Reaper, J.A., Waterston, S.W. & Ahya, T. (2000b) ABO blood groups and Achilles tendon rupture in the Grampian region of Scotland. *Clinical Journal of Sport Medicine* **10**, 269–271.

Maffulli, N., Waterston, W., Squair, J., Reaper, J. & Douglas, A.S. (1999a) Changing incidence of Achilles tendon rupture in Scotland: a 15 year study. *Clinical Journal of Sports Medicine* **9**, 157–160.

Mathiak, G., Wening, J.V., Mathiak, M., Neville, L.F. & Jungbluth, K. (1999b) Serum cholesterol is elevated in patients with Achilles tendon rupture. *Archives of Orthopaedics, Trauma and Surgery* **119**, 280–284.

McGonagle, D., Marzo-Ortega, H., Benjamin, M. & Emery, P. (2003) Report on the Second international Enthesitis Workshop. *Arthritis and Rheumatism* **48**, 896–905.

Mehm, W.J., Pimsler, M., Becker, R.L. & Lissner, C.R. (1988) Effect of oxygen on *in vitro* fibroblast cell proliferation and collagen biosynthesis. *Journal of Hyperbaric Medicine* **3**, 227–234.

Mokone, G.G., Gajjar, M., September, A.V., *et al.* (2005) The guanine-thymine dinucleotide repeat polymorphism within the tenascin-C gene is associated with Achilles tendon injuries. *American Journal of Sports Medicine* **33**, 1016–21.

Mokone, G.G., Schwellnus, M.P., Noakes, T.D. & Collins, M. (2006) The COL5A1 gene and Achilles tendon pathology. *Scandinavian Journal of Medicine & Science in Sports* **16**, 19–26.

Molloy, T., Wang, Y. & Murrell, G. (2003) The roles of growth factors in tendons and ligament healing. *Sports Medicine* **33**, 381–394.

Movin, T., Gad, A., Guntner, P, Foldhazy, Z. & Rolf, C. (1997a) Pathology of the achilles tendon in association with ciprofloxacin treatment. *Foot and Ankle International* **18**, 297–299.

Movin, T., Gad, A., Reinholt, F.P. & Rolf, C. (1997b) Tendon pathology in long-standing achillodynia. Biopsy findings in 40 patients. *Acta Orthopaedica Scandinavia* **68**, 170–175.

Moyer, K.E., Saba, A.A., Hauck, R.M. & Ehrlich, H.P. (2003) Systemic vanadate ingestion modulates rat tendon repair. *Experimental and Molecular Pathology* **75**, 80–88.

Murrell, G.A., Szabo, C., Hannafin, J.A., *et al.* (1997) Modulation of tendon healing by nitric oxide. *Inflammation Research* **46**, 19–27.

Nirschl, R.P. (1992) Elbow tendinosis/tennis elbow. *Clinics in Sports Medicine* **11**, 851–870.

O'Brien, M. (1997) Structure and metabolism of tendons. *Scandinavian Journal of Medicine and Science in Sports* **7**, 55–61.

Ohberg, L. & Alfredson, H. (2002) Ultrasound guided sclerosis of neovessels in painful chronic Achilles tendinosis: pilot study of a new treatment. *British Journal of Sports Medicine* **36**, 173–177.

Ohberg, L., Lorentzon, R. & Alfredson, H. (2001) Neovascularisation in Achilles tendons with painful tendinosis but not in normal tendons: an ultrasonographic investigation. *Knee Surgery, Sports Traumatology, Arthroscopy* **9**, 233–238.

Olivieri, L., Gemignani, G., Gherardi, S., Grassi, L. & Ciompi, M.L. (1987) Isolated HLA B-27 associated Achilles tendinitis. *Annals of Rheumatic Diseases* **46**, 626–627.

Orchard, J.W. (2001) Intrinsic and extrinsic risk factors for muscle strains in Australian football. *American Journal of Sports Medicine* **29**, 300–303.

Ozgurtas, T., Yildiz, C., Serdar, M., Atesalp, S. & Kutluay, T. (2003) Is high concentration of serum lipids a risk factor for Achilles tendon rupture? *Clinica Chimica Acta* **331**, 25–28.

Paoloni, J., Appleyard, R. & Murrell, G.A.C. (2003) Topical nitric oxide application in the treatment of chronic extensor tendinosis at the elbow: a randomized, double-blinded, placebo-controlled clinical trial. *American Journal of Sports Medicine* **31**, 915–20.

Prasad, S., Lee, A., Clarnette, R. & Faull, R. (2003) Spontaneous bilateral patellar tendon rupture in a woman with previous Achilles rupture and systemic lupus erythematosus. *Rheumatology* **42**, 905–906.

Provenzano, P.P., Hayashi, K., Kunz, D.N., Markel, M.D. & Vanderby, R. Jr. (2002) Healing of subfailure ligament injury: comparison between immature and mature ligaments in a rat model. *Journal of Orthopaedic Research* **20**, 975–983.

Pufe, T., Petersen, W., Kurz, B., Tsokos, M., Tillmann, B. & Mentlein, R. (2003) Mechanical factors influence the expression of endostatin: an inhibitor of angiogenesis—in tendons. *Journal of Orthopaedic Research* **21**, 610–616.

Rempel, D. & Abrahamsson, S.O. (2001) The effects of reduced oxygen tension on cell proliferation and matrix synthesis in synovium and tendon explants from the rabbit carpal tunnel: an experimental study *in vitro*. *Journal of Orthopaedic Research* **19**, 143–148.

Ritty, T.M. & Herzog, J. (2003) Tendon cells produce gelatinases in response to type I collagen attachment. *Journal of Orthopaedic Research* **21**, 442–450.

Rufai, A., Ralphs, J.R. & Benjamin, M. (1995) Structure and histopathology of the insertional region of the human Achilles tendon. *Journal of Orthopaedic Research* **13**, 585–593.

Schmid, M.R., Hodler, J., Cathrein, P., Duewell, S., Jacob, H.A. & Romero, J. (2002) Is impingement the cause of jumper's knee? Dynamic and static magnetic resonance imaging of patellar tendinitis in an open-configuration system. *American Journal of Sports Medicine* **30**, 388–395.

Scott, A., Khan, K., Heer, J., Cook, J.L., Lian, O. & Duronio, V. (2005) High strain mechanical loading rapidly induces tendon apoptosis: an *ex vivo* rat tibialis anterior model. *British Journal of Sports Medicine* **39**, e25.

Shalaby, M. & Almekinders, L.C. (1999) Patellar tendinitis: The significance of magnetic resonance imaging findings. *American Journal of Sports Medicine* **27**, 345–349.

Shirakura, K., Ciarelli, M.J., *et al.* (1995) Deformation induced calcium signaling in tenocytes *in situ*. Combined Orthopaedic Research Societies Meeting, San Diego, California.

Smith, R.K.W., Birch, H.L., Goodman, S., Heinegard, D. & Goodship, A.E. (2002) The influence of ageing and exercise on tendon growth and degeneration: hypotheses for the initiation and prevention of strain-induced tendinopathies. *Comparative Biochemistry and Physiology Part A* **133**, 1039–1050.

Sullo, A., Maffulli, N., Capasso, G. & Testa, V. (2001) The effects of prolonged peritendinous administration of PGE$_1$ to the rat Achilles tendon: a possible animal model of chronic Achilles tendinopathy. *Journal of Orthopaedic Science* 6, 349–357.

Ta, K.T., Eidelman, D. & Thomson, J.G. (1999) Patient satisfaction and outcomes of surgery for de Quervain's tenosynovitis. *Journal of Hand Surgery. American volume* 24A, 1071–1077.

Terslev, L., Qvistgaard, E., Torp-Pedersen, S., Laetgaard, J., Danneskiold-Samsoe, B. & Bliddal, L. (2001) Ultrasound and power Doppler findings in jumper's knee: preliminary findings. *European Journal of Ultrasound* 13, 183–189.

Thomopoulos, S., Williams, G.R., Gimbel, J.A., Favata, M. & Soslowsky, L.J. (2003) Variation of biomechanical, structural, and compositional properties along the tendon to bone insertion site. *Journal of Orthopaedic Research* 21, 413–419.

Tsai, W.C., Tang, F.T., Wong, M.K. & Pang, J.H. (2003) Inhibition of tendon cell migration by dexamethasone is correlated with reduced alpha-smooth muscle actin gene expression: a potential mechanism of delayed tendon healing. *Journal of Orthopaedic Research* 21, 265–271.

Tuite, D.J., Renstrom, P.A. & O'Brien, M. (1997) The aging tendon. *Scandinavian Journal of Medicine & Science in Sports* 7, 72–77.

Uhthoff, H.K. & Matsumoto, F. (2000) Rotator cuff tendinopathy. *Sports Medicine and Arthroscopy Review* 8, 56–68.

van Griensven, M., Zeichen, J., Skuten, M., Barkhausen, T., Krettek, C. & Bosch, U. (2003) Cyclic mechanical strain induces NO production in human patellar tendon fibroblasts: a possible role for remodelling and pathological transformation. *Experimental and Toxilogical Pathology* 54, 335–338.

Wang, M.X., Wei, A., Yuan, J., *et al.* (2001) Antioxidant enzyme peroxiredoxin 5 is upregulated in degenerative human tendon. *Biochemical and Biophysical Research Communications* 284, 667–673.

Wilson, A.M. & Goodship, A.E. (1994) Exercise-induced hyperthermia as a possible mechanism for tendon degeneration. *Journal Biomechanics* 27, 899–905.

Witvrouw, E., Bellemans, J., Lysens, R., Danneels, L. & Cambier, D. (2001) Intrinsic risk factors for the development of patellar tendinitis in an athletic population: a two-year prospective study. *American Journal of Sports Medicine* 29, 190–195.

Woo, S.L-Y., Gomez, M.A., Woo, Y.K. & Akeson, W.H. (1982) Mechanical properties of tendons and ligaments. II. The relationship between immobilization and exercise on tissue remodelling. *Biorheology* 19, 397–408.

Woo, S.L-Y., Maynard, J. *et al.* (1988) Ligament, tendon and joint capsule insertions to bone. In: *Injury and Repair of the Musculoskeletal Soft Tissues* (Woo, S.L-Y. & Buckwalter, J.A., eds.) American Academy of Orthopedic Surgeons, Park Ridge, IL: 133–166.

Yuan, J., Murrell, G.A., Trickett, A. & Wang, M.X. (2003) Involvement of cytochrome c release and caspase-3 activation in the oxidative stress-induced apoptosis in human tendon fibroblasts. *Molecular Cell Research* 1641, 35–41.

Yuan, J., Murrell, G.A., Wei, A.Q. & Wang, M.X. (2002) Apoptosis in rotator cuff tendonopathy. *Journal of Orthopaedic Research* 20, 1372–1379.

Zamora, A.J. & Marini, J.F. (1988) Tendon and myotendinous junction in an overloaded skeletal muscle of the rat. *Anatomy and Embryology* 179, 89–96.

Zanetti, M., Metzdorf, A., Kundert, H.P., *et al.* (2003) Achilles tendons: clinical relevance of neovascularization diagnosed with power Doppler US. *Radiology* 227, 556–560.

Zehntner, M.K., Reitamo, R., Mordasini, R. & Ledermann, M. (1984) Traumatic ruptures of the Achilles tendon and hyperlipidaemia. *Unfallheilkunde* 87, 226–229.

Chapter 3

The Molecular Biology of Tendinopathy: Signaling and Response Pathways in Tenocytes

ALBERT J. BANES, MARI TSUZAKI, MICHELLE WALL, JIE QI, XI YANG, DONALD BYNUM, SPERO KARAS, DAVID A. HART, ALLISON NATION, ANN MARIE FOX, AND LOUIS C. ALMEKINDERS

Pathologic states of flexor, and sometimes extensor tendons, have been classified as variations of acute "tendonitis" or, more popularly, tendinosis. These conditions are described as painful but usually lacking inflammatory cells, presenting with edema and capillary enlargement in the epitenon and/or endotenon. Emphasis has been placed on an inciting event such as a traumatic injury or an overuse pattern which may result in classic signs including erythema, swelling, tenderness, and pain. Although data from recent reports speak against classic inflammation, an inciting event may involve brief activation of a classic inflammatory pathway with elaboration of mediators, limited recruitment of inflammatory cells, vascular involvement, and cellular inflammation. However, non-classic inflammatory pathways may dominate in the etiology of tendinopathy. It is hypothesized that tenocytes themselves are stimulated by cytokines to produce catabolic proteases which weaken the matrix. Tenocytes can also secrete neuroactive mediators which affect pain or mechanoreceptors. Local concentrations of neurotransmitters such as Ca^{2+}, adenosine triphosphate (ATP), substance P, neuropeptide Y, glutamate, or even prostaglandin E_2 (PGE_2) may contribute to increased pain. Cytokines, such as tumor necrosis factor α (TNF-α) and interleukin-1β (IL-1β) from the circulation immune cells, or from tenocytes themselves, induce matrix metalloproteinases (MMP) in tenocytes, which, when activated, degrade collagen and proteoglycan, resulting in tendon rupture. Continued mechanical loading superposed on tendon pathology drive shared pathways that are modulatory, and may be synergistic or antagonistic. A unifying model of inciting events for tenocytes is presented, which is hypothesized to lead to a tendinopathy. The involvement of Ca^{2+} as a signaling mediator inside the cell, as well as a regulator of a load response as an exogenous mediator, underscores the importance of extracellular calcium concentration as well as ion channels that regulate its movement. Other mediators, such as ATP or adenosine diphosphate (ADP) as load response modulators, particularly of IL-1β-induced MMP expression, emphasize both positive and negative modulation of these pathways. Overall, tenocytes have options in their responses to mechanical load and mediators. These options include cell migration, proliferation, cytoskeletal changes, alteration of cell modulus, matrix reorganization and/or remodeling, matrix metabolism, change in biomechanical strength, and tenocyte death. Pain, matrix disruption, and, ultimately, tendon failure are the results of chronic tendinopathy.

Introduction

Tendons join striated skeletal muscle at an origin, an extensively integrated myotendinous junction that is biased towards tendon infiltration and/or interdigitation into the muscle body with an accompanying trellis or sheet-like epimysium at the muscle surface (Purslow 2002). A tendon joins distally with bone where fibrous collagens in the tensile load-bearing segment transform into a more cartilaginous matrix with variations on the angle of insertion into bone, depending on the tendon location, to form an osseotendinous junction (Benjamin *et al.* 2002). Tendons mandate a more complex architecture and symbiosis with communicating structures to accomplish force transmission involved in limb movement. Tendons are comprised of or interact with special structures, such as aponeuroses and other tendons, bursas, pulleys, and sheaths in the hand and wrist, and incorporate vinculae in digital tendons, as conduits for vessels and nerves (O'Brien 2005). In addition, vessels, nerves, and component cells contend with the shear created during excursion, compression where tendons travel through soft tissue pulleys or over bone, and tensile forces transferred from muscle to the tendon matrix. Tenocytes can also generate their own traction forces as they remodel the matrix (Stopak & Harris 1982). Blood vessels and nerves cannot invade or function along the full extent of a long tendon, likely because of the pressures exerted through muscle force but also as a result of grasping, body weight, ground reaction forces, and even swelling. Moreover, in thick tendons, such as the Achilles tendon, diffusion of nutrients from blood vessels becomes more difficult because of distance, leaving diffusion as the principal means of nutrient transfer to cells. These anatomic points underlie functional issues and design limitations that evolve into pathologies as use paradigms are pushed to the maximum and aging phenomena exacerbate the intrinsic limitations.

Injuries to tendons most often occur in the digital flexor tendon in the hand as a result of traumatic lacerations and tendon–pulley mismatch. Intrinsic, non-penetrating injuries are most common in patellar tendon in the knee, Achilles, and posterior tibialis tendons in the lower leg, common extensor tendon at the elbow, and supraspinatus tendon in the shoulder. A total of 120 000 patients per year undergo tendon or ligament repairs in the USA (Langer & Vacanti 1993). Chronic overuse of a tendon may lead to tendon pain, loss of function, and ultimately failure. There are two principal patient scenarios associated with tendon injury that result in an examination and procedure by a doctor: an acute incident during an activity such as running, lifting, or upper body work/sports activities resulting in sudden pain and loss of function of a limb, or a chronic pain that worsens, resulting in inability to perform work or sports at a normal level. The subjective analysis of Repetitive Motion Disorder is graded 1–6, where 1 is the ability to function normally and 6 is an inability to function at all or with extreme pain and weakness (Curwin & Stanish 1984). The supraspinatus tendon in the shoulder and flexor tendon of the hand usually present with an entrapment problem where the tendon impinges or is swollen and cannot glide easily through its tunnel, pulley, or extratendinous tissue. The posterior tibialis tendon generally becomes painful as a result of abnormal gait or strain from an overuse activity. The patellar tendon may avulse from bone, whereas the Achilles tendon tears at mid-substance about 1.7–7 cm from the insertion into bone (Åström & Rausing 1995).

Tendon pathologies can be classified as:
1 tendinitis, an inflammation of the paratenon with pain and swelling;
2 tendinosis, a defect in the tendon matrix without inflammation but with pain and swelling; or
3 a traumatic injury involving a partial or complete rupture of the tendon.

Rupture results in bleeding, clotting, and release of platelet-derived growth factor (PDGF) and transforming growth factor β (TGF-β) from platelets, release of hormones such as epinephrine and norepinephrine from blood vessels and/or nerves, release of ATP, activation of insulin-like growth factor 1 (IGF-1) from plasma and tendon matrix and TGF-β from matrix at the wound site. Inflammation can occur with influx of white cells, swelling, expression of cytokines, such as IL-1β, and metalloproteinases, such as MMP-1, MMP-2, MMP-3, and MMP-13, respectively (Guyton *et al.* 2000). Within hours to several days, cell migration from the paratenon and epitenon into the wound site occurs followed by cell division and then matrix synthesis (Banes *et al.* 1981). Results of microscopy studies of chronic Achilles tendinopathy indicate that pathologic regions contain less collagen, loss of fibrillar structure, more glycosaminoglycans (GAG) and hemosiderin deposits from red blood cells indicating a vascular compromise (Movin *et al.* 1997). Passive or active motion speeds recovery and promotes increased range of motion, but the mechanisms by which this phenomenon occurs remain conjectural (Gelberman *et al.* 1983).

Results of light and transmission electron microscopy studies have shown that cells in both the epitenon and the internal compartment of whole tendon are physically connected to each other (Chaplin & Greenlee 1975; McNeilly *et al.* 1996). It is through these junctions that tenocytes signal load stimuli via inositol 1,4,5-triphosphate (IP_3) movement and increased intracellular calcium ions (Boitano *et al.* 1992). Epitenon cells and internal fibroblasts *in vivo* are layered in longitudinal syncytia that seem optimal for rapid and repeated chemical and electrical coupling. Cells within tendon and *in vitro* are coupled and respond to a plasma membrane indentation by releasing intracellular calcium stores and propagating a calcium wave to adjacent cells for up to 4–7 cell diameters (Banes 1993). *In vivo*, tendons fixed with glutaraldehyde under tension contain cells that are dramatically indented, like marshmallows squeezed between rods (Merrilees & Flint 1980). Avian tendon cells express connexin (cx) gap junctions (Banes *et al.* 1999). Avian tendon cells have at least three forms of cx43: a 42-kD non-phosphorylated form and two intermediate forms of 44–47 kD that are phosphorylated at serine (Musil *et al.* 1990). Quiescent tendon surface cells (TSC) have predominantly the non-phosphorylated form of cx43 but have phosphorylated forms during log phase (Banes *et al.* 1998). TSC and tendon internal fibroblasts (TIF) express mRNA for cx42, 43, 45, and 45.5 detected by polymerase chain reaction and confirmed by cloning and sequencing, but cx43 is the only form detected by Northern analysis, underscoring its role as the major gap junction species expressed by tendon cells (Tsuzaki *et al.* 1997; Banes *et al.* 1999). However, cx26, 32, and 43 have been detected by Western blots. Cx32 and 43 have been visualized by scanning confocal microscopy and cx37 has been detected by gene array analysis (Banes *et al.* 1999). However, cx43 appears to predominate.

Tissues and cells *in vivo* are subjected to ground reaction forces, gravity, barometric pressure, vibration, and contact with bodies, resulting in dynamic mechanical stimulation. Cells can sense mechanical stimuli in diverse ways. They respond to "outside-in" mechanical signals through stretch-activated and other ion channels as the plasma membrane is deformed, through integrin linkages from the matrix to the cytoskeleton, and with cadherins or desmosomes in cell–cell connections (Banes *et al.* 1995, 2003). Ion channels, particularly calcium channels, have an important role in the signal transduced from the mechanical stimulus to a chemical signal, such as an increase in intracellular calcium concentration which can be blocked by removal of extracellular calcium (Wall *et al.* 2004). Subsequently, intracellular pathway activation initiates phosphorylation events and protein–protein associations, including association of integrin β subunits with the cytoskeleton and associated proteins, including focal adhesion kinase (FAK), paxillin, filamin, integrin-linked kinase (ILK), vinculin, and talin. Phospholipases A and C (PLA, PLC), adenyl cyclase, guanyl cyclase, inducible nitric oxide synthase (iNOS), and other enzymes are activated producing the second messengers: cyclic adenosine monophosphate (cAMP), cyclic guanosine monophosphate (cGMP), ATP, guanosine triphophate (GTP), nitric oxide (NO), PGE_2, IP_3, and diacyglycerol (DAG), which act in autocrine and paracrine fashion. Furthermore, specific pathways may be activated that drive mitogenesis (MEK/MAPK), a stress response (JAK/STAT and JNK/SAPK), apoptosis, or other responses (Banes *et al.* 1981; Lavignino *et al.* 2003; Arnoczky *et al.* 2004; Lavagnino & Arnoczky 2005). The signal can be transduced from cell to cell by mediator secretion or through gap junctions.

Relevance to tendinopathy

Pathways that have an impact on driving tenocytes toward tendinopathy include high intracellular calcium, which can lead to cell death through apoptosis (Arnoczky *et al.* 2002). High NO concentrations have also been associated with activating an apoptotic pathway (Murrell 2002). If both intracellular calcium and NO were in high concentration at the cell level, apoptosis would occur, resulting in local cell death, a high ATP concentration, and perhaps a focal necrotic lesion. Other destructive pathways may be activated by cytokines that drive matrix destruction.

Methods

Cell culture

Avian tendon internal fibroblasts (ATIF) were isolated from the flexor digitorum profundus tendons of 52-day-old White Leghorn chickens. Chicken feet were obtained from a Purdue processing plant (Robbins, NC). Legs were washed with soap and cold water prior to tendon isolation. The flexor digitorum profundus tendons were removed from the middle toes after transection at the proximal portion of the metatarsal and distal portion of the tibiotarsus. Using sterile technique, tendons were dissected from their sheath and placed in a sterile dish of phosphate buffered saline (PBS) with 20 mmol HEPES, pH 7.2 with 1× penicillin/streptomycin (100 units penicillin·100 μg streptomycin per ml, 1× PS). Cells from patients were obtained from tissues discarded at surgery. Cells were subsequently isolated by sequential enzymatic digestion and mechanical disruption (Banes *et al.* 1988). Either TSC or TIF were used in these experiments. Cells were cultured until confluent in Dulbecco Minimum Essential Media-High glucose (DMEM-H) with 10% fetal calf serum (FCS), 20 mmol HEPES, pH 7.2, 100 μmol ascorbate-2-phosphate and antibiotics (100 units penicillin·100 μg streptomycin per ml, 1× PS).

Strain application to rat tail tendon fascicles

Rats were euthanized by CO_2 asphyxiation in an approved device that did not unduly stress the animals (Institutional Animal Care and Use Committees [IACUC] regulations). Tendon fascicles were harvested from the tails of 4–6-month-old Sprague–Dawley rats weighing approximately 0.3–0.4 kg. A Tendon Loading Device (TLD) was used to apply strain to tendon fascicles. It consisted of a stainless steel plate with a stainless steel reservoir mounted on top. Inside the reservoir was a track along which two grips with ball-bearing bases could slide. One grip was adjusted to remain in a stationary position to simulate the osteotendinous junction, while the other grip was attached to a movable, small diameter steel cable through which forces were administered, simulating the myotendious junction. The cable was attached to a linear screw actuator with a 0.1-μm resolution (Encoded Linear Actuator 842, Siskiyou Design Instruments, Inc., Grants Pass, OR), and equipped with a Sensotec 5 lb load cell (Model 31, Sensotec, Columbus, OH). The actuator was mounted to an XYZ-axis stage (Crossed Roller Translation Stage, 1600 Series, Siskiyou Design Instruments, Inc., Grants Pass, OR) which was manually adjustable to maintain linearity among the actuator, cable, and gripped fascicle. All components were mounted to a rigid base so that tensile load from the actuator could be applied to the sample in the grips with minimal slippage in the system. The actuator was controlled by a closed loop, four axis motion controller (MC2000, Siskiyou Design Instruments, Inc., Grants Pass, OR) using a laptop computer with a custom LabVIEW software interface for direct input of increases or decreases in actuator position. The load cell was connected to an additional laptop computer with a second custom LabVIEW software interface which was used to collect load data every second. Tendon fascicles in warm PBS were washed with calcium-free Earles' balanced salt solution (EBSS) before being incubated in 5 mmol Fura 2-AM at room temperature (25°C) for 1 hour. After 1 hour, the fascicles were washed in EBSS to remove excess Fura 2-AM. EBSS was added with a calcium concentration of 1.80 mmol and the fascicles were allowed to incubate for another hour.

Tendon fascicles were placed in the TLD such that a crimp pattern was still visible when observed through the 20× objective lens of an Olympus BX 51 ratiometric calcium imaging microscope (Olympus, Melville, NY). The microscope was connected to a Lambda DG-4 light source (Sutter Instruments, Novato, CA), and fluorescent images of the cells were captured using a Photometrics Cool Snap FX digital camera (Roper Scientific, Trenton, NJ). RatioTool software (ISEE Imaging Systems, Raleigh, NC) was used to quantitate the intracellular calcium. A ratio-dye method, with 340/380 nm excitation and 510 nmol and above emission was used to convert the fluorescence intensity of the cells to intracellular calcium concentration based on known calcium standards.

The reservoir was filled with an EBSS bath of 1.80 mmol calcium concentration. A 60-s baseline was recorded. Each tendon fascicle was stretched only once to a static strain of 3–10%. A strain rate of 1.7 µm·s was used to keep the cells in focus while the fascicle was being deformed. After each trial, the EBSS bath was replaced with fresh EBSS.

Human tenocytes in 2D culture ± IL-1β ± ATP—human tenocytes were cultured as above, plated in six well, collagen-bonded BioFlex® culture plates, and grown to quiescence by reducing the serum concentration by 50% in DMEM on days 3 and 5 post-plating. Groups included: control cells with no treatment, cells + 10 or 100 µmol ATP, cells mechanically loaded at 1% elongation for 2 hours at 1 Hz, and collected at 18 hours post-load. Gene expression for IL-1β, cyclo-oxygenase 2 (COX-2), and MMP-3 was semi-quantitated by reverse transcription polymerase chain reaction (RT-PCR) and compared with a β-actin standard ($n = 4$ patients; $n = 6$ replications) (Tsuzaki et al. 1999).

Fabrication of bioartificial tendons (BATs), IL-1β treatment, and MMP assays

Human tendon internal fibroblasts were enzymatically and mechanically disaggregated, washed in PBS, then plated in a type I collagen gel (Vitrogen, Cohesion Technologies, Palo Alto, CA) mixed with growth media, FCS, and neutralized to pH 7.0 with 1 mol sodium hydroxide. A total of 200 k cells/170 µL of the collagen mixture were dispensed to each well of TissueTrain™ culture plate (Banes et al. 1988). Linear, tethered, bioartificial tendons (BATs) as 3D cell-populated matrices were formed by placing the TissueTrain™ culture plate atop a four-place gasketed baseplate with planar-faced cylindrical posts with centrally located, rectangular cut-outs (six-place Loading Station™ with TroughLoaders™) beneath each flexible well base. The TroughLoaders™ had vertical holes in the floor of the rectangle through which a vacuum could be applied to deform the flexible membrane into the trough. The trough provided a space for delivery of cells and matrix. The baseplate was transferred to a 5% CO_2 humidified incubator at 37°C, where the construct was held in position under vacuum for 1.5 hours

until the cells and matrix formed a gelatinous material connected to the anchor stems (Garvin et al. 2003, Triantiafillopolous et al. 2004). BATs were then covered with 3 mL per well growth medium and cultures digitally scanned in the incubator. Cytokine-treated cultures received IL-1β (100 pmol) in the bathing media, which was refreshed daily. MMP-1, MMP-2, and MMP-3 assays were conducted using enzyme-linked immunosorbent assay (ELISA) kits per the manufacturer's protocol (R&D Systems, Minneapolis, MN).

Mechanical loading to bioartificial tendons (BATs)

BATs were uniaxially loaded by placing Arctangular™ loading posts (rectangle with curved short ends) beneath each well of the TissueTrain™ plates in a gasketed baseplate and applying vacuum to deform the flexible membranes downward at east and west poles (Garvin et al. 2003). The flexible but inelastic anchors deformed downwards along the long sides of the Arctangular™ loading posts, thus applying uniaxial strain along the long axis of each of the BATs. The loading regime was 30 min·day at 1% elongation and 1 Hz using a Flexercell™ Strain Unit to control the regimen.

Gene array analyses of human tenocytes ± IL-1β

Normal human tenocytes from the carpiradialis and flexor digitorum profundus tendons from these patients at passage three were cultured to quiescence then treated with 1 pmol·hour IL-1β for 6 hours. Cells were harvested in lysis buffer and RNA purified using Qiagen columns. RNA was checked for quality by assessing 18 s and 28 s ratio and peak shape. Then RNA was reverse transcribed to cDNA with Cyan 3 and Cyan 5 dyes conjugated to CTP in control (no IL-1β) and test (+IL-1β). cDNAs were mixed and hybridized to Agilent human 44-k gene array chips, washed, scanned, and graded using an Agilent scanner. DNA arrays were prepared in triplicate. The UNC database for microarrays program was used to determine fold changes in a given gene as well as a mean and a standard deviation (SD) for each value. The significance analysis of microarrays (SAM) technique was used to find significant genes in the microarray data (Tusher *et al.* 2001). The mean values of triplicate measurements for each gene from each patient were used as input data for the SAM program to compare the response variable, Il-1β-treated to the non-treated control cells. SAM computes a statistic d_i for each gene i, measuring the strength of the relationship between gene expression and the response variable. Permutations of the data are used to determine if the expression of any genes are significantly related to the response. The cut-off for determining a significance level is achieved by "tuning" a delta parameter to minimize a false positive rate. In addition, a fourfold change in gene expression was selected to filter out potential false positive results.

Statistics

Results in each experiment were performed in triplicate. Experiments involving patients have the patient number given with each experiment. Statistical methods used to analyze data included analysis of bovine (ANOVA) with a Student's *t*-test to determine level of significance in a given group.

Results

Rat tenocyte signaling response to tensile strain

Rat tail tendon fascicles subjected to 1% strain and above sustained a significant increase in intracellular calcium concentration when bathed in 1.80 mmol extracellular calcium-containing EBSS (Fig. 3.1a). When no extracellular calcium was present, there was no significant increase in intracellular calcium above baseline until strains of 8% were administered (Fig. 3.1b). Strains of 8–10% resulted in failure of the fascicle and release of cellular calcium ions, which likely contributed to the intracellular calcium rise in surviving cells.

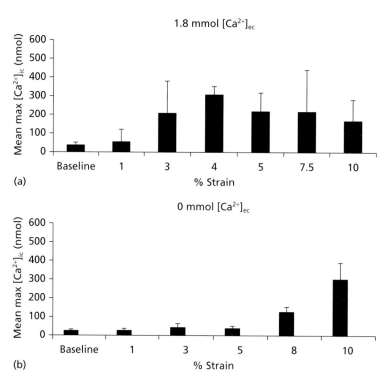

Fig. 3.1 Data in (a) indicate that in the absence of extracellular calcium ion ($[Ca^{2+}]_{ec}$), tenocytes in a rat tail tendon fascicle do not signal to a static strain of 3–8% by increasing $[Ca^{2+}]_{ic}$. When calcium ion is present at 1.8 mmol, cells signal to strain by increasing intracellular calcium (b).

Human tenocytes in 2D culture, MMP response to load, IL-1β and blockade by ATP

Human tenocytes treated with IL-1β in 2D culture expressed MMP-1, MMP-3, and MMP-13, ADAMTS-4 (aggrecanase), IL-1β, and COX-2 (Fig. 3.2a) (Tsuzaki *et al.* 2003b). The IL-1β receptor message was constitutively expressed with or without IL-1β. Expression of TIMPS-1 and TIMPS-2 was unchanged. In a subsequent experiment, cyclic substrate strain stimulated expression of MMP and COX-2 but ATP reduced the effect of load to stimulate gene expression (Fig. 3.2b) (Tsuzaki *et al.* 2003a).

Human tenocytes in 3D bioartificial tendons: response to load and IL-1β

Normal human tendon internal fibroblasts seeded in 3D collagen gels formed linear $3 \times 3 \times 25$ mm BATs whose ends attached to polar anchors in a special TissueTrain™ culture plate (Garvin *et al.* 2003). The BAT™s began to contract the collagen

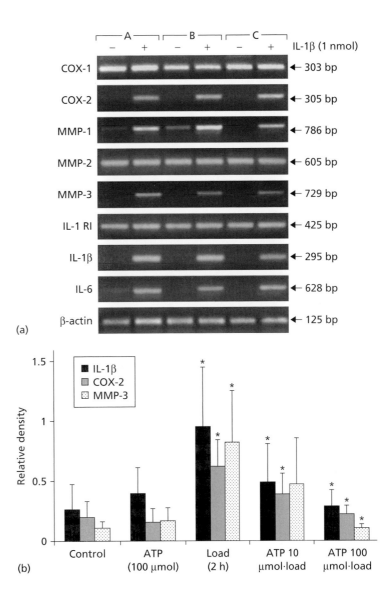

Fig. 3.2 Data in (a) indicate the effect of 100 pmol interleukin-1β (IL-1β) on human tenocytes (epitenon surface cells, TSC). Cyclo-oxygenase 1 (COX-1) was constitutively expressed as were matrix metalloproteinase-2 (MMP-2) and the IL-1 receptor (IL-1 R1). However, expression of COX-2, MMP-1, and MMP-3, as well as IL-1β and IL-6, were increased after 16 incubation with IL-1β. Reprinted with permission from the *Journal of Orthopaedic Research* (2003) **21**, 256–264. Data in (b) indicate that cyclic load at 3% strain for 2 hours increased gene expression for MMP and COX-2. Treatment with ATP decreased load-induced expression. Reprinted with permission from the *Journal of Cellular Biochemistry* (2003) **89**, 556–562.

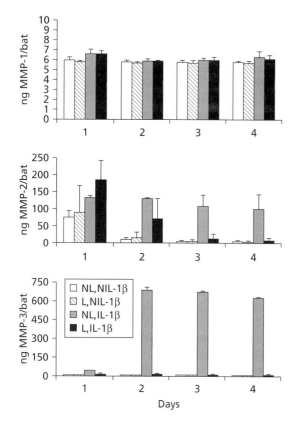

Fig. 3.3 Data indicate the effects of cyclic load (L) and/or IL-1β-treatment (IL-1β) on MMP-1, MMP-2, or MMP-3 protein production and secretion into the medium in human tenocytes grown in 3D bioartificial tendon (BATs) cultures *in vitro* compared to non-loaded or non-IL-1β-treated controls (NL, NIL-1β). Production of MMP-1 protein was unaffected by either treatment during days 1–4. MMP-2 amount was increased by IL-1β beginning on day 1 but was downregulated by load throughout 4 days of treatment. MMP-3 production/secretion was most dramatically downregulated by load, beginning on day 1 and continuing through day 4.

gel matrix within hours of seeding. BATs treated with IL-1β expressed MMP-1, MMP-2, and MMP-3 (Fig. 3.3). BATs that received mechanical loading at 1 Hz, 1% strain for 30 min/day suppressed MMP-2 and MMP-3 protein expression, even when BATs were stimulated with IL-1β.

Genes up- or downregulated by IL-1β in human tenocytes

Results of gene array experiments involving tenocytes cultured from tendons of three patients and treated with IL-1β, indicated that expression of 501 genes of 44,000 genes tested (Agilent 44 K chip) were statistically upregulated while 457 genes were statistically downregulated after 18 hours' treatment (twofold or greater increase or decrease in expression respectively, SAM plot analysis). Further data reduction revealed that 72 genes were upregulated by IL-1β and 283 were downregulated at the fourfold level. Table 3.1 contains a select list of genes that were upregulated by at least fourfold in IL-1β-treated tenocytes. It is noteworthy that the IL-1β gene itself was upregulated as it was found in other experiments previously published by our laboratory (Tsuzaki *et al.* 2003b). Two genes also induced by TNF-α (TNF-α inducible protein 6, 8) were upregulated. Expression of an epidermal growth factor-like gene, epiregulin, was also upregulated as were genes for hyaluronan binding protein 2, FGF$_2$, a K channel, and cx37. Interestingly, expression of a gene called ninjurin 1, or nerve damage-induced factor 1, was increased. This protein is a cell adhesion molecule previously isolated as a gene induced in Schwann cells after nerve injury (Araki & Milbrandt 1996).

Table 3.2 lists select genes of 283 that were downregulated by at least fourfold by IL-1β in human tenocytes. The leading genes that were downregulated included a pleckstrin homology domain, an ATP-binding cassette protein and an integrin β1 binding protein, among others. Interestingly, an apoptosis-inhibitor gene was strongly downregulated by IL-1β, which could contribute to increased cell death. Numerous transcription related proteins were downregulated, including MADS transcription factor enhancer factor 2, PHD finger protein 15, doublesex and mab-3-related TF 3, upstream TF 2, fos interacting, among others. TGF-β3 and FGF13 were downregulated, indicating a negative regulation point for matrix (TGF-β). FGF13 is a novel protein that has a role in the peripheral nervous system (Hartung *et al.* 1997). Its role in human tenocytes is unknown but may contribute to neuron-like properties, given the expression of ninjurin 1 and neuroligin 1 are also expressed by neurons in the central nervous system (CNS). Several genes for potassium and calcium channels were also downregulated.

Table 3.1 Genes upregulated in human tenocytes by interleukin-1β (IL-1β). Data indicate the human internal fibroblast tenocyte (hTIF) genes whose expression was induced at least fourfold in a gene array experiment, by 100 pmol IL-1β for 6 hours.

Gene	Name	Score (log twofold change)
TNFAIP6	Tumor necrosis factor alpha-induced protein 6	5.07
CXCL3	Chemokine CXC motif ligand 3	4.45
IL-1β	Interleukin-1β	4.1
CCL8	Chemokine cc motif ligand 8	3.66
ARHGDIG	Rho GDP dissociation inhibitor GDI gamma	3.54
FST	Follistatin	3.40
CXCL3	Chemokine cxc motif ligand 3	3.38
SPHAR	S phase response cyclin related	3.35
NPPB	Natriuretic peptide predursor B	3.10
EREG	Epiregulin	3.09
AUP1	Ancient ubiquitous protein 1	3.05
LIN7C	Lin-7 homolog C (C. elegans)	3.01
ZNF271	Zinc finger protein 271	3.00
HABP2	Hyaluronan binding protein 2	2.95
FGF2	Fibroblast growth factor 2	2.93
TNFAIP8	Tumor necrosis factor alpha-induced protein 8	2.84
MT1X	Metallothionein	2.84
KCNG4	Potassium voltage gated channel subfamily G, 4	2.77
GJA4	Gap junction protein, Alpha 4, 37kDa (connexin 37)	2.66
NINJ1	Ninjurin 1	2.56
MYO1D	Myosin 1D	2.57
IFNA8	Interferon, alpha 8	2.53
COL8A1	Collagen type VIII, alpha 1	2.50
RCD8	Autoantigen	2.49
CDK6	Cyclin-dependent kinase 6	2.48
TIAM2	T-cell lymphoma invasion and metastasis 2	2.48
PLA2G3	Phospholipase A2, group III	2.42

Discussion

Extracellular calcium

Calcium ion outside the cell is a powerful mediator of a load response in tenocytes (Knutson 2003). Removal of Ca^{2+} from the bathing medium ablates a cell's ability to respond to a deformation such as a membrane indentation or strain event (Knutson 2003). Rat tail tenocytes *ex vivo* in stretched tendon fascicles signaled with an increase in intracellular calcium at as little as 0.5% strain in the presence of 1.7 mmol Ca^{2+} in the bathing medium. However, if exogenous calcium ion was not present, cells did not respond significantly until up to 8% strain, at the failure point of the fascicle. It is likely that cell membrane integrity was compromised and intracellular calcium was released, which became available as extracellular calcium. The signaling response to strain could be regained if Ca^{2+} ion was added to fascicles. One might expect that tenocytes in swollen Achilles tendons might be bathed in a higher concentration of exogenous calcium as capillaries leak plasma into the extracellular space. Increased $[Ca^{2+}]_{ec}$ might increase the mechanosensitivity of tenocytes as well as increase neurogenic pain.

Cytokines

Cartilage cells, annulus cells, and periodontal tissue respond to IL-1β by increasing metalloproteinases

Table 3.2 Genes downregulated in human tenocytes by interleukin-1β (IL-1β). Data indicate the human internal fibroblast tenocyte (hTIF) genes whose expression was repressed at least fourfold in a gene array experiment, by 100 pmol IL-1β for 6 hours.

Gene	Name	Score (log twofold change)
PHLDA 1	Pleckstrin homology-like domain, family A, member 1	−7.95
ABCG2	ATP-binding cassette, sub-familky G, member 2	−7.82
ZSCAN 2	Zinc finger and SCAN domain containing 2	−7.59
CBLN 4	Cerebellin 4 precursor	−7.51
ERBB4	V-erb-a erthyroblastic leukemia viral oncogene homolog 4	−7.46
MLLT6	Myeloid/lymphoid or mixed lineage leukemia	−7.37
EFCBP1	EF hand calcium binding protein 1	−7.35
FLOT2	Flotillin 2	−7.32
ITGB1BP2	Integrin beta 1 binding protein (melusin) 2	−7.26
PMP2	Peripheral myelin protein 2	−7.22
FGF13	Fibroblast growth factor 13	−7.22
PIN4	Protein (peptidyl-prolyl *cis/trans* isomerase) NIMA 4, (parvulin)	−7.22
GPR157	G protein coupled receptor 157	−7.16
PRG-3	Plasticity-related gene	−7.51
MEF2A	MADS box transcription enhancer factor 2	−7.14
FKSG2	Apoptosis inhibitor	−7.11
MLANA	Melan-A	−6.91
CPN2	Carboxypeptidase N	−6.87
ADA	Adenosine deaminase	−6.86
ILF5	Interleukin 1 family member 5 (delta)	−6.83
DKK3	Dickkopf homolog 3	−6.8
TLE4	Transducin-like enhancer of split 4	−6.73
CSF3	Colony stimulating factor 3 (granulocyte)	−6.72
TGFB3	Transforming growth factor beta 3	−6.62
ATP5H	ATP synthase, H transporting, mitochondrial FO complex, subunit d	−6.57
NPL4	Nuclear protein localization 4	−6.55
ADPRH	ADP-ribosylarginine hydrolase	−6.51
GSC	Goosecoid	−6.48
KRTCAP3	Kerastinocyte-associated protein 3	−6.45
IL3RA	Interleukin-3 receptor, alpha low affinity	−6.41
PPEF1	Protein phosphatase, EF hand calcium binding domain 1	−6.40
DMRT3	Doublesex and mab-3 related transcription factor 3	−6.37
TLR4	Toll-like receptor 4	−6.36
STK24	Serine/threonine kinase 24	−6.35
NOTCH2NL	Notch homolog 2	−6.18
KCNJ1	Potassium inwardly rectifying channel, subfamily J, member 1	−6.11
LCP1	Lymphocyte cytosolic protein 1 (L-plastin)	−6.07
SDC2	Syndecan 2 (heparin sulfate PG 1, fibroglycan	−5.95
NLGN1	Neuroligin 1	−5.56

and stimulating matrix degradation (Bonassar *et al.* 1996). A similar result occurs in intervertebral disc tissue (Nachemson 1996). Results of RT-PCR experiments on total RNA isolated from whole human or rabbit Achilles or flexor digitorum profundus tendons and their isolated cells indicate that tendon cells express two isoforms of mRNA for IL-1β receptor: RI, the functional receptor, and RII, the decoy receptor, which is not linked to an intracellular signaling pathway (Tsuzaki *et al.* 1997). These cells also respond to IL-1β by increasing intracellular calcium (Guyton *et al.* 2000). Therefore, tendon cells respond to this cytokine by activating an intracellular signaling pathway involving an increase in intracellular calcium (Guyton *et al.* 2000). A cAMP response element (CRE) and activated CREBs are likely responsible for activation after IL-1β binds to its receptor (Chandra *et al.* 1995). Moreover, both whole tendon and isolated cells upregulate COX-2 message and message for MMP-1, MMP-3, and MMP-13 in response to as little as 10 pmol IL-1β (Tsuzaki *et al.* 1999). PGE$_2$ secretion also increases in tendon cells exposed to IL-1β and may be involved in a pain response, although glutamate has been found in tendon fluids and may be linked to a pain response (Tsuzaki *et al.* 1999). In addition, human tendon cells *in vitro* secrete PGE$_2$ and upregulate MMP-1 and MMP-3 mRNA in response to IL-1β (Tsuzaki *et al.* 2000).

Additional data from our laboratory indicate that IL-1β mRNA is also induced by IL-1β, suggesting that a destructive positive feedback loop may occur (Tsuzaki *et al.* 2003b; unpublished results of microarray data). This result underscores the potential for IL-1β to be induced locally, in turn inducing MMP and resulting in a focal necrotic lesion in the tendon that could lead to a tendon rupture. However, simultaneous, upregulation of tissue inhibitors of metalloproteinases may occur, although data indicate that in cultured human FDP tendon cells, this does not occur in response to IL-1β (Tsuzaki *et al.* 2003b). Recent data from experiments by Archambault *et al.* (2002a) have indicated that tendon cells respond synergistically to fluid-induced shear stress or tension and IL-1β by increasing expression of MMP-3. This costimulation response of tendon cells links an inflammatory cytokine to mechanical loading and belies a potential etiology for tendon damage, particularly in repetitive motion disorder (Archambault *et al.* 2002a). Lastly, preliminary data indicate that rabbit Achilles tendons prelabeled with ^{3}H-proline to make radioactive collagen then incubated in IL-1β release significantly more labeled matrix into the supernatant fluid than did control tendons (Bowman *et al.* 2005). Taken together, these *in vitro* and *ex vivo* results indicate that IL-1β is a prime cytokine candidate stimulating matrix destruction leading to tendonitis and tendinosis *in vivo*.

Substantiating the latter thought, results of gene array experiments conducted with mRNAs from degenerate Achilles tendons (two painful and two ruptured specimens; 11 painful with paired "normal" specimens from the same patient) and two control normal cadaver tissue (expired 2 days) showed similar results to those with patient's cells (Ireland *et al.* 2001). mRNAs for collagens I and II were elevated in two painful Achilles samples and one ruptured sample but other collagens (collagen types 4, 6, 8, 9, 11, 16, and 18) were either unchanged or data not interpretable because of lack of controls (Ireland *et al.* 2001). Results with MMP expression (MMP 1, 2, 3, 7–9, 10, 11, 13–17, and 19) indicated that MMP-2 and MMP-14 might have been increased but others unchanged, undetected or data uninterpretable). Data from five paired pathologic specimens and four controls indicated a trend of downregulation in MMP-3 message in pathologic Achilles specimens (4/5) (Alfredson *et al.* 2003). However, two of four control specimens were also decreased to the same extent as the values for the pathologic specimens; three of six pathologic specimens assayed for MMP-2 were downregulated but did not meet the twofold criteria for a significant change (Ireland *et al.* 2001). TIMP expression did not show an altered trend.

Experiments of the latter type with human tissue are difficult to perform because of sample collection problems, lack of acceptable paired controls, age differences, cost, and statistical variation. However, results showing increased MMP expression, based on tissue specimens, are concordant with those findings *in vitro*. A subsequent experiment by Riley *et al.* (2002) was aimed at quantifying the MMP activity in Achilles specimens. Supraspinatus tendons from patients with ruptures (Banes 1993) were compared with non-ruptured supraspinatus tendons (Ireland *et al.* 2001) as well as with biceps brachii tendons (Franke *et al.* 1998; Riley *et al.* 2002). MMP-1 was the most active candidate enzyme in ruptured specimens (2.7-fold elevated), MMP-2 activity was 28% of control and that for MMP-3 was 16% of control, but the control value had an SD as large as the mean (Riley *et al.* 2002). Conclusions were that gelatinolytic and MMP-3 activities were lower in normal biceps brachii and ruptured tendons than in normal supraspinatus tendons but

MMP-1 activity was greater in supraspinatus than the others. These results are somewhat different from those with IL-1β-treated patient's cells where MMP-1 is unchanged but MMP-2 and MMP-3 are elevated (Tsuzaki *et al.* 2003b). In addition, the aspartic acid content, a measure of protein stability (i.e. lack of turnover) was greatest in the biceps brachii tendon, indicating low turnover rates and low degradation, and least in normal supraspinatus and even lower in ruptured tendons (Riley *et al.* 2002). MMP-1, MMP-2, and MMP-3 increased with age in control supraspinatus tendons compared with values in biceps brachii tendons (Riley *et al.* 2002). Tibialis, supraspinatus, FDP, and Achilles tendon specimens obtained at surgery and treated with IL-1β also increase expression of MMP-3 and release MMP-3 into the medium (Guyton *et al.* 2000). Likewise, cells cultured from the same patient specimens and treated with IL-1β had an even more dramatic stimulation of MMP-3 expression and protein release (up to 17-fold increased protein release by ELISA detection).

Taken together, these results indicate that matrix destruction occurs *in vivo* and is likely related to the activity of MMP. It is difficult to prove this aspect with the patient's specimens to date because of timing of specimen collection and disease staging problems. However, results of *ex vivo* and *in vitro* experiments, both with protease assays and message detection, implicate MMP as causative enzymes in tendon matrix degradation. A leading candidate cytokine that is at the heart of the problem is IL-1β because it can robustly induce the genes for COX-2 that cause PGE_2 production and pain, as well as the MMP which causes matrix destruction (particularly MMP-1, MMP-3, and MMP-13 that can activate MMP-1 and degrade matrix). In addition, MMP-3 (i.e. stromelysin-1) degrades aggrecan, an important proteoglycan expressed in tendon, whereas MMP-13 can degrade both collagen 1 and aggrecan. It can also activate MMP-1, or collagenase that degrades type I collagen, the principal collagen in tendons (Tsuzaki *et al.* 1993). Treatment strategies that block COX-2 and MMP production or activity should ameliorate some of the symptoms and even matrix sequelae in tendinopathies.

Tenocyte modulating agents

Recently, our laboratory reported the expression of adrenergic receptors on avian and human tenocytes that respond to norepinephrine (NE) (Wall *et al.* 2004). Tenocytes increased $[Ca^{2+}]_{ic}$ when NE was applied and also increased expression of cx43 and were better coupled when given NE and a regimen of cyclic loading (Wall *et al.* 2004). These data indicate that NE supplied by nerve endings or from the blood supply can synergize with a mechanical loading regimen, likely through a cAMP pathway, to upregulate genes, particularly cx43, involved in cell–cell communication.

ATP is another ligand that modulates not only a load response but also downregulates MMP expression (Tsuzaki *et al.* 2003a). Tenocytes respond to ATP by increasing intracellular calcium ($[Ca^{2+}]_{ic}$ (Franke *et al.* 1998). Tenocytes secrete ATP particularly in response to fluid shear or stretch (Tsuzaki *et al.* 2003a). These nucleotides activate $P2Y_2$ purinoceptors (Tsuzaki *et al.* 2003a). ATP and uridine triphosphate (UTP) likely act to amplify a load response because they activate a common pathway through an increase in $[Ca^{2+}]_{ic}$ (Tsuzaki *et al.* 2003a). Tenocytes from $P2Y_2$ knockout mice that lack the receptor for ATP do not respond to substrate strain by increasing $[Ca^{2+}]_{ic}$ (Fox *et al.* 2004, 2005). Therefore, ATP or a breakdown product such as ADP or adenosine may act as a stop, or modulating signal(s) for some genes impacted by mechanical load. Stop, or inhibitory signals, are equally as important as "go", or stimulatory signals (Banes *et al.* 2003). It is hypothesized that a cell must be able to attenuate its response to load by utilizing a stop or otherwise modulatory signal. ADP may be a stop signal acting at $P2Y_1$ receptors. Tenocytes from $P2Y_1$ knockout mice that lack the receptor for ADP have a heightened response to a plasma membrane indentation or stretch stimulus and increase intracellular calcium to a greater degree than *wt* controls (Fox *et al.* 2005). Moreover, one group has hypothesized that low-amplitude strain may be anti-inflammatory while high-level strain may be pro-inflammatory in connective tissue (Xu *et al.* 2000). Therefore, certain load regimens may stimulate catabolism through endogenous IL-1β or

TNF-α, which then stimulate expression of MMP (Xu *et al.* 2000).

Signaling and outcome pathways in tendinopathies

Figure 3.4 addresses the relationships between events that incite a tendinopathy, pathways that are activated, and the ultimate outcomes. The initiators may include a traumatic event such as a tendon rupture, a crush injury, or a repetitive motion injury. An acute inciting event resulting in release of mediators such as ATP, UTP, PGE_2, NO, and growth factors such as PDGF, IGF-1, TGF-β, or cytokines, such

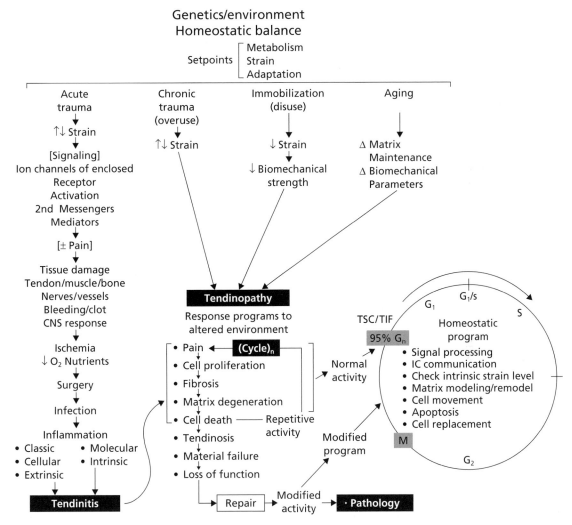

Fig. 3.4 A general outline of events that may result in tendinopathy. Events include acute trauma leading to a change in strain, second messenger signaling, pain, tissue damage, and ischemia. Surgical correction may result in infection and inflammation. Both classic and molecular inflammation pathways are listed, leading to a transient tendonitis. This condition flows into a tendinopathy scenario instigated by chronic trauma, immobilization or aging superposed on genetic factors. In each case, the tendon follows a repair paradigm that flows into a homeostatic program resulting in "normal" function. If the tendon cannot enter a homeostatic program, a pathologic state occurs that is a tendinopathy.

as IL-1β or TNF-α from plasma, platelets, leukocytes, or local sources, stimulate receptors and activate cell recruitment and migration. A cell migration–mitogenic cycle is then activated, which likely involves a signaling pathway through mitogen-activated protein kinases (MAPK) (Banes *et al.* 1995b). This process will drive cell migration followed by proliferation to a limited extent, perhaps 2–5 proliferation cycles, depending on growth factor concentration, availability, and receptor regulation (Banes 1993). Note that a tendon with a region of proliferating cells may be biomechanically weak compared with a mature tendon in homeostasis. Next, some of these same factors (IGF-1, TGF-β1), if present for an extended period, may stimulate fibrosis by increasing expression of matrix proteins, particularly collagen I and proteoglycans, as well as MMPs (Tsuzaki *et al.* 2000). This may lead to nodule formation within a tendon and adhesions at the surface, causing pain and loss of function by limiting range of motion and use. This cycle favors net matrix deposition. However, because MMPs are not only expressed but are stored as pro-enzymes in the matrix, they require activation to initiate a cascade of matrix destruction, perhaps even in the absence of many cells (Tsuzaki *et al.* 2003b). Cytokines such as IL-1β, originating from leukocytes or from endogenous tenocytes, stimulate expresson of COX-2 producing PGE_2, resulting in pain, as well as MMP, particularly MMP-3 which can activate MMP-1 and degrades collagen and proteoglycans simultaneously (Tsuzaki *et al.* 2003b). Moreover, loss of use may lead to increased MMP expression, further driving a modeling–remodeling pathway, resulting in matrix degradation and reduced biomechanical strength (Archambault *et al.* 2002b). Lastly, mediators such as NO, reactive oxygen species, or elevated temperature can drive the NF-κB pathway that leads to apoptosis and cell death (Fig. 3.5) (Smith 2000). The result is loss of function, reduced biomechanical strength, material failure, and eventual tendon rupture. At this point, a surgeon may intervene and excise pathologic tissue and/or rejoin the ruptured ends as in repair of the FDP, supraspinatus, Achilles, or biceps tendons. If the patient follows a physical therapy regimen, they may return to a modified normal homeostatic state. If the patient continues an overuse paradigm, then they will regress to a pathologic state of chronic tendinopathy with a high likelihood of a second failure. The term tendinosis applies to the outcomes that encompass matrix degradation, cell death, fibrosis, and matrix failure. These outcomes meet in a final common pathway embodied by pain, loss of biomechanical strength, material failure, rupture, and loss of function. The clinical relevance and significance section includes a synopsis of what we know about the cell and molecular biology of tendon cells in relation to these tendinopathy outcomes.

Clinical relevance and significance

Tendinopathy in the athlete is a recognized pathology thought to be caused by overuse activities. Its molecular etiology is unclear but likely involves cell death as well as cytokine-induced expression and activation of COX-2, elaboration of pain mediators, and MMPs. Once activated, MMPs degrade collagens and proteoglycans. Initiators of apoptosis result in cell death. The end result is a weak tendon with a decreased useful lifetime. Non-steroidal anti-inflammatory drugs (NSAIDs) are often prescribed as analgesics to relieve pain, even those known to block COX-2. During the initial phase of tendon injury, cells are driven by exogenous growth factors and cytokines to migrate, produce MMP, hydrolyze, and reorganize matrix. During convalescence and healing, tendons regain control of cell division and maintenance functions as net matrix synthesis exceeds matrix destruction. However, chronic tendon pain, loss of range of motion, and even loss of strength are associated with recognized disorders such as impingement, tendon tears, and "inflammation." Treatment for these clinical entities includes rest, ice, elevation, and dosing with NSAIDs as the treatment strategies of choice. Practically speaking, there is no formalized staging of tendinitis or tendinosis, but the diseases are treated as if they were acute or chronic inflammatory processes. The hypothesis is that a cause of tendinosis is a response to a cytokine such as IL-1β and extensive exercise. Chronic exposure to this cytokine and motion results in a feedback loop that perpetuates its production followed by MMP induction, activation,

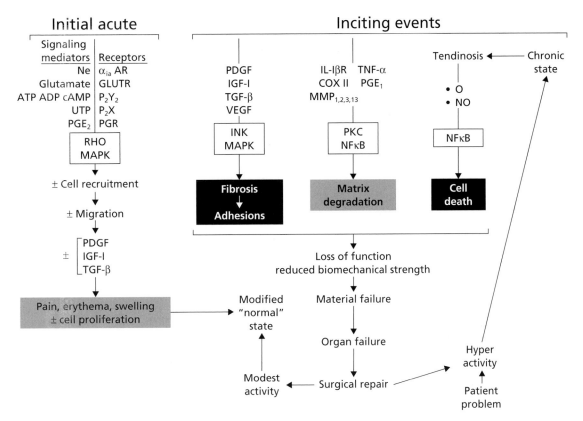

Fig. 3.5 Signaling pathways in tendinopathy demonstrates that an initial response of tenocytes to an acute event involves signaling mediators and pathway activation, leading to cell recruitment to an area, cell migration with accompanying pain, swelling, erythema, and perhaps cell proliferation. Further inciting events of an increasing number (*n*), activate adhesion formation, matrix degradation, and cell death. Events result in a tendinopathy and, ultimately, tendon rupture.

and matrix degradation. The use of specific inhibitors of the load detection mechanisms in tendon cells may indicate a specific pathway that is involved in the etiology of RMD.

Future directions

What we need to know:

1 *Tendon transcriptome* Develop biomarkers from gene array data for a "tendinome" (i.e. a tendon transcriptome for normal and pathologic tendons based on tendon expression during development) in mediator, cytokine, thermally or hypoxic-treated tendons and in recognized stages of human tendon pathology.

2 *Diagnostic markers: biomarker identification in normal and pathologic tendons* Use biomarkers in a dia-

gnostic manner to identify and stage tendinopathy in patients by imaging a marker or from tendon fluid, tendon biopsy, urine, or blood. Question: is the etiology of activity-induced tendinopathy cell death and/or matrix destruction?

3 *Animal model of exercise-induced tendinopathy and staging of disease* Use the rat supraspinatus model of Soslowsky *et al.* or develop a large animal model of tendon damage and monitor biomarkers with invasive and non-invasive techniques to stage progression of the disease.

4 *Tendinopathy staging in patients* Staging of tendinopathy may be monitored non-invasively by imaging a well-characterized biomarker. Address the question of existence and definition of inflammation in tendon. Can effects of tendinopathy be reversed or corrected?

5 *Drug targets and treatment strategies* Can symptoms be ameliorated based on use of biomarkers of disease, treatment of pain, altered physical activity, and new drugs developed to treat tendinopathy? Can we develop drugs that reverse or correct tendinopathy? Can we develop a tendon replacement material?

How do we get to a new knowledge base in tendinopathy?

1 *Genomics, proteomics, and metabolomics* Utilize the latest techniques to identify genes, proteins, and/or metabolic markers to predict which patients will develop a tendon problem or stage the disease in patients who already have tendinoses.

2 *Small and large animal model: for tendinopathy* Utilize the rat supraspinatus model and a larger animal model to study at the cell and tissue level, ± mediators, cytokines, heat, hypoxia, and overuse.

3 *Human normal and pathologic tendons* Utilize

patients to define stages in tendinopathy. Define stages with biomarker-based imaging techniques.

4 *Develop pharmacologies to treat new drug targets* If the etiology of tendinopathy does not involve "bad" cytokines, COX-2, or MMPs, then what are the mechanisms and drug targets?

5 *Develop tendon treatment and/or tendon replacement strategies* Use novel synthetic replacement materials and tissue-engineered constructs to treat damaged tendons so that tendons heal and patients can function at or beyond expected levels. Develop an engineered tendon replacement.

Acknowledgments

This work was supported by NIH AR38121, the Hunt Foundation and Flexcell® International Corporation. AJB is President of Flexcell® International Corporation and receives compensation as such.

References

Alfredson, H., Lorentzon, M., Backman, S., Backman, A. & Lerner, U.H. (2003) CDNA-arrays and real-time quantitative PCR techniques in the investigation of chronic Achilles tendinosis. *Journal of Orthopaedic Research* **21**, 970–975.

Araki, T. & Milbrandt, S. (1996) Ninjurin, a novel adhesion molecule, is induced by nerve injury and promotes axonal growth. *Neuron* **17**, 353–361.

Archambault, J., Elfervig-Wall, M., Tsuzaki, M., Herzog, W. & Banes, A.J. (2002a) Rabbit tendon cells produce MMP-3 response to fluid flow without significant calcium transients. *Journal of Biomechanics* **35**, 303–309.

Archambault, J., Tsuzaki, M., Herzog, W. & Banes, A.J. (2002b) Stretch and interleukin-1β induce matrix metalloproteinases in rabbit tendon cells *in vitro. Journal of Orthopaedic Research* **20**, 36–39.

Arnoczky, S., Tian, T., Lavagnino, M., Gardener, K., Schuler, P. & Morse, P. (2002) Activation of stress-activated protein kinases (SAPK) in tendon cells following cyclic strain: the effects of strain frequency, strain magnitude, and cytosolic calcium. *Journal of Orthopaedic Research* **20**, 947–952.

Arnoczky, S., Lavagnino, M., Gardner, K., Tian, T., Vaupel, Z.M. & Stick, J.A. (2004)

Ex vivo static tensile loading inhibits MMP-1 expression in rat tail tendon cells through a cytoskeletally based mechanotrasduction mechanism. *Journal of Orthopaedic Research* **22**, 328–333.

Åström, M. & Rausing, A. (1995) Chronic Achilles tendinopathy: a survey of surgical and hisopathologic findings. *Clinical Orthopaedics* **316**, 151–164.

Banes, A.J. (1993) Mechanical strain and the mammalian cell. In: *Physical Forces and the Mammalian Cell* (Frangos J., ed.) Academic Press: 81–123.

Banes, A.J., Enterline, D., Bevin, A.G. & Salisbury, R.E. (1981) Repair of flexor tendon: effects of trauma and devascularization on collagen synthesis. *Journal of Trauma* **21**, 505–512.

Banes, A.J., Donlon, K., Link, G.W., *et al.* (1988) Cell populations of tendon: a simplified method for isolation of synovial cells and internal fibroblasts: confirmation of origin and biologic properties. *Journal of Orthopaedic Research* **6**, 83–94.

Banes, A.J., Tsuzaki, M., Hu, P., *et al.* (1995a) Cyclic mechanical load and growth factors stimulate DNA synthesis in avian tendon cells. *Journal of Biomechanics* **28**, 1505–1513.

Banes, A.J., Tsuzaki, M., Yamamoto, J., Fischer, T., Brown, T. & Miller, L. (1995b)

Mechanoreception at the cellular level: the detection, interpretation and diversity of responses to mechanical signals. *Special Issue on Cytomechanics, Biochemistry and Cell Biology* **73**, 349–365.

Banes, A.J., Tsuzaki, M., Yang, X., *et al.* (1998) Equibiaxial strain activates Ap-1 and Cre transcription factors but not NF-κB or SSRE and upregulates Cx43 MRNA in tendon cells *in vitro. Orthopaedic Research Society* **25**, 182.

Banes, A.J., Horesovsky, G., Tsuzaki, M., *et al.* (1999) Connexin 43 is mechanosensitive in avian flexor tendon cells. In: *The Biology of the Synovial Joint* (Caterson, B., Archer, C., Benjamin, M. & Ralphs, J., eds.) Harwood Academic Publishers, Amsterdam, the Netherlands: 279–299.

Banes, A.J., Qi, J., Maloney, M., Almekinders, L. & Bynum, D. (2004) A model 3D system for testing tenocyte responses to drugs, cytokines and mechanical load *ex vivo. Tissue Engineering in Musculoskeletal Practice* **25**.

Benjamin, M., Kumai, T., Milz, S., Boszczyk, B.M. & Ralphs, J.R. (2002) The skeletal attachment of tendons: tendon "enthuses". *Comparative Biochemistry and Physiology. Part A: Molecular & Integrative Physiology* **133**, 931–945.

Boitano, S., Dirksen, E.R., Sanderson, M.J. (1992) Intercellular propagation of calcium waves mediated by inositol triphosphate. *Science* **258**, (5080), 292–295.

Bonassar, L.J., Stinn, J.L., Paguino, C.G., *et al.* (1996) Activation and inhibition of endogenous matrix metalloproteinases in articular cartilage: effects on composition and biophysical properties. *Archives of Biochemistry and Biophysics* **333**, 359–367.

Bowman, K., Guyton, G., Spencer, K., *et al.* (2002) IL-1β-induced MMPs degrade collagen in rabbit Achilles tendon explants. *Orthopaedic Research Society* **27**, 0591.

Chandra, G., Cogswell, J.P., Miller, L.R., *et al.* (1995) Cyclic AMP signaling pathways are important in IL-1β transcriptional regulation. *Journal of Immunology* **155**, 4535–4543.

Chaplin, D.M. & Greenlee, T.K. (1975) The development of human digital tendons. *Journal of Anatomy* **120**, 253–274.

Curwin, S.L. & Stanish, W.D. (1984) *Tendinitis: Its Etiology and Treatment.* Collamore Press, Lexington, MA.

Fox, A.M., Jones, B., Koller, B.H. & Banes, A.J. (2005) Reduced load response in tenocytes from P2y1/P2y2 purinoreceptor null mice. *Orthopaedic Research Society* **30**, 0059.

Francke, E., Sood, A., Kenamond, C., *et al.* (1998) ATP stimulates an increase in intracellular calcium in human tendon cells via purinergic receptors. ATP temporally blocks gap junction signaling. In: *Orthopaedic Research Society* **23**.

Garvin, J., Qi, J., Maloney, M. & Banes, A.J. (2003) A novel system for engineering linear or circular bioartificial tissues (BATS) and application of mechanical load. *Tissue Engineering* **9**, 967–979.

Gelberman, R.H., Vandeberg, J.S., Lundborg, G.N. & Akeson, W.H. (1983) Flexor tendon healing and restoration of the gliding surface: an ultrastructural study in dogs. *Journal of Bone and Joint Surgery. American volume* **65**, 70–80.

Guyton, G., Francke, E., Elfervig, M., Tsuzaki, M., Bynum, D. & Banes, A.J. (2000) IL-1β receptor activation signals through the Ca++ messenger pathway in human tendon cells. In: *Orthopaedic Research Society* **25**, 0808.

Hartung, H., Feldman, B., Lovec, H., Coulier, F., Birnbaum, D. & Goldfarb, M. (1997) Murine Fgf-12 and Fgf-13: expression in embryonic nervous stestem, connective tissue and heart. *Mechanical Devices* **64**, 31–39.

Ireland, D., Harrall, R., Curry, V., *et al.* (2001) Multiple Changes in gene expression in chronic human Achilles tendinopathy. *Matrix Biology* **20**, 159–169.

Knutson, J. (2003) Rat tail tenocytes respond to uniaxial strain. Master's Thesis. University of North Carolina at Chapel Hill, Chapel Hill, NC.

Langer, R. & Vacanti, J.P. (1993) Tissue engineering. *Science* **260**, 920–926.

Lavagnino, M. & Arnoczky, S. (2005) In vitro alterations in cytoskeletal tensional homeostasis control gene expression in tendon cells. *Journal of Orthopaedic Research* **23**, 1211–1218.

Lavagnino, M., Arnoczky, S., Tian., T. & Vaupel, Z.M. (2003) Effect of amplitude and frequency of cyclic tensile strain on the inhibition of MMP-1 MRNA Expression in tendon cells: an in vitro study. *Connective Tissue Research* **44**, 1–7.

McNeilly, C., Benjamin, M., Banes, A.J. & Ralphs, J. (1996) Immuochemical localization of multiple connexins in flexor tendons. *Journal of Anatomy* **189**, 593–600.

Merrilees, M.J. & Flint, M.H. (1980) Ultrastructural study of tension and pressure zones in a rabbit flexor tendon. *American Journal of Anatomy* **157**, 87–106.

Movin, T., Gad, A., Gunter, P., Foldhazy, Z. & Rolf, C. (1997) Pathology of the Achilles tendon in association with ciprofloxacin treatment. *Foot & Ankle International* **18**, 297–299.

Murrell, G.A. (2002) Understand tendinopathies. *British Journal of Sports Medicine* **36**, 392–393.

Musil, L.S., Beyer, E.C. & Goodenough, D.A. (1990) Expression of the gap junction protein connexin43 in embryonic chick lens: molecular cloning, ultrastructural localization, and post-translational phosphorylation. *Journal of Membrane Biology* **116**, 163–175.

Nachemson, A. (1996) The load on lumbar disks in different positions of the body. *Clinical Orthopaedics* **45**, 107–122.

O'Brien, M. (2005) Anatomy of tendons. In: *Tendon Injuries* (Maffulli, N., Renstrom, P. & Leadbetter, W.B., eds.) Springer, London: 3–13.

Purslow, P.P. (2002) The structure and functional significance of variations in the connective tissue within muscle. *Comparative Biochemistry and Physiology. Part A: Molecular & Integrative Physiology* **133**, 647–666.

Riley, G.P., Curry, V., DeGroot, J., *et al.* (2002) Matrix metalloproteinase activities and their relationship with collagen remodelling in tendon pathology. *Matrix Biology* **21**, 185–195.

Smith, L.L. (2000) Cytokine hypothesis of overtraining: a physiological adaptation to excessive stress? *Medicine & Science in Sports and Exercise* **32**, 317–331.

Stopak, D. & Harris, A.K. (1982) Connective tissue morphogenesis by fibroblast traction. I. Tissue culture observations. *Developmental Biology* **90**, 383–398.

Triantafillopoulos, I.K., Banes, A.J., Bowman, K.F. Jr., Maloney, M. Garret, W.F. Jr., Karas, S.G. (2004) Nandrolone decanoate and load increase remodeling and strength in human supraspinatus bioartficial tendon. *American Journal of Sports Medicine* **32(4)**, 934–3.

Tsuzaki, M., Bynum, D., Almekinders, L., Yang, X., Faber, J. & Banes, A.J. (2003a) ATP modulates load-inducible IL-1β, COX 2 and MMP-3 gene expression in human tendon cells. *Journal of Cell Biochemistry* **89**, 556–562.

Tsuzaki, M., Guyton, G., Garrett, W., *et al.* (2000) Interleukin-1β stimulates expression of COX II and MMP I in human tendon epitenon cells. In: *Orthopaedic Research Society* **25**, 0019.

Tsuzaki, M., Guyton, G., Garrett, W., *et al.* (2003b) IL-1 induces COX2, MMP-1, -3 and -13, ADAMTS-4, IL-1 beta and IL-6 in human tendon cells. *Journal of Orthopaedic Research* **21**, 256–264.

Tsuzaki, M., Xiao, H., Brigman, B., *et al.* (1999) IGF-I is expressed by avian flexor tendon cells. *Journal of Orthopaedic Research* **18**, 546–556.

Tsuzaki, M., Yamauchi, M. & Banes, A.J. (1993) Tendon collagens: extracellular matrix composition in shear stress and tensile componets of flexor tendon. *Connective Tissue Research* **29**, 141–152.

Tsuzaki, M., Yang, X.J.B., Benjamin, M., *et al.* (1997) Avian tendon cells express multiple connexins but acute mechanical load reduces cell–cell coupling. In: *Orthopaedics Research Society*: 712.

Tusher, V., Tibshirani, R. & Chu, C. (2001) Siginificant analysis of microarrays applied to conizing radiation response. *Proceedings of the National Academy of Sciences* **98**, 5116–5121.

Wall, M.E., Faber, J., Yang, X., Tsuzaki, M. & Banes, A.J. (2004) Norepinephrine-induced calcium signaling and expression of adrenoceptors in avain tendon cells. *American Journal of Physiology. Cell Physiology* **287**, C912–918.

Xu, Z., Buckley, M.J., Evans, C. & Agarwal, S. (2000) Cyclic tensile strain acts as an antagonist of IL-1β actions in chondrocytes. *Journal of Immunology* **165**, 453–460.

Chapter 4

The Response of Tendon Cells to Changing Loads: Implications in the Etiopathogenesis of Tendinopathy

STEVEN P. ARNOCZKY, MICHAEL LAVAGNINO, AND MONIKA EGERBACHER

While much clinical information currently exists on the pathologic changes associated with tendinopathy, the precise etiopathogenesis of this condition remains a topic of controversy and confusion. Classically, the etiology of tendinopathy has been linked to the performance of repetitive activities (so-called overuse injuries). This has led many investigators to explore the effect(s) of repetitive loading on the metabolic response of tendon cells *in vitro*. Although numerous studies have shown that tendon cells are able to respond to various loading conditions when cultured on an artificial matrix, few studies have examined the *in situ* response of tendon cells within their normal extracellular matrix to various loading situations.

For the past several years, our research laboratory has used a rat tail tendon model to investigate how loading affects the gene response of tendon cells *in situ*. We have shown that the response of tendon cells to load is both frequency and amplitude dependent and that tendon cells appear to be "programmed" to sense a certain level of stress. In addition, we have shown that the absence of stress has a profound effect on the catabolic response of tendon cells. To that end we have forwarded the hypothesis that the catabolic cascade associated with tendinopathy is initiated by understimulation of the tendon cells secondary to altered cell–matrix interactions rather than overstimulation.

In this chapter we discuss our research involving the response of tendon cells to changing load conditions and examine the implications of these responses as a potential etiopathogenic mechanism for the onset of tendinopathy.

Introduction

The ability of tendons cells to respond to load is central to the concept of mechanotransduction and the subsequent maintenance of tissue homeostasis (Wang & Ingber 1994; Banes *et al.* 1995b; Ingber 1997). A plethora of *in vitro* studies have demonstrated a wide-ranging array of gene expression in tendon cells following exposure to mechanical strain (Almekinders *et al.* 1993; Banes *et al.* 1999; Archambault *et al.* 2002; Lavagnino *et al.* 2003; Tsuzaki *et al.* 2003; Wang *et al.* 2003; Arnoczky *et al.* 2004). While the precise level (magnitude, frequency, and duration) of mechanobiologic stimulation required to maintain normal tendon homeostasis is not currently known, it is very likely that an abnormal level(s) of stimulation may have a role in the etiopathogenesis of tendinopathy (Józsa & Kannus 1997; Arnoczky *et al.* 2002a).

Numerous investigators have suggested that overstimulation of tendon cells, secondary to repetitive loading, results in a pattern of gene expression that can lead to tendinopathy (Almekinders *et al.* 1993; Banes *et al.* 1995a, 1999; Skutek *et al.* 2001; Archambault *et al.* 2002; Tsuzaki *et al.* 2003; Wang *et al.* 2003; Bhargava *et al.* 2004). Overstimulation of tendon and ligament cells *in vitro* has been shown to induce increases in inflammatory cytokines and degradative enzymes (Almekinders *et al.* 1993; Banes *et al.* 1995a, 1999; Archambault *et al.* 2002; Tsuzaki *et al.* 2003; Wang *et al.* 2003; Bhargava *et al.* 2004). However, many of these investigations have utilized non-physiologic strain patterns (high strain amplitudes and frequencies as well as long durations) (Almekinder *et al.* 1993; Wang *et al.* 2003; Bhargava *et al.* 2004) or the addition of external factors (Archambault *et al.* 2002; Tsuzaki *et al.* 2003) to elicit these cell responses. Thus, the clinical relevance of these studies must be called into question.

Experimental studies from our laboratory have shown that *mechanobiologic understimulation* of tendon cells can also produce a pattern of catabolic gene expression that results in extracellular matrix degradation and subsequent loss of tendon material properties (Lavagnino *et al.* 2003, 2005, 2006a,b; Arnoczky *et al.* 2004; Lavagnino & Arnoczky 2005). We have also shown that at the extremes of physiologic loading, isolated fibril damage can occur in tendons, which alters normal cell–matrix interactions in this damaged area (Lavagnino *et al.* 2006b). The inability of the damaged fibrils to transmit extracellular matrix loads to the tendon cells results in an understimulation of these cells which, in turn, initiates a catabolic response that can weaken the tendon, making it more susceptible to damage from subsequent loading (Lavagnino *et al.* 2006b).

In this chapter we examine the mechanobiologic response of tendon cells to changing loading patterns and forward the hypothesis that it is a mechanobiologic understimulation and *not* an overstimulation of tendon cells that is the etiopathogenic stimulus for a degradative cascade that can lead to tendinopathy.

What we know

How do cells sense load?

Mechanoresponsiveness is a fundamental feature of all living tissues and tendons are no exception. (Banes *et al.* 1995b; Ingber 1997; Lavagnino & Arnoczky 2005; Wang 2006). The ability of tendon cells to sense load is mediated through a mechano-electrochemical sensory system(s) which detects mechanical load signals through the deformation of the cellular membrane and/or the cytoskeleton (Ben-Ze'Ev 1991; Watson 1991; Adams 1992; Wang *et al.* 1993, 1994; Banes *et al.* 1995b; Ingber 1997; Brown *et al.* 1998; Wang 2006). Cellular deformation produces changes in tension in the cytoskeleton which can be sensed by the cell nucleus through

a mechanosensory tensegrity system to elicit a response (Ben-Ze'ev 1991; Watson 1991; Adams 1992; Wang *et al.* 1993, 1994; Banes *et al.* 1995b; Ingber 1997; Arnoczky *et al.* 2002a; Wang 2006).

Studies from our laboratory have demonstrated *in situ* deformation of rat tail tendon cells in response to tensile load (Arnoczky *et al.* 2002a). Using confocal laser microscopy we were able to demonstrate a significant, albeit weak, correlation between cellular (nuclear) strain and tendon strain (Fig. 4.1). This is most likely because of differential tissue strains within the same local area of the tendon resulting from the sequential straightening and loading of individual crimped collagen fibrils in response to tensile loading (Kastelic *et al.* 1978, 1980; Viidik 1980; Woo *et al.* 1982). The relationship between changes in cell morphology and tissue strain is thought to occur through the binding of the cell to extracellular matrix proteins such as collagen and fibronectin (Banes *et al.* 1995b; Rosales *et al.* 1995; Sung *et al.* 1996). These connections are mediated by the integrin family of cell surface receptors which link the extracellular matrix to the interior of the cell through the cytoskeleton (Ingber 1991; Wang *et al.* 1993; Banes *et al.* 1995a; Janmey 1998).

Deformation of the cellular membrane can also open or close stretch-activated ion channels which control the influx of second-messenger molecules such as calcium and inositol triphosphate (IP_3) (Sachs 1988; Banes *et al.* 1995b). These second messengers, in turn, can activate a wide array of cellular machinery including DNA synthesis, mitosis, cell differentiation, and gene expression (Sachs 1988; Banes *et al.* 1995b). Our laboratory has demonstrated an increase in cytosolic calcium in tendon cells in response to *in situ* deformation (Shirakura *et al.* 1995). In this study, rat tail tendon cells were labeled *in situ* with a fluorescent indicator of calcium (Fluo-3-AM, Molecular Probes, Eugene, OR) (Kao *et al.* 1989) and subjected to various levels (0, 2%, 4%, and 6%) of tendon strain (grip-to-grip strain) using a previously described low-load tensile testing apparatus (Arnoczky *et al.* 2002a). The testing apparatus was attached to the stage of a Zeiss 10 laser scanning confocal microscope (Carl Zeiss, Inc., Thornwood, NY) and fluorescent images of targeted cells were captured at each tissue strain

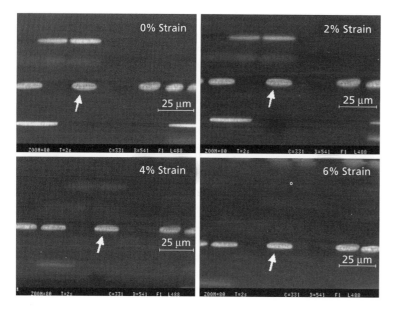

Fig. 4.1 Confocal images of a rat tail tendon illustrating the *in situ* deformation of a tendon cell (arrow) at 0, 2%, 4%, and 6% grip-to-grip tendon strain. Note how some of adjacent tendon cells fall out of the plane of focus as the tendon is strained.

level. Fluorescent intensity of each cell was measured using image processing software (NIH Images, http://rsb.info.nih.gov/nih-image). The major diameter of each targeted cell (cell longitudinal length) and minor diameter (cell height) were also measured. A repeated measures ANOVA was performed to determine if significant ($P < 0.05$) changes in cell dimensions or fluorescent intensity occurred at each of the whole tendon strain levels tested. Measurements at each of the four strain levels were made on cells from nine separate tendons.

The results of the study demonstrated that upon application of tensile load there was a significant increase in cytosolic calcium levels at 0–2% of whole tendon strain (Fig. 4.2). While the average fluorescent intensity also increased at 2–4% strain, this was

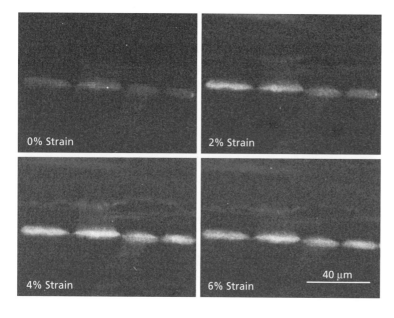

Fig. 4.2 Confocal images of rat tail tendon cells *in situ*. The cells were pre-labeled with a fluorescent indicator of cytosolic calcium (Fluo-3 AM Molecular Probes, Eugene, OR). Note the increase in fluorescence as the tendon is strained and the cells are deformed.

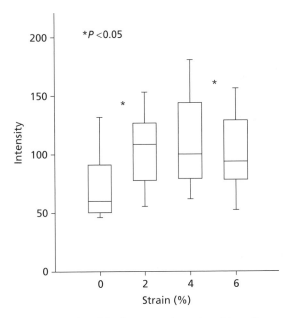

Fig. 4.3 Box plot of the fluorescent intensity of the cells as a function of tendon strain. There was a significant increase in fluorescent intensity (cytosolic calcium levels) as the tendon was strain from 0 to 2%. While the fluorescent intensity also appeared to increase between 2% and 4% strain this was not statistically significant. The significant drop in intensity in fluorescence between 4% and 6% strain was attributed to photobleaching of the specimen.

not significant. However, a significant decrease in fluorescent intensity was noted at 4–6% (Fig. 4.3). This decrease in fluorescence was attributed to photo-bleaching during the time required to sequentially strain each specimen because previous experiments demonstrated a qualitative decrease in fluorescent intensity over time. Whole tendon straining from 0% to 2% to 4% also produced a significant increase in cell elongation. No significant increase in cell length was found at 4–6% strain and no significant changes in cell height were found at any strain levels. The increase in cytosolic calcium associated with cell deformation supports a calcium channel mediated signaling system in tendon cells that is responsive to load.

How does tendon loading affect gene expression in tendon cells?

Tendon cells are able to detect mechanical signals from deformation of their cellular membrane and/or cytoskeleton through a mechanoelectrochemical sensory system(s) resulting in specific cellular responses (Banes *et al.* 1995b). A plethora of *in vitro* studies have demonstrated a wide-ranging array of gene expression in tendon cells following exposure to mechanical strain (Almekinders *et al.* 1993; Banes *et al.* 1995a, 1999; Archambault *et al.* 2002; Arnoczky *et al.* 2002b; Tsuzaki *et al.* 2003; Wang *et al.* 2003). However, the majority of these *in vitro* studies are based on the response of tendon cells cultured on artificial substrates to mechanical loading (Almekinders *et al.* 1993; Banes *et al.* 1995a, 1999; Archambault *et al.* 2002; Arnoczky *et al.* 2002b; Tsuzaki *et al.* 2003; Wang *et al.* 2003). In these culture systems, large numbers of cells are subjected to the same loading regime. While this permits analysis of large amounts of cellular material and cellular products, it may not replicate the normal *in situ* environmental conditions of tendon cells within a three-dimensional collagenous matrix. Because mechanotransduction signals are known to be mediated through the pericellular matrix to the nucleus via integrin-based cell–matrix connections (Sachs 1988; Ingber 1991; Watson 1991; Wang *et al.* 1993; Banes *et al.* 1995b; Ritty *et al.* 2003) it is not clear how, or even if, these complex cell–matrix interactions are maintained or recreated in cell cultures. In addition, tendons are known to exhibit non-homogeneous strain patterns in response to tensile load (Kastelic *et al.* 1978), therefore it is impossible to determine precise amplitudes of strain experienced by the cells based on overall tendon strain. Studies have shown that in rat tail tendons even local tissue strain is non-homogenous throughout the depth of the tendon (Arnoczky *et al.* 2002a; Hanson *et al.* 2002). Therefore, to better understand how the mechanotransduction response of tendon cells affects gene expression, our laboratory has utilized an *in situ* rat tail tendon model in an effort to maintain the tendon cells' natural matrix interactions and strain fields (Arnoczky *et al.* 2004; Lavagnino *et al.* 2003, 2006a,b).

Experimental studies have shown that tendon cells are calibrated to respond to a specific level of strain (Lavagnino *et al.* 2003, 2005; Arnoczky *et al.* 2004). Stress-deprivation of tendon cells *in situ* results in an immediate upregulation of rat inter-stitial collagenase via a cytoskeletally based mechanotransduction system (Lavagnino *et al.* 2003; Arnoczky *et al.* 2004). *In vivo* studies have reported similar findings in immobilized ligaments and tendons (Goomer *et al.* 1999; Majima *et al.* 2000). Removing tendons from their normal mechanical environment could significantly alter the homeo-static tension within the cytoskeletal tensegrity system and be responsible for the upregulation of collagenase mRNA expression seen following 24 hours of stress deprivation. Conversely, applying static tensile load to the tendon produces a dose-dependent inhibition of interstitial collagenase mRNA expression; presumably through the same cytoskeletally based mechanism (Arnoczky *et al.* 2004). However, this inhibition was incomplete at the physiologic stresses examined (Arnoczky *et al.* 2004). This amplitude-dependent inhibition of col-lagenase expression appears to correlate with the progressive loss of collagen crimp and the increase in fiber recruitment reported in tendon fascicles with increasing stresses (Hanson *et al.* 2002). Thus, sequential increases in substrate strain likely result in an increasing number of cells being deformed (Arnoczky *et al.* 2002). However, because collage-nase mRNA expression was only inhibited and not totally eliminated with what would appear to be physiologic levels of static stress, substrate deforma-tion may not be the sole factor, or even the most important factor, involved in tendon cell signaling and subsequent gene expression with tensile load.

Transmission of tissue strain to the extracellular matrix and cells is believed to have two potential modes: substrate (extracellular matrix) strain and fluid flow (Watson 1991; Banes *et al.* 1995b; You *et al.* 2000). In an effort to more closely represent physio-logic loading conditions and the effects of fluid flow, cyclic strains within the normal functional range of tendons were applied to rat tail tendons (Lavagnino *et al.* 2003). Applying a low cyclic strain amplitude of 1% at 0.017 Hz resulted in a significant, but incomplete inhibition of collagenase expression (Lavagnino *et al.* 2003). Increasing the cyclic ampli-tude to 3% or 6% strain at 0.017 Hz or increasing the cyclic frequency to 0.17 or 1.0 Hz at 1% strain completely eliminated collagenase expression

(Lavagnino *et al.* 2003). The inhibitory effect of cyclic tensile loading on collagenase expression and syn-thesis was eliminated when the actin cytoskeleton was chemically disrupted (Lavagnino *et al.* 2003). The results of this study demonstrated that col-lagenase mRNA expression in tendon cells *in situ* can be modulated by cyclic tensile strain in a dose-dependent manner (both amplitude and frequency), presumably through a cytoskeletally based mechanotransduction pathway (Lavagnino *et al.* 2003). The inhibitory effect of cyclic loading on collagenase mRNA expression seen in our *in vitro* model is similar to that reported in an *in vivo* study (Majima *et al.* 2000).

These results suggest that tendon cells, like bone cells, may have a threshold, or set point, with regard to their mechanoresponsiveness to tensile loading (Frost 1987). It is probable that cytoskeletal tensional homeostasis is the mechanism by which tendon cells establish and attempt to maintain their mech-anostat set point. A previously described collagen gel matrix model system (Eastwood *et al.* 1996; Brown *et al.* 1998; Grinnell *et al.* 1999) was used to investigate if changes in the cytoskeletal tensional homeostasis of tendon cells are related to the con-trol of gene expression and to determine the ability of tendon cells to re-establish their cytoskeletal tensional homeostasis in response to a changing mechanical environment (Lavagnino & Arnoczky 2005). In this system, tendon cells seeded into the collagen gels were able to establish a cytoskeletal tensional homeostasis through an isometric contrac-tion against collagen gel matrices left attached to their culture dishes (Lavagnino & Arnoczky 2005). This was characterized by the presence of organ-ized stress fibers within the cytoskeleton and an upregulation of an anabolic gene (α1(I) collagen) (Lavagnino & Arnoczky 2005). Changes in cyto-skeletal tension control a reciprocal expression of anabolic and catabolic genes by tendon cells (Lavagnino & Arnoczky 2005). Loss of cytoskeletal organization through chemical disruption or a detachment of the gel resulted in an upregulation in the expression of the catabolic gene (interstitial collagenase) and an inhibition in the expression of the anabolic gene (α1(I) collagen) (Lavagnino & Arnoczky 2005). Previous studies have also shown that alterations in cell shape, secondary to cell detachment, or loss of extracellular matrix tension produce an increase in interstitial collagenase expression and a decrease in collagen production (Unemori & Werb 1986; Mauch *et al.* 1989; Lambert *et al.* 1992; Prajapati *et al.* 2000).

The apparent ability of the tendon cells to re-establish their baseline level of internal cytoskeletal tension (as evidenced by a return to baseline gene expression) following the loss of opposing external forces offered by the collagen matrices upon release is a significant finding (Lavagnino & Arnoczky 2005). It suggests that tendon cells can have an active role in "recalibrating" their sens-itivity to changes in external stresses. While this "recalibration" was accomplished by a gross re-organization and contraction of pliable collagen gel matrices, such alteration in cell–matrix interactions may be more localized (i.e. the pericellular matrix) (Egerbacher *et al.* 2006) and/or require more time (chronic exposure to altered matrix strain) in a mature connective tissue setting. However, the upper and lower limits of the external forces against which the cell can maintain tensional homeostasis are likely dependent on a myriad of factors includ-ing cell type and local extracellular matrix composi-tion as well as the frequency and rate of external stress application.

Can altered cell loading patterns have a role in the etiopathogenesis of tendinopathy?

A proposed algorithm for the onset of overuse tendinopathy involves altered cell–matrix inter-actions in response to repetitive loading (Fig. 4.4) (Archambault *et al.* 1995). In this scenario, the tendon cells are not able to maintain the extra-cellular matrix of the tendon which leads to a degeneration of the matrix and a transient weakness of the tissue making it more susceptible to damage from continued loading. This damage then ac-cumulates until tendinopathy (overuse injury) develops (Archambault *et al.* 1995). While this is a feasible algorithm for the development of overuse tendinopathy, the precise mechanism(s) of the altered cell–matrix interactions have not been described.

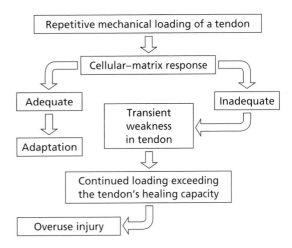

Fig. 4.4 Proposed algorithm of the etiopathogenesis of tendinopathy. After Archambault *et al.* (1995).

An increasing body of clinical material has sug-gested that tendons from tendinopathy patients exhibit an increase in degradative enzymes (matrix metalloproteinases) as well as an induction of apop-tosis (Ireland *et al.* 2001; Fu *et al.* 2002; Riley *et al.* 2002; Yuan *et al.* 2002, 2003; Alfredson *et al.* 2003; Lo *et al.* 2004; Riley 2004; Hosaka *et al.* 2005; Magra & Maffulli 2005; Sharma & Maffulli 2005; Tuoheti *et al.* 2005). Therefore, many investigators have focused on inducing expression of these molecular "markers" by exposing tendon cells to various loading regimes (Almekinders *et al.* 1993; Banes *et al.* 1995a, 1999; Skutek *et al.* 2001; Archambault *et al.* 2002; Lavagnino *et al.* 2003, 2005, 2006a; Tsuzaki *et al.* 2003; Wang *et al.* 2003; Arnoczky *et al.* 2004). Numerous studies have suggested that overstimu-lation of tendon cells, secondary to repetitive load-ing, results in a pattern of gene expression that can lead to tendinopathy (Almekinders *et al.* 1993; Banes *et al.* 1995a, 1999; Skutek *et al.* 2001; Archambault *et al.* 2002; Tsuzaki *et al.* 2003; Wang *et al.* 2003). However, the strain magnitudes and durations required to achieve an upregulation in the expres-sion of these inflammatory and catabolic genes may not be clinically relevant. Some of these studies have used a sustained application of cyclic strains in excess of 8% to elicit catabolic and inflammatory gene expression in tendon and ligament cells cultured on artificial substrates (Almekinders *et al.*

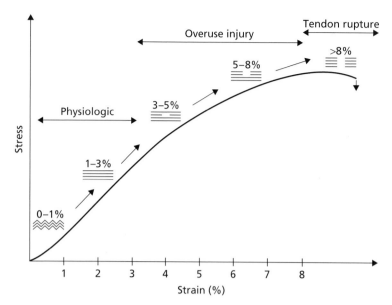

Fig. 4.5 Schematic drawing of a load deformation curve illustrating the mechanical response of a tendon to tensile loading. Modified from Józsa and Kannus (1997).

1993; Wang *et al.* 2003; Bhargava *et al.* 2004). Because tendon cell strain *in situ* has been shown to be significantly less than whole tendon strain (Arnoczky *et al.* 2002a), it is unlikely that such high levels of repetitive tendon cell strain could be reached and maintained *in vivo* without significant damage occurring within the extracellular matrix of the tendon (Woo *et al.* 1982).

Previous biomechanical studies have suggested that isolated collagen fibril damage occurs near the end of the linear portion of the load deformation curves of ligaments and tendons (Fig. 4.5) (Viidik & Ekholm 1968; Viidik 1972, 1980; Woo *et al.* 1982; Józsa & Kannus 1997). The ability to produce isolated fibril failure within an otherwise intact tendon is likely attributable to the multicomposite structure of the tissue (Kastelic *et al.* 1980; Viidik 1980). The sequential straightening and loading of crimped collagen fibrils, as well as interfibrillar sliding and shear between fibers and/or fibrils, produce a non-linear, load-deformation behavior of tendons that may put certain fibrils "at risk" for damage before others (Fig. 4.6) (Viidik 1980). While this damage may not affect the ultimate tensile strength of the tissues (Panjabi *et al.* 1996), it could alter the cell–matrix interactions within the damaged portion of the tendon. A previous study has demonstrated that following isolated fibrillar damage in

tendons the damaged fibrils relax (Knorzer *et al.* 1986). This would suggest an inability of these fibrils to transmit load and therefore maintain a homeostatic mechanobiologic stimulus to those cells associated with the damaged fibrils.

Based on the above findings, our laboratory has forwarded the hypothesis that an alteration of cell–matrix interaction secondary to isolated fibrillar damage could result in a mechanobiologic *understimulation* of tendon cells, which has been shown to result in an upregulation of collagenase mRNA expression and protein synthesis (Lavagnino *et al.* 2003, 2005; Arnoczky *et al.* 2004; Lavagnino & Arnoczky 2005). This, in turn, causes a decrease in material properties of the tendon (Fig. 4.7) and could put more of the extracellular matrix at risk for further damage with subsequent loading (Lavagnino *et al.* 2005).

Recently, our laboratory has demonstrated that creation of isolated tendon fibrillar damage within an otherwise intact tendon fascicle results in an upregulation of collagenase mRNA expression and protein synthesis by only those tendon cells associated with the damaged fibrils (Figs 4.8 & 4.9) (Lavagnino *et al.* 2006b). This would suggest a loss of load-transmitting function in the damaged fibril(s) and a subsequent altered cell–matrix interaction within the affected area. Previous studies

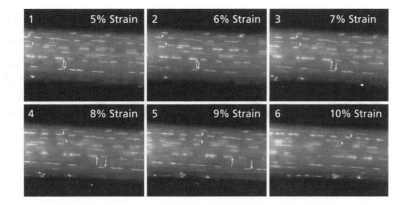

Fig. 4.6 Time-lapse confocal images of a rat tail tendon being strained at a rate of 20 μm/second. The cell nuclei have been stained with acridine orange and the pairs of short and long arrows identify cell nuclei used as fiduciary markers to identify fibril sliding. At 7% strain (image 3) the lower (long) pair of arrows can be seen separating indicating fiber slippage. This separation continues to increase with increasing strain (images 4 and 5). After 8% strain (image 4) the upper (short) pair of arrows begin to get closer and pass over one another at 9% strain (image 5). This slippage continues to increase at 10% strain (image 6). In both instances fibril slippage occurred in advance of complete tendon rupture.

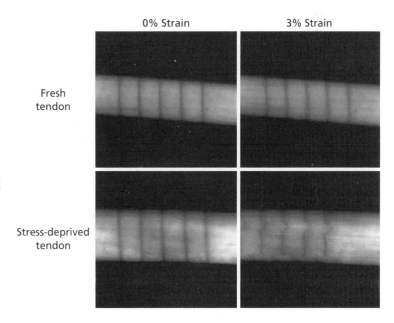

Fig. 4.7 Confocal images of a fresh and 21-day stress-deprived rat tail tendon. Parallel registration lines have been photobleached onto the surface of the tendons. When strained to 3% (grip-to-grip strain) the registration lines on the fresh tendon remain parallel. This is in contrast to the 21-day stress-deprived tendon that demonstrated an altered strain pattern due to breakdown of the extracellular matrix by collagenase which is upregulated in these tendons following stress deprivation.

from our laboratory have shown that loss of a homeostatic tensile load on tendon cells *in situ* results in an immediate upregulation of collagenase mRNA expression and protein synthesis (Lavagnino *et al.* 2003; 2005; Arnoczky *et al.* 2004; Lavagnino & Arnoczky 2005). The presence of increased levels of collagenase protein in these injured tendons is similar to what has been reported in clinical cases of tendinopathy (Fu *et al.* 2002; Riley *et al.* 2002; Lo *et al.* 2004; Magra & Maffulli 2005; Sharma & Maffulli 2005).

A clinical study examining matrix metalloproteinase (MMP) activity in ruptured human tendons demonstrated an altered expression and activity of

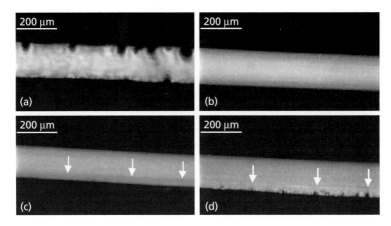

Fig. 4.8 Images of a rat tail tendon fascicle at various points throughout the testing protocol: (a) prior to loading (the crimp pattern is clearly visible); (b) during loading in the linear portion of the stress–strain curve demonstrating the elimination of the crimp pattern; (c) onset of fibrillar damage as manifested by a change in the reflectivity of the damaged fibrils (arrows); and (d) unloading of the tendon to 100 g and the reoccurrence of the crimp pattern within the damaged fibrils (arrows) (bar = 200 μm). (From Lavagnino, M., Arnoczky, S.P., Egerbacher, M., Gardner, K., Burns, M.E. (2006b) Isolated fibrillar damage in tendons stimulates local collagenase mRNA expression and protein synthesis. *Journal of Biomechanics* **39**, 2355–2362; with permission from Elsevier.)

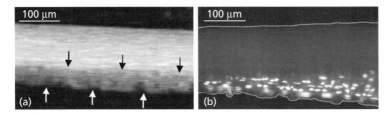

Fig. 4.9 Representative images of a rat tail tendon fascicle following fibrillar damage. (a) Presence of the crimp pattern on the bottom of the tendon fascicle (arrows) indicates the site of isolated fibrillar damage. (b) *In situ* hybridization of the tendon fascicle reveals interstitial collagenase mRNA expression in those cells associated with the damaged fibril(s). The borders of the tendon fascicle are delineated by lines (bar = 100 μm). (From Lavagnino, M., Arnoczky, S.P., Egerbacher, M., Gardner, K., Burns, M.E. (2006b) Isolated fibrillar damage in tendons stimulates local collagenase mRNA expression and protein synthesis. *Journal of Biomechanics* **39**, 2355–2362; with permission from Elsevier.)

several members of the MMP family (Riley *et al.* 2002). MMP-1 levels were significantly higher in ruptured tendons compared with normal controls, whereas MMP-2 and MMP-3 levels were reduced, possibly representing a failure in the normal remodeling process (Riley *et al.* 2002; Riley 2004). This increase in collagenase activity was associated with a deterioration in the quality of the collagen network. In addition, MMP expression was stimulated in rabbit tendon *in vivo* by extended periods of cyclic loading, although there was no sign of injury upon histologic examination (Archambault *et al.* 2001). Increased expression of MMP-1 was also found in human patellar tendinosis tissue (Fu *et al.* 2002).

The result of this MMP-mediated degradation of the extracellular matrix is reflected in the histopathologic findings in tendinosis which reveal irregular orientation of collagen, fiber disruption, change in fiber diameter, a decrease in the overall density of collagen, and an upregulation of collagen type III production (Józsa *et al.* 1990; Kannus & Józsa, 1991; Järvinen *et al.* 1997). Another study that examined the histopathology of ruptured and tendinopathic Achilles tendons suggested that while the ruptured tendons were significantly more degenerated than the tendinopathic tendons, the general pattern of degeneration was common to both groups (Tallon *et al.* 2001). Areas of acellularity or hypocellularity, interspersed with regions of hypercellularity with no evidence of inflammation, have been found in degenerative tendon tissue (Järvinen *et al.* 1997).

In addition to the documented increase in collagenase activity seen in clinical cases of tendinopathy, other studies have suggested that apoptosis may have a role in the pathogenesis of tendinopathy (Yuan *et al.* 2002, 2003; Hosaka *et al.* 2005). Studies on the pathogenesis of rotator cuff disorders demonstrate a significant increase in the number of apoptotic cells detected in degenerative supraspinatus tendons compared to normal control tendons (Yuan *et al.* 2002; Tuoheti *et al.* 2005). It is theorized that the increased number of apoptotic cells seen in the degenerative tissues of tendinopathy patients could adversely affect the rate of collagen synthesis and the potential for repair (Yuan *et al.* 2003). Apoptosis was also detected in samples of inflamed superficial digital flexor tendon in the horse possibly resulting in tendon weakness and increased risk of tendinopathy (Hosaka *et al.* 2005). However, at present it is still unknown whether apoptosis is the result or the cause of tendon degeneration.

Experimental studies from our laboratory have documented an increase in caspase-3 mRNA expression and protein synthesis as well as an increase in the number of apoptotic cells (demonstrated by detection of single-stranded DNA) following 24 hours of stress deprivation in our rat tail tendon model (unpublished data). While another *ex vivo* study was able to induce apoptosis in tendon cells following exposure to high strains (20% strain for 6 h at 1 Hz), it is probable that the high strains utilized in this investigation damaged tendon fibers or fibrils (Scott *et al.* 2005). This could result in the understimulation of the tendon cells associated with the damaged fibers or fibrils and the subsequent induction of apoptosis secondary to the release of cellular tension (Grinnell *et al.* 1999). Thus, these experimental and clinical studies point to a possible effect of mechanical stimulus, or lack thereof, on the induction of apoptosis in tendon cells. However, the precise mechanism(s) that trigger programmed cell death under these conditions must still be defined.

Clinical relevance and significance

The etiology of tendinopathy remains unclear, and many causes have been theorized (Józsa & Kannus 1997; Sharma & Maffulli 2005). Central to these theories is the concept that excessive loading of tendons during vigorous physical activity is the main pathologic stimulation for degeneration of the extracellular matrix (Selvanetti *et al.* 1997). Some investigators have suggested that it is the tendon cells' mechanobiologic response to excessive loading that initiates the degenerative cascade of events that leads to tendinopathy (Skutek *et al.* 2001; Archambault *et al.* 2002; Tsuzaki *et al.* 2003; Wang *et al.* 2003). The idea being that prolonged mechanical stimuli of tendon cells induce production of degradative cytokines and inflammatory prostaglandins which are thought to be mediators of tendinopathy (Sharma & Maffulli 2005). However, as noted above, the level of stimuli required to elicit these cellular responses is not clinically relevant and has, to date, only been demonstrated in cultured cells on artificial substrates (Almekinder *et al.* 1993; Wang *et al.* 2003; Bhargava *et al.* 2004).

We contend that it is actually an absence of mechanical stimuli, secondary to microtrauma, that is the mechanobiologic stimulus for the degradative cascade that leads to tendinopathy. Numerous investigators have postulated that during excessive, repetitive loading, microtrauma occurs within the tendon matrix (Archambault *et al.* 1995; Józsa & Kannus 1997; Sharma & Maffulli 2005; Wang *et al.* 2006). If this microtrauma is not balanced by an active repair response from the tenocytes, it will result in cumulative damage and, ultimately, degradation of the tendon (Ker 2002). Our research supports the concept that isolated fibril damage can occur during the extremes of physiologic loading (Lavagnino *et al.* 2006a). This damage alters cell–matrix interactions (mechanobiologic signaling) in the area causing an upregulation in collagenase and a weakening of the collagen structure

(Lavagnino *et al.* 2005, 2006a). This could make the tendon more susceptible to damage from additional loading at lower strains. We have also shown that mechanobiologic understimulation can induce apoptosis in these understimulated cells (unpublished research). This loss of cells could further compromise the tendon's ability to repair itself or even maintain its local extracellular matrix.

While mechanobiologic understimulation of tendon cells is a feasible explanation for the increase in apoptosis and collagenase reported in clinical cases of tendinopathy (Ireland *et al.* 2001; Fu *et al.* 2002; Riley *et al.* 2002; Yuan *et al.* 2002, 2003; Alfredson *et al.* 2003; Lo *et al.* 2004; Riley 2004; Hosaka *et al.* 2005; Magra & Maffulli 2005; Sharma & Maffulli 2005; Tuoheti *et al.* 2005), the question remains as to the role of repetitive strain in the etiopathogenesis of tendinopathy. As we have demonstrated in our model system, a single high load event was able to cause sufficient fibril damage to initiate a cell-mediated response as a result of mechanobiologic understimulation (Lavagnino *et al.* 2006a). Tendon microtrauma can also result from a non-uniform stress occurring within a tendon producing abnormal loading concentrations and localized fiber damage (Ker 2002). Therefore, it is possible that during a series of repetitive loading cycles a single abnormal loading cycle could produce strains sufficient enough to induce isolated fibril damage but not cause clinical injury (Fig. 4.10). This abnormal loading cycle could be a result of muscle fatigue and/or altered kinematics that can occur with the

performance of repetitive activities. It has long been suggested that mental fatigue (and altered neuromuscular responses) may also have a role in tendinopathy (Darling 1899a,b).

Thus, while repetitive loading, per se, may not be responsible for initiating the cascade of events that lead to tendinopathy, it is likely that continued loading of the compromised tissues has a significant role in the progression of the pathologic process. Additional research is needed to determine the magnitude of tendon forces experienced in activities that are often associated with the development of tendinopathy (jumping, running, throwing). In addition, the effect of muscle fatigue and/or altered kinematics on these tendon forces must be determined to gain insight into the mechanobiologic mechanism(s) that may have a role in the etiopathogenesis of tendinopathy.

Future directions

The response of tendon cells to changing loading conditions has significant implications in unraveling the etiopathogenesis of tendinopathy. While the knowledge base regarding the potential role(s) of tendon cell mechanobiology in tendon, health, injury, and repair is continuing to expand (Wang 2006), additional research is required to determine how changes (mechanical, chemical, and structural) in the *in situ* extracellular environment affects the mechanotransduction response(s) of tendon cells. In addition, we must determine how (or if) tendon cells can adapt to these changing loading conditions and/or changes in extracellular matrix composition.

Finally, we must assure that these *in vitro* investigations into tendon cell mechanobiology are clinically relevant so that the basic science data gleaned from these studies can be appropriately translated into the clinical situation. To do this we must have a comprehensive understanding of what is happening to tendons (on both a structural and material level) during actual *in vivo* activities.

What do we need to know?

• What is (are) the effect(s) of extremes of loading on the mechanostat set point of tendon cells?

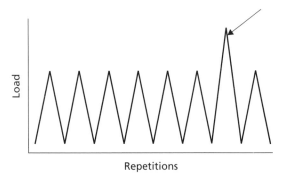

Fig. 4.10 Schematic representation of the concept of a single abnormal loading event during a series of repetitive activities.

- Are tendon cells able to adapt (change their mechanostat set point) in response to large changes in loads over time? If so, by what mechanism(s)?
- Are the degradative effects of mechanobiologic understimulation of tendon cells on the extracellular matrix reversible?
- What are the actual *in vivo* tendon forces experienced in repetitive loading activities?
- Are these forces sufficient to cause isolated fibril damage?
- How are these forces altered with muscle fatigue and/or poor kinematics?

How do we get there?

- Develop *in vivo* animal models that allow us to precisely control the degree of tendon loading.
- Use this *in vivo* model to examine (subfailure) extremes of loading conditions on the mechanotransduction response of tendon cells.
- Use this *in vivo* model to create isolated fibril damage and monitor the progression and/or reversability of the expected degenerative response.
- Develop anthropomorphic-based computer models to determine tendon loads based on joint angle, jumping/landing forces, and muscle activation.
- Develop monitoring technologies that allow real time gathering of the above variables during the "real life" performance of repetitive activities.
- Use this data to identify "at risk" variables that can result in abnormal tendon forces and isolated fibril damage.

Conclusions

The role of the mechanobiologic response of tendon cells in the etiopathogenesis of tendinopathy remains a point of controversy and debate. In this chapter we have presented an argument for mechanobiologic *understimulation* of tendon cells, secondary to microtrauma and isolated collagen fibril damage, as a predisposing factor for the pathologic changes (collagen disruption, increased MMP levels, and apoptosis) reported in clinical cases of tendinopathy. While our basic science data supports this hypothesis, additional translational research is needed to determine how, or even if, these proposed mechanobiologic mechanisms are involved in the etiopathogenesis of clinical tendinopathy.

References

Adams, D.S. (1992) Mechanisms of cell shape change: the cytomechanics of cellular response to chemical environment and mechanical loading. *Journal of Cell Biology* **117**, 83–93.

Alfredson, H., Lorentzon, M., Bäckman, S., Bäckman, A. & Lerner, U.H. (2003) cDNA arrays and real time qualitative PCR techniques in the investigation of chronic Achilles tendinosis. *Journal of Orthopaedic Research* **21**, 970–975.

Almekinders, L.C., Banes, A.J. & Ballenger, C.A. (1993) Effects of repetitive motion on human fibroblasts. *Medicine and Science in Sports and Exercise* **25**, 603–607.

Archambault, J.M., Hart, D.A. & Herzog, W. (2001) Response of rabbit Achilles tendon to chronic repetitive loading. *Connective Tissue Research* **42**, 13–23.

Archambault, J., Tsuzaki, M., Herzog, W. & Banes, A.J. (2002) Stretch and interleukin-1beta induce matrix metalloproteinases in rabbit tendon cells *in vitro*. *Journal of Orthopaedic Research* **20**, 36–39.

Archambault, J.M., Wiley, J.P. & Bray, R.C. (1995) Exercise loading of tendons and the development of overuse injuries. *Sports Medicine* **20**, 77–89.

Arnoczky, S.P., Lavagnino, M., Whallon, J.H. & Hoonjan, A. (2002a) *In situ* cell nucleus deformation under tensile load: a morphologic analysis using confocal laser microscopy. *Journal of Orthopaedic Research* **20**, 29–35.

Arnoczky, S.P., Tian, T., Lavagnino, M., Gardner, K., Schuler, P. & Morse, P. (2002b) Activation of stress-activated protein kinases (SAPK) in tendon cells following cyclic strain: the effects of strain frequency, strain magnitude, and cytosolic calcium. *Journal of Orthopaedic Research* **20**, 947–952.

Arnoczky, S.P., Tian, T., Lavagnino, M. & Gardner, K. (2004) *Ex vivo* static tensile loading inhibits MMP-1 expression in rat-tail tendon cells through a cytoskeletally based mechanotransduction mechanism. *Journal of Orthopaedic Research* **22**, 328–333.

Banes, A.J., Horesovsky, G., Larson, C., *et al.* (1999) Mechanical load stimulates expression of novel genes *in vivo* and *in vitro* in avian flexor tendon cells. *Osteoarthritis and Cartilage* **7**, 141–153.

Banes, A.J., Tsuzaki, M., Hu, P., *et al.* (1995a) Cyclic mechanical load and growth factors stimulate DNA synthesis in avian tendon cells. *Journal of Biomechanics* **28**, 1505–1513.

Banes, A.J., Tsuzaki, M., Yamamoto, J., *et al.* (1995b) Mechanoreception at the cellular level: the detection, interpretation, and diversity of responses to mechanical signals. *Biochemistry and Cell Biology* **73**, 349–365.

Ben-Ze'ev, A. (1991) Animal cell shape changes and gene expression. *Bioessays* **13**, 207–212.

Bhargava, M., Attia, E. & Hannafin, J.A. (2004) The effect of cyclic tensile strain on MMPs, collagen, and casein degrading activities of fibroblasts isolated from anterior cruciate and medial collateral ligaments. *Transactions of the Orthopaedic Research Society* **29**, 110.

Brown, R.A., Prajapati, R., McGrouther, D.A., Yannus, I.V. & Eastwood, M. (1998) Tensional homeostasis in dermal fibroblasts: mechanical responses to mechanical loading in three dimensional substrates. *Journal of Cellular Physiology* **175**, 323–332.

Darling, E.A. (1899a) The effects of training: a study of the Harvard crews. *Boston Medical and Surgical Journal* **141**, 205–209.

Darling, E.A. (1899b) The effects of training: a study of the Harvard crews. *Boston Medical and Surgical Journal* **141**, 229–233.

Eastwood, M., Porter, R., Khan, U., McGrouther, G. & Brown, R. (1996) Quantitative analysis of collagen gel contractile forces generated by dermal fibroblasts and the relationship to cell morphology. *Journal of Cellular Physiology* **166**, 33–42.

Egerbacher, M., Arnoczky, S.P., Gardner, K., Caballero, O. & Gartner, J. (2006) Stress-deprivation of tendons results in alterations in the integrin profile and pericellular matrix of tendon cells. *Transactions of the Orthopaedic Research Society* **31**, 1100.

Frost, H.M. (1987) Bone "mass" and the "mechanostat": a proposal. *Anatomical Record* **219**, 1–9.

Fu, S.C., Chan, B.P., Wang, W., Pau, H.M., Chan, K.M. & Rolf, C.G. (2002) Increased expression of matrix metalloproteinase 1 (MMP-1) in 11 patients with patellar tendinosis. *Acta Orthopaedica Scandinavica* **73**, 658–662.

Goomer, R.S., Basava, D., Maris, T., Kobayashi, K., Harwood, F. & Amiel, D. (1999) Effect of stress deprivation on MMP-1 gene expression and regulation of MMP-1 promoter in medial collateral and anterior cruciate ligament (MCL, ACL) and patellar tendon. *Transactions of the Orthopaedic Research Society* **24**, 45.

Grinnell, F., Zhu, M., Carlson, M. & Abrams, J. (1999) Release of mechanical tension triggers apoptosis of human fibroblasts in a model of regressing granulation tissue. *Experimental Cell Research* **248**, 608–619.

Hanson, K.A., Weiss, J.A. & Barton, J.K. (2002) Recruitment of tendon crimp with applied tensile strain. *Journal of Biomechanical Engineering* **124**, 72–77.

Hosaka, Y., Teraoka, H., Yamamoto, E., Ueda, H. & Takehana, K. (2005) Mechanism of cell death in inflamed superficial digital flexor tendon in the horse. *Journal of Comparative Pathology* **132**, 51–58.

Ingber, D.E. (1991) Integrins as mechanochemical transducers. *Current Opinion in Cell Biology* **3**, 841–848.

Ingber, D.E. (1997) Tensegrity: the architectural basis of cellular mechanotransduction. *Annual Review of Physiology* **59**, 575–599.

Ireland, D., Harrall, R., Curry, V., *et al.* (2001) Changes in gene expression in chronic human Achilles tendinopathy. *Matrix Biology* **20**, 159–169.

Janmey, P.A. (1998) The cytoskeleton and cell signaling component localization and mechanical coupling. *Physiology Review* **78**, 763–781.

Järvinen, M., Józsa, L., Kannus, P., Järvinen T.L., Kvist, M. & Leadbetter, W. (1997) Histopathological findings in chronic tendon disorders. *Scandinavian Journal of Medicine & Science in Sports* **7**, 86–95.

Józsa, L.G. & Kannus, P. (1997) *Human Tendons: Anatomy, Physiology, and Pathology*. Human Kinetics, Champaign, IL: 164–253.

Józsa, L.G., Reffy, A., Kannus, P., Demel, S. & Elek, E. (1990) Pathological alterations in human tendons. *Archives of Orthopaedic and Trauma Surgery* **110**, 15–21.

Kannus, P. & Józsa, L.G. (1991) Histopathological changes preceding spontaneous rupture of a tendon. A controlled study of 891 patients. *Journal of Bone and Joint Surgery. American volume* **73**, 1507–1525.

Kao, J.P.Y., Harootunian, A.T. & Tsien, R.Y. (1989) Photochemically generated cytosolic calcium pulses and their detection by Fluo-3. *Journal of Biological Chemistry* **264**, 8179–8184.

Kastelic, J., Galeski, A. & Baer, E. (1978) The multicomposite structure of tendon. *Connective Tissue Research* **6**, 11–23.

Kastelic, J., Palley, I. & Baer, E. (1980) A structural mechanical model for tendon crimping. *Journal of Biomechanics* **13**, 887–893.

Ker, R.F. (2002) The implications of the adaptable fatigue quality of tendons for their construction, repair, and function. *Comparative Biochemistry and Physiology. Part A, Molecular and Integrative Physiology* **133**, 987–1000.

Knorzer, E., Folkhard, W., Geercken, W., *et al.* (1986) New aspects of the etiology of tendon rupture. An analysis of time-resolved dynamic-mechanical measurements using synchrotron radiation. *Archives of Orthopaedic and Trauma Surgery* **105**, 113–120.

Lambert, C., Soudant, E., Nusgens, B. & Lapiere, C. (1992) Pretranslational

regulation of extracellular matrix macromolecules and collagenase expression in fibroblasts by mechanical forces. *Laboratory Investigation: a journal of technical methods and pathology* **66**, 444–451.

Lavagnino, M. & Arnoczky, S.P. (2005) *In vitro* alterations in cytoskeletal tensional homeostasis control gene expression in tendon cells. *Journal of Orthopaedic Research* **23**, 1211–1218.

Lavagnino, M., Arnoczky, S.P., Caballero, O., Robertson, E.M. & Nashi, S.M. (2006a) *In vitro* stress-deprivation alters the mechanostat set point of tendon cells. *Transactions of the Orthopaedic Research Society* **31**, 329.

Lavagnino, M., Arnoczky, S.P., Egerbacher, M., Gardner, K. & Burns, M.E. (2006b) Isolated fibrillar damage in tendons stimulates local collagenase mRNA expression and protein synthesis. *Journal of Biomechanics* **39**, 2355–2362.

Lavagnino, M. Arnoczky, S.P., Frank, K. & Tian, T. (2005) Collagen fibril diameter distribution does not reflect changes in the mechanical properties of *in vitro* stress-deprived tendons. *Journal of Biomechanics* **38**, 69–75.

Lavagnino, M., Arnoczky S.P., Tian, T. & Vaupel, Z. (2003) Effect of amplitude and frequency of cyclic tensile strain on the inhibition of MMP-1 mRNA expression in tendon cells: *in vitro* study. *Connective Tissue Research* **44**, 181–187.

Lo, I.K.Y., Marchuk, L. & Hollinshead, R. (2004) Matrix metalloproteinases and tissue inhibitors of metalloproteinases mRNA are specifically altered in torn rotator cuff tendons. *American Journal of Sports Medicine* **32**, 1223–1229.

Magra, M. & Maffulli, N. (2005) Matrix metalloproteases: a role in overuse tendinopathies. *British Journal of Sports Medicine* **39**, 789–791.

Majima, T., Matchuk, L.L., Shrive, N.G., Frank, C.B. & Hart, D.A. (2000) *In vitro* cyclic tensile loading of an immobilized and mobilized ligament autograft selectively inhibits mRNA levels for collagenase (MMP-1). *Journal of Orthopaedic Science: official journal of the Japanese Orthopaedic Association* **5**, 503–510.

Mauch, C., Adelmann-Grill, B., Hatamochi, A. & Krieg, T. (1989) Collagenase gene expression in fibroblasts is regulated by a three-dimensional contact with collagen. *Federation of European Biochemical Societies (FEBS) Letters* **250**, 301–305.

Panjabi, M.M., Yoldas, E., Oxland, T.R. & Crisco 3rd, J.J. (1996) Subfailure injury of the rabbit anterior cruciate ligament. *Journal of Orthopaedic Research* **14**, 24–31.

Prajapati, R.T., Chavally-Mis, B., Herbage, D., Eastwood, M. & Brown, R.A. (2000) Mechanical loading regulates protease production by fibroblasts three-dimensional collagen substrates. *Wound Repair and Regeneration: official publication of the Wound Healing Society and the European Tissue Repair Society* **8**, 226–237.

Riley, G.P. (2004) The pathogenesis of tendinopathy: a molecular perspective. *Rheumatology* **43**, 131–142.

Riley, G.P., Curry, V., DeGroot, J., *et al.* (2002) Matrix metalloproteinase activities and their relationship with collagen remodeling in tendon pathology. *Matrix Biology* **21**, 185–195.

Ritty, T.M., Roth, R. & Heuser, J.E. (2003) Tendon cell array isolation reveals a previously unknown fibrillin-2-containing macromolecular assembly. *Structure* **11**, 1179–1188.

Rosales, C., O'Brien, V., Kornberg, L. & Juliano, R. (1995) Signal transduction by cell adhesion receptors. *Biochimica et Biophysica Acta* **1242**, 77–98.

Ruoslahti, E. (1997) Stretching is good for a cell. *Science* **276**, 1345–1346.

Sachs, F. (1988) Mechanical transduction in biological systems. *Critical Reviews in Biomedical Engineering* **16**, 141–169.

Scott, A., Khan, K.M., Heer, J., Cook, J.L., Lian, O. & Duronio, V. (2005) High strain mechanical loading rapidly induces tendon apoptosis: an *ex vivo* rat tibialis anterior model. *British Journal of Sports Medicine* **39**, e25.

Selvanetti, A., Cipolla, M. & Puddu, G. (1997) Overuse tendon injuries: basic science and classification. *Operative Techniques in Sports Medicine* **5**, 110–117.

Sharma, P. & Maffulli, N. (2005) Tendon injury and tendinopathy: healing and repair. *Journal of Bone and Joint Surgery* **87A**, 187–202.

Shirakura, K., Ciarelli, M., Arnoczky, S.P. & Whallon, J.H. (1995) Deformation induced calcium signaling. *Transactions of the Combined Orthopaedic Research Societies* **2**, 94.

Skutek, M., van Griensven, M., Zeichen, J., Brauer, N. & Bosch, U. (2001) Cyclic mechanical stretching enhances secretion of interleukin 6 in human tendon fibroblasts. *Knee Surgery Sports Traumatology and Arthroscopy* **9**, 322–326.

Sung, K.-L.P., Whittemore, D.E., Yang, L., Amiel, D. & Akeson, W.H. (1996) Signal pathways and ligament cell adhesiveness. *Journal of Orthopaedic Research* **14**, 729–735.

Tallon, C., Maffulli, N. & Ewen, S.W. (2001) Ruptured Achilles tendons are significantly more degenerated than tendinopathic tendons. *Medicine and Science in Sports and Exercise* **33**, 1983–1990.

Tsuzaki, M., Bynum, D., Almekinders, L., Yang, X., Faber, J. & Banes, A.J. (2003) ATP modulates load-inducible IL-1β, COX 2, and MMP3 gene expression in human tendon cells. *Journal of Cellular Biochemistry* **89**, 556–562.

Tuoheti, Y., Itoi, E., Pradhan, R.L., *et al.* (2005) Apoptosis in the supraspinatus tendon with stage II subacromial impingement. *Journal of Shoulder and Elbow Surgery* **14**, 535–541.

Unemori, E.N. & Werb, Z. (1986) Reorganization of polymerized actin: a possible trigger for induction of procollagenase in fibroblasts cultured in and on collagen gels. *Journal of Cell Biology* **103**, 1021–1031.

Viidik, A. (1972) Interdependence between structure and function in collagenous tissues. In: *Biology of Collagen* (Viidik, A. & Vaust, J., eds). Academic Press, New York: 257–280.

Viidik, A. (1980) Mechanical properties of parallel-fibered collagenous tissues. In: *Biology of* Collagen (Viidik, A. & Vuust, J., eds). Academic Press, London: 237–255.

Viidik, A. & Ekholm, R. (1968) Light and electron microscopic studies of collagen fibers under strain. *Zeitschrift für Anatomie und Entwicklungsgeschichte* **127**, 154–164.

Wang, J.H.-C. (2006) Mechanobiology of tendon. *Journal of Biomechanics* **39**, 1563–82.

Wang, J.H.-C., Iosifidis, M.I. & Fu, F.H. (2006) Biomechanical basis for tendinopathy. *Clinical Orthopaedics and Related Research* **443**, 320–332.

Wang, J.H.-C., Jia, F., Yang, G., *et al.* (2003) Cyclic mechanical stretching of human tendon fibroblasts increases the production of prostaglandin E2 and levels of cyclooxygenase expression: a novel *in vitro* model study. *Connective Tissue Research* **44**, 128–133.

Wang, N., Butler, J.P. & Ingber, D.E. (1993) Mechanotransduction across the cell surface and through the cytoskeleton. *Science* **260**, 1124–1127.

Wang, N. & Ingber, D.E. (1994) Control of cytoskeletal mechanics by extracellular matrix, cell shape, and mechanical tension. *Biophysical Journal* **66**, 2181–2189.

Watson, P.A. (1991) Function follows form: generation of intracellular signals by cell deformation. *Federation of American Societies for Experimental Biology (FASEB) Journal* **5**, 2013–2019.

Woo, S. L-Y., Gomez, M.A., Woo, Y.K. & Akeson, W.H. (1982) Mechanical properties of tendons and ligaments. I. Quasistatic and nonlinear viscoelastic properties. *Biorheology* **19**, 385–396.

You, J., Yellowley, C.E., Donahue, H.J., Zhang, Y., Chen, Q. & Jacobs, C.R. (2000) Substrate deformation levels associated with routine physical activity are less stimulatory to bone cells relative to loading-induced oscillatory fluid flow. *Journal of Biomechanical Engineering* **122**, 387–393.

Yuan, J., Murrell, G.A., Wei, A.Q. & Wang, M.X. (2002) Apoptosis in rotator cuff tendinopathy. *Journal of Orthopaedic Research* **20**, 1372–1379.

Yuan, J., Wang, M.X. & Murrell, G.A. (2003) Cell death and tendinopathy. *Clinics in Sports Medicine* **22**, 693–701.

Chapter 5

How Alive are Tendons? Metabolic and Circulatory Activity Associated with Exercise in Humans

MICHAEL KJÆR, HENNING LANGBERG, ROBERT BOUSHEL, SATU KOSKINEN, BENJAMIN MILLER, KATJA HEINEMEIER, JENS L. OLESEN, METTE HANSEN, PHILIP HANSEN, AND S. PETER MAGNUSSON

Exercise results in increased metabolic and circulatory activity of the tendons in humans. With loading, the tendon and peritendinous blood flow can be demonstrated to increase up to sevenfold. This seems adequate in relation to the metabolic activity of the tendon, and no clear tissue ischemia can be found in tendons during loading. In fact, a close correlation exists between tendon blood flow and declining oxygen tissue saturation, and tendon flow is not simply a function of skeletal muscle blood flow but represents a separate regulatory system. Several vasodilatory substances are released locally (e.g. prostaglandin, bradykinin) during exercise, and flow during exercise is regulated—at least partly—by cyclo-oxygenase 2 pathways during exercise. Tendon collagen synthesis rises and tissue concentrations of degrading metalloprotease enzymes are increased for several days after an acute bout of exercise. Training results in a chronic elevation of collagen turnover, and dependent on the type of collagen also to some degree of net collagen synthesis. These changes will modify the mechanical properties of the tissue and thereby lower the tendon stress, but require a prolonged period of adaptation. Several growth factors are found within and around the loaded tendon, and interstitial concentrations of these (interleukin-1 [IL-6], transforming growth factor β [TGF-β], and insulin-like growth factor 1 [IGF-1] binding proteins) were found to be elevated after a bout of exercise. Human tendon tissue responds to mechanical loading both with a rise in metabolic and circulatory activity as well as with an increased extracellular matrix synthesis. These changes contribute to the training-induced adapta-

tion in mechanical properties whereby resistance to loading is altered and tolerance towards strenous exercise can be improved and injuries avoided.

Introduction

So far, the adaptive changes of tendon as a result of exercise with regards to tissue blood flow, and turnover of the extracellular matrix have been thought to be of limited magnitude. Thus, prolonged stimulation is required to create even moderate changes in tissue characteristics (Kjær 2004). However, the metabolism of collagen and the connective tissue network is known to respond dynamically to altered levels of physical activity, in that biosynthesis decreases with reduced activity (Kovanen 1989). Conversely, exercise accelerates formation and degradation of connective tissue in both muscle and tendon, which may reflect both physiologic adaptation and repair of damage of extracellular matrix structures (Kovanen 1989; Langberg et al. 1999c, 2001; Koskinen et al. 2000, 2001). It is therefore likely that in human tendon far more dynamic processes occur than hitherto thought, but this area of research has been limited by the abilty to measure relevant parameters in vivo. Such limitations have been in sharp contrast to the long-term interest and expertise in in vitro studies of tendon relevant cells and structures (e.g. Banes et al. 1995). However, human models have been developed to allow for more real time in vivo determinations of metabolism, blood flow, inflammatory activity, and collagen turnover in relation to human tendon tissue and its environment during and after exercise (Langberg *et al.* 1999a–d; Boushel *et al.* 1999, 2000, 2001). These methods together with ultrasound determination of mechanical properties of human tendon during muscular activity (Magnusson *et al.* 2001, 2003a) and magnetic resonance imaging (MRI) are promising regarding coupling of tissue metabolism to the viscoelastic properties and thus to function of the human tendon.

Methods and results

Tendon blood flow and metabolic activity with exercise

The use of the microdialysis technique allows for *in vivo* determination of biochemical substances in various local tissues, and has been applied to the peritendinous space of the Achilles tendon in runners before, immediately after, and 72 hours after 36 km of running (Langberg *et al.* 1999c). With this technique it was demonstrated that acute exercise induces changes in metabolic and inflammatory activity (Langberg *et al.* 1999b), and that the peritendinous changes reflect changes occuring also within the tendon (Langberg *et al.* 2002a). It can furthermore be demonstrated that human tendon increases its oxygen uptake with loading (Boushel *et al.* 2001), and that glucose uptake increases with muscle contraction (Kaliokoski *et al.* 2005).

Tendons have a limited vasculature (approximately 0.2–2% of the tendon cross-sectional area) (Petersen *et al.* 2000; Marsolais *et al.* 2003) and thus it has been speculated that overloading and injury to tendons are at least partly coupled to insufficient blood flow and lack of oxidative metabolism with muscular contraction. However, resting tendon has a resting flow of 30–40% of that in skeletal musculature and in animals an increase in tendon blood flow with exercise has been demonstrated (Bakman *et al.* 1991). It has been possible to determine peritendinous blood flow in humans during muscular contraction by the use of radiolabeled ^{133}Xe-washout placed immediately ventral to the Achilles tendon, and it was demonstrated that blood flow in the peritendon region increased 3–4-fold during heel raising exercise or during static intermittent calf muscle exercise (Langberg *et al.* 1998, 1999a)

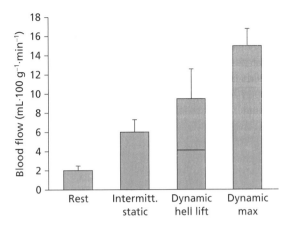

Fig. 5.1 Blood flow in the peritendinous and core Achilles region in exercising humans performing either isometric or dynamic exercise of the calf with increasing work load. Data from Langberg *et al.* (1998, 1999a) and Boushel *et al.* (1999, 2000).

(Fig. 5.1). In addition, a dynamic ergometer model has been developed by which the Achilles tendon can be studied during standardized dynamic exercise loading. By the use of this model, blood flow in the Achilles peritendinous region has been shown to rise up to sevenfold during intense plantar flexion exercise compared to values obtained at rest (Boushel *et al.* 1999, 2000) (Fig. 5.1). Taken together, these findings indicate that flow in the peritendinous region is increased with exercise in an exercise-dependent manner, and in parallel with muscle perfusion during calf muscle contraction. Interestingly, a simultaneous use of near-infrared spectroscopy (NIRS) (Boushel *et al.* 1999) indicated that oxygen extraction rose in parallel with exercise in both the peritendinous and muscle region. In addition, the parallel rise in total hemoglobin volume in both muscle and peritendon regions and the concomitant drop in oxygen saturation, indicates the presence of vasodilation during intense exercise that is coupled to tissue oxygenation in the peritendinous region (Fig. 5.2). It is clear from these experiments that although the increase in tendon blood flow is somewhat restricted, there is no indication of any major ischemia in the tendon region during exercise. Furthermore, tendon flow is not only a function of skeletal muscle flow but most likely has a separate regulatory system.

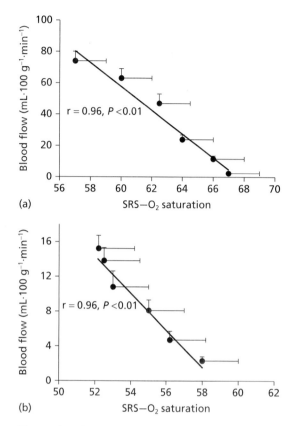

(a)

(b)

Fig. 5.2 Correlation between spatially resolved near-infrared spectroscopy (SRS) oxygen saturation and blood flow in both calf muscle (top) and in the peritendinous Achilles region (bottom) at rest and during graded dynamic plantar flexion exercise to exhaustion ($n = 8$). Spearmann test was used to determine correlation significance. Data from Boushel et al. (1999, 2000).

The question remains as to how blood flow to the tendon region is regulated. Several candidates for regulation of flow in skeletal muscle (nitric oxide [NO]), adenosine, endothilium-derived hyperpolarizing factor [EDHF], and prostaglandins) have been proposed, and it cannot be excluded that similar substances and metabolites are also vasoactive in the tendon region (Langberg et al. 2002b,c). One candidate—bradykinin—attracts specific interest because of its simultaneous vasodilatory and nociceptive properties. As bradykinin is known to activate prostaglandin and NO-dependent pathways, it may be important not only in relation to

regulation of flow to the normal tendon, but also to the overused, sore, and hyperperfused tendon. With the use of microdialysis it has been demonstrated that both in muscle and tendon tissue, there is detectable bradykinin present in the tissue, and that the interstitial concentration of bradykinin increases with exercise (Langberg et al. 2002c). In addition, interstitial adenosine concentrations rose during exercise not only in muscle but also in the peritendinous tissue (Langberg et al. 2002c). To what extent this has a role for the vasodilatory response is not yet proven, but exercise-induced changes in bradykinin levels are in the range that in vitro will cause a vasodilatory effect on the endothelium (Rosen et al. 1983). Other substances of potential relevance for nociception in tendon such as substance P and glutamine have been demonstrated in animal tendon and human tendon, respectively (Alfredson et al. 1999; Ackermann et al. 2001).

Role of prostaglandins for flow and inflammation in human tendon

In vitro models have demonstrated an increased production of prostaglandins after repetitive motion of human mesenchymal tendon cells in cultures (Almekinders et al. 1993). This response was blocked by indometacin and was unrelated to any microscopically visible cellular damage of repeated stretching. This indicates that inflammatory mediators are secreted in response to normal loading of connective tissue. In line with this, with the use of the microdialysis technique, release of prostaglandin and thromboxane could be demonstrated in response to exercise both in muscle and in peritendinous tissue (Langberg et al. 1999b; Karamouzis et al. 2001). In the resting tendon with long-term symptoms of overuse, no elevated levels of prostaglandins could be detected (Alfredson et al. 1999), whereas an exaggerated response of interstitial prostaglandin concentration could be detected in association with exercise in overused versus healthy tendon (unpublished observation). This points to a more vulnerable state with chronic injury, which results in a more pronounced inflammatory response upon stimulation. The exact location of the prostaglandin production cannot be stated, but

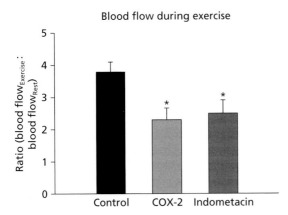

Fig. 5.3 Tendon region blood flow increases with 30 min of dynamic plantar flexion exercise, either with preceding intake of placebo or drugs inhibiting cyclo-oxygenase 1+2 (COX-1+2) or only COX-2 induced prostaglandin formation. Data from Langberg *et al.* (2003).

whereas muscle static contraction was not sufficient and considerable dynamic activity was needed to release prostaglandin, only moderate isometric contraction was needed to elicit a response in tendon-associated tissue. The inflammatory response was only transient and it remains unclear to what extent this response is coupled to collagen synthesis and degradation. Interestingly, it can be shown that the exercise-induced increase in tendon flow is inhibited 40% by a blockade of prostaglandin secretion with cyclo-oxygenase blockers. This indicates that prostanoids have an important role for vasodilation in tendon tissue with exercise (Langberg *et al.* 2003) (Fig. 5.3), but it remains unknown to what extent it has a role in inflamed tendons, and in recovery after overuse. However, it is notable that there is an important seperate role for prostaglandins in flow regulation during exercise in tendon (Langberg *et al.* 2003), which contrasts that in muscle where reduction in exercise flow is seen only when a blockade of several pathways is carried out (Boushel *et al.* 2002).

Synthesis and degradation of collagen in human tendon with exercise

The cleavage of the carboxypeptide allows for indirect determination of collagen type I formation. Development of assays for such markers of type 1

collagen synthesis (the carboxyterminal propeptide of type 1 collagen [PICP]) and degradation (the carboxyterminal telopeptide region of type 1 collagen [ICTP]) has made it possible to study the effect of exercise on collagen type I turnover. When detected in circulating blood, these markers have been shown to be relatively insensitive to a single bout of exercise, whereas prolonged exercise or weeks of training were shown to result in increased type I collagen turnover and net formation (Langberg *et al.* 2000). However, as bone is the main overall contributor of procollagen markers for collagen type I turnover in the blood, and as serum levels of PICP and ICTP do not allow for the detection of the location of the specific type of region or tissue in which changes in turnover are taking place, it cannot be concluded from these studies whether changes in collagen turnover of tendon-related tissue occurs. In addition, acute exercise caused increased local formation of type I collagen in the recovery process, suggesting that acute physical loading leads to adaptations in tendon-related collagen in humans (Langberg *et al.* 1999c). It has been shown that this response is dose–response related, as 1 hour of exercise also resulted in increased interstitial levels of PICP after 3 days, but to a lesser degree than after 36 km of running (Heinemeier *et al.* 2003) (Fig. 5.4). More recently, the use of stable isotopes (^{13}C or ^{15}N-proline) with subsequent sampling of human

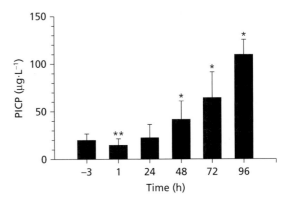

Fig. 5.4 Changes in peritendinous interstitial levels of procollagen C-terminal propeptide (PICP) with exercise of 3 hours' duration. Data collected from microdialysis fluid obtained peritendinously to the loaded Achilles tendon. Data from Langberg *et al.* (1999c).

muscle and tendon tissue has allowed for direct determination of collagen synthesis in human tendon and skeletal muscle (as well as in ligament, skin, and bone). From these studies it can be shown that tendon, ligament, and skeletal muscle collagen synthesis seems to be in the range of 2–3% (fractional synthesis rate) per day (24 hours) (Babraj et al. 2005). Furthermore, the exercise-induced increase in synthesis of collagen is present 3 days after an acute exercise bout (1 hour), as evaluated from incorporated proline into patella tendon tissue (Miller et al. 2005).

When type I collagen synthesis and degradation in connective tissue of the Achilles peritendinous space was studied before and after 4 and 11 weeks of intense physical training, an adaptive response of the collagen type I metabolism of the peritendinous tissue around human Achilles tendon was found in response to physical training (Langberg et al. 2001). The increase in interstitial concentrations of PICP rose within 4 weeks of training and remained elevated thereafter for the entire training period, indicating that collagen type I synthesis was chronically elevated in response to training. As blood values for PICP did not change significantly over the training period, it is likely that the increased collagen type I formation occurs locally in non-bone tendon connective tissue rather than reflecting a general rise in formation of collagen type I throughout the body. Also, tissue ICTP concentrations rose in response to training, but the rise was transient, and interstitial levels of ICTP returned to baseline levels with more prolonged training. Taken together, the findings indicate that the initial response to training is an increase in turnover of collagen type I, and that this is followed by a predomination of anabolic processes resulting in an increased net synthesis of collagen type I in non-bone connective tissue such as tendons (Langberg et al. 2001). The pattern of stimulation of both synthesis and degradation with the anabolic process dominating in response to exercise in tendon-related connective tissue is a pattern that is in accordance with events occuring with connective tissue (as well as with other muscle proteins) and in muscle tissue in response to loading (Han et al. 1999).

Stretch-induced hypertrophy of chicken skeletal muscle has been shown to increase muscle collagen turnover using tracer methods (Laurent et al. 1985), which is in accordance with the present findings on humans where collagen synthesis increased markedly at the beginning of training. It was in the study by Laurent et al. (1985) concluded that a large amount of newly synthesized collagen was wasted, resulting in a disproportionate high collagen turnover rate compared to the magnitude of true net synthesis of collagen. Likewise, in human muscle, type IV collagen degradation—as indicated by an increase in matrix metalloprotease 2 (MMP-2)—increased over a period of 1 year with electrical stimulation of spinal cord injured individuals, without any detectable change in total type IV content, indicating an increased collagen turnover rate with no or very little net synthesis (Koskinen et al. 2000). Early changes after exercise indicating increased MMP activity and increased collagen synthesis in skeletal muscle has been shown in animal muscle (Koskinen et al. 2001). In human peritendinous tissue it has been shown that MMP-9 increases early and MMP-2 late after an acute bout of 60 min running exercise (Koskinen et al. 2004) and while the exact source of this release remains to be demonstrated, both fibroblasts and leukocytes are likely candidates. The present studies in humans and animals support the idea of a simultaneous activation of both formation and degradation in collagen of both muscle and tendon tissue in response to loading. Interestingly, for type I collagen in tendon, this is timewise followed by a more pronounced imbalance in favor of formation and resulting in a net collagen synthesis.

Acute exercise has been shown to cause an increase in collagen catabolism as determined across an exercising human leg (Brahm et al. 1996). Furthermore, in the peritendinous space of the Achilles tendon, collagen formation was depressed immediately in response to acute exercise and followed by a rise in synthesis rate (Langberg et al. 1999c). As individuals in the latter training study were training on a daily basis, it is difficult to differentiate effects of each bout of acute exercise from the chronic training adaptation. It has been demonstrated that acute exercise elevates collagen type I formation for at least 3–4 days post-exercise

(Langberg *et al.* 1999c) (Fig. 5.4). Therefore, previous acute bouts of exercise will influence the outcome of each subsequent one. This probably explains why highly trained runners (training up to 12 hours per week) in one study had high basal levels of interstitial levels of PICP (Langberg *et al.* 1999c). Thus, it cannot be excluded that the effect on collagen metabolism found during a program with daily training simply reflects an effect on collagen formation from the last training bout, rather than any more chronic effect of training. On the basis of these findings it can be concluded that both an increased collagen turnover is observed in response to training, and that with prolonged training a net synthesis of collagen type I is to be expected.

Do tendons grow in response to training?

It is far from clear whether a net synthesis of collagen type I is transformed into morphologically detectable increases in tendon size. However, in accordance with this view it has been demonstated in animal models that prolonged training results in enlargement of tendon diameter. It has to be noted that in most animal studies the overall increase in tendon cross-sectional area after prolonged training was preceded by a transient decrease in tendon diameter in the initial period of training (Woo *et al.* 1982; Sommer 1987; Birch *et al.* 1999), suggesting a pivotal response to increased loading. Recent cross-sectional observations in trained runners versus sedentary humans have shown that MRI-determined Achilles tendon cross-sectional area was enlarged in trained individuals compared to untrained controls (Rosager *et al.* 2002), whereas a shorter period of training (longitudinal study) did not result in any significant increase in tendon cross-sectional area (Hansen *et al.* 2003). On this basis it can be speculated that training initially results in an increased turnover of collagen type I to allow for reorganization of the tissue, while more prolonged training results in a net increase in tendon tissue and probably alterations in tissue diameter and strength. Such an increase in tendon area can potentially be beneficial in reducing the stress upon the tendon when exercised. Interestingly, the amount of tendon tissue in the elderly is increased even though they are less active and have a smaller maximal muscle strength than their younger counterparts (Magnusson *et al.* 2003b). The increased cross-sectional area in the elderly might compensate for reduced tendon quality and tensile strength of the tendon tissue by increasing the amount of tendon tissue to ensure a sufficient safety margin to avoid tendon rupture (Magnusson *et al.* 2003b).

Regulation of collagen synthesis with exercise: results from human studies

Several growth factors in tendon change with mechanical loading *in vitro* (Banes *et al.* 1995), but their exact role in collagen synthesis of human tendon and muscle in relation to physiologic loading remains to be elucidated. It has been shown that mechanical loading of human tendon results in a rise in interstitial concentraton of both TGF-β (Heinemeier *et al.* 2003), IGF-1 and its binding protein IGF-BP 4 and IL-6 (Langberg *et al.* 2002b). The effect of specific growth factors or serum components in combination with mechanical loading on procollagen synthesis and PCP gene regulation indicate a synergy between signaling pathways in regards to procollagen gene expression and processing, similar to what has been documented in cardiac fibroblasts (Butt & Bishop 1997). Currently, it is not completely understood how the growth factors regulate collagen synthesis and interact with the mechanotransduction *in vivo* during and after exercise as well as with loading of the tendon and the intramuscular connective tissue.

Clinical relevance and significance

The very dynamic changes in blood flow and metabolism with acute exercise, and the adaptability of tendon tissue to physical training in human tissue, have recently been shown with the use of techniques that allow both a close description of normal adaptation as well as detailing events occuring with overloading. It has been shown that connective tissue such as tendon not only responds to exercise by small "mechanical ruptures" but undergo dynamic proteolysis and protein synthesis in the period following training as a part of the normal physiologic response. This is relevant for sports activities in several ways. First, it may show us what kind of training is best suited for strengthening tendons and provide information on the relevant recovery time between training bouts. Second, it may teach us to identify the border between healthy training adaptation and unhealthy overloading and subsequent injury. This may lead to the identification of biomarkers for overuse injury. Third, the tools we have now may help us to identify which individuals can resist high amounts of training and those who should be more careful. Finally, the current findings may help us to understand how to optimize recovery after overuse injury, and how training and pharmacologic treatment should be combined in order to return the athlete to regular training.

Future directions

Tendons display increased blood flow and metabolic activity with exercise. These pathways are likely to involve an interplay with growth factors and cytoskeletal tissue damage, as well as inflammatory and vasoactive/angiogenetic substances released locally. The fact that prostanoid synthesis and release of prostacyclin and prostaglandin is involved in physiologic control of tendon blood flow increase with exercise raises the question whether it is advantageous or detrimental to use anti-inflammatory pharmalogic treatment or other attempts to reduce tendon flow in the case of overuse injury. Are we actually interrupting a

mechanism that is required for optimal adaptation of the tissue? However, it is still puzzling why the subjective feeling of tendon pain in association with overuse injury is only a weak marker of what in fact goes on in the tissue. Both equine and human experiments seem to show that overuse of tendons can be associated with site-specific degenerative and pathologic changes in the core of the tendon, a localization that is poor in afferent nerves and nociceptive substances. With advancements both within *in vitro* and *in vivo* methodologies, tools are now available to study tissue adaptation and its function in relation to varying degrees of physical activity in detail, and several explanations are to be expected within a short period. The traditional pragmatic view that overuse injury of tendons should be treated with rest and that they are always signs of small partial ruptures of tendon is now outdated. Rather, efforts should be made to take advantage of methodologic capacities of several fields of science and incorporate these with applied and clinical sports medicine to bridge the gap between clinical presentation of tendon injury and to provide treatment in an evidence-based way.

Acknowledgements

Grant support from the Danish Medical Research Foundation, Danish Ministry of Culture Foundation for Exercise Research, Copenhagen University Hospital (HS) Foundation, NOVO Nordisk Foundation, and Michaelsen Foundation is greatly acknowledged.

References

Ackermann, W.P., Spetea, M., Nylander, I., Ploj, K., Ahmed, M. & Kreicsberg, A. (2001) An opioid system in connective tissue: A study of Achilles tendon in the rat. *Journal of Histochemistry and Cytochemistry* **49**, 1387–1396.

Alfredson, H., Thorsen, K. & Lorentzon, R. (1999) *In situ* microdialysis in tendon tissue: High levels of glutamate but not prostaglandin E₂ in chronic Achilles tendon pain. *Knee Surgery, Sports Traumatology, Arthroscopy* **7**, 378–381.

Almekinders, L., Banes, A.J. & Ballenger, C.A. (1993) Effects of repetitive motion

on human fibroblasts. *Medicine and Science in Sports and Exercise* **25**, 603–607.

Babraj, J.A., Cuthbertson, D.J., Smith, K., et al. (2005) Collagen synthesis in human musculoskeletal tissues and skin. *American Journal of Physiology* **243**, 80–87.

Bakman, C.L., Friden, J. and Widmark, A. (1991) Blood flow in chronic Achilles tendinosis. Radioactive microsphere study in rats. *Acta Orthopaedica Scandinavica* **62**, 386–387.

Banes, A.J., Tsuzaki, M., Hu, P., et al. (1995) PDGF-BB, IGF-1, and mechanical load stimulate DNA synthesis in avian

tendon fibroblast *in vitro*. *Journal of Biomechanics* **28**, 1505–1513.

Birch, H.L., McLaughlin, L., Smith, R.K. & Goodship, A.E. (1999) Treadmill exercise-induced tendon hypertrophy: Assessment of tendons with different mechanical functions. *Equine Veterinary Journal* **30**, 222–226.

Boushel, R., Langberg, H., Green, S., Skovgaard, D., Bülow, J. & Kjær, M. (1999) Blood flow and oxygenation in peritendinous tissue and calf muscle during dynamic exercise. *Journal of Physiology* **524**, 305–313.

Boushel, R., Langberg, H., Olesen, J., et al. (2000) Regional blood flow during exercise in humans measured by near-infrared spectroscopy and indocyanine green. Journal of Applied Physiology 89, 1868–1876.

Boushel, R., Langberg, H., Olesen, J., Gonzales-Alonso, J., Bülow, J. & Kjær, M. (2001) Monitoring tissue oxygen availability with near infrared spectroscopy (NIRS) in health and disease. Scandinavian Journal of Medicine and Science in Sports 11, 213–222.

Boushel, R., Langberg, H., Gemmer, C., et al. (2002) Combined blockade of nitric oxide and prostaglandins reduces human skeletal muscle blood flow during exercise. Journal of Physiology 543, 691–698.

Brahm, H., Piehl-Aulin, K. & Ljunghall, S. (1996) Biochemical markers of bone metabolism during distance running in healthy regularly exercising men and women. Scandinavian Journal of Medicine and Science in Sports 6, 26–30.

Butt, R.P. & Bishop, J.E. (1997) Mechanical load enhances the stimulatory effect of serum growth factors on cardiac fibroblast procollagen synthesis. Journal of Molecular and Cellular Cardiology 29, 1141–1151.

Han, X.Y., Wang, W., Komulainen, J., et al. (1999) Increased mRNAs for procollagens and key regulating enzymes in rat skeletal muscle following downhill running. Pflügers Archives 437, 857–864.

Hansen, P., Aaagaard, P., Kjær, M., Larsson, B. & Magnusson, SP. (2003) Effect of habitual Achilles tendon load-deformation properties and cross sectional area. Journal of Applied Physiology 95, 2375–2380.

Heinemeier, K., Langberg, H., Olesen, J.L. & Kjær, M. (2003) Role of transforming growth factor beta-1 in relation to exercise-induced type I collagen synthesis in human tendinous tissue. Journal of Applied Physiology 95, 2390–2397.

Kalliokoski, K.K., Langberg, H., Ryberg, A.K., et al. (2005) The effect of dynamic knee-extension exercise on patellar tendon and quadriceps femoris muscle glucose uptake in humans studied by positron emission tomography. Journal of Applied Physiology 99, 1189–1192.

Karamouzis, M., Langberg, H., Skovgaard, D., Bülow, J., Kjær, M. & Saltin, B. (2001) In situ microdialysis of intramuscular prostaglandin and thromboxane in contracting skeletal muscle in humans. Acta Physiology Scandinavica 171, 71–76.

Kjær, M. (2004) Conversion of mechanical loading into functional adaptation of tendon and skeletal muscle: a role for extracellular matrix. Physiolical Review 84, 649–698.

Koskinen, S.O.A., Kjær, M., Mohr, T., Biering Sørensen, F., Suuronen, T. & Takala, T.E.S. (2000) Type IV collagen and its degradation in paralyzed human muscle: effect of functional electrical stimulation. Muscle and Nerve 23, 580–589.

Koskinen, S.O.A., Wang, W., Ahtikoski, A.M., et al. (2001) Turnover of basement membrane type IV collagen in exercise-induced skeletal muscle injury. American Journal of Physiology 280, R1292–R1300.

Koskinen, S.O.A., Heinemeier, K.M., Olesen, J.L., Langberg, H., & Kjær, M. (2004) Physical exercise can influence local levels of matrix metalloproteinases and their inhibitors in tendon related connective tissue. Journal of Applied Physiology 96, 861–864.

Kovanen, V. (1989) Effects of ageing and physical training on rat skeletal muscle. Doctoral thesis. Acta Physiologica Scandinavica 135 (Suppl. 577), 1–56.

Langberg, H., Bülow, J. & Kjær, M. (1998) Blood flow in the peritendinous space of the human Achilles tendon during exercise. Acta Physiologica Scandinavica 163, 149–153.

Langberg, H., Bülow, J. & Kjær, M. (1999a) Standardized intermittent static exercise increases peritendinous blood flow in human leg. Clinical Physiology 19, 89–93.

Langberg, H., Skovgaard, D., Karamouzis, M., Bülow, J. & Kjær, M. (1999b) Metabolism and inflammatory mediators in the peritendinous space measured by microdialysis during intermittent isometric exercise in humans. Journal of Physiology 515, 919–927.

Langberg, H., Skovgaard, D., Petersen, L.J., Bülow, J. & Kjær, M. (1999c) Type-1 collagen turnover in peritendinous connective tissue after exercise determined by microdialysis. Journal of Physiology 521, 299–306.

Langberg, H., Skovgaard, D., Bülow, J. & Kjær, M. (1999d) Negative interstitial pressure in the peritendinous region during exercise. Journal of Applied Physiology 87, 999–1002.

Langberg, H., Skovgaard, D., Asp, S. & Kjær, M. (2000) Time pattern of exercise-induced changes in type-I collagen turnover after prolonged endurance exercise in humans. Calcified Tissue International 67, 41–44.

Langberg, H., Rosendal, L. & Kjær, M. (2001) Training induced changes in peritendinous type I collagen turnover determined by microdialysis in humans. Journal of Physiology 534, 397–402.

Langberg, H., Olesen, J., Bülow, J. & Kjær, M. (2002a) Metabolism in and around the Achilles tendon measured by microdialysis in pigs. Acta Physiologica Scandinavica 174, 377–380.

Langberg, H., Olesen, J.L., Gemmer, C. & Kjær, M. (2002b) Substantial elevation of interleukin-6 concentration in peritendinous tissue, but not in muscle, following prolonged exercise in humans. Journal of Physiology 542, 985–990.

Langberg, H., Bjørn, C., Boushel, R., Hellsten, Y. & Kjær, M. (2002c) Exercise-induced increase in interstitial bradykinin and adenosine concentrations in skeletal muscle and peritendinous tissue in humans. Journal of Physiology 542, 977–983.

Langberg, H., Boushel, R., Risum, N. & Kjær, M. (2003) Cyclooxygenase 2 mediated regulation of exercise induced blood flow increase in human tendon tissue. Journal of Physiology 551, 683–689.

Laurent, G.J., McAnulty, R.J. & Gibson, J. (1985) Changes in collagen synthesis and degradation during skeletal muscle growth. American Journal of Physiology 249, C352–C355.

Magnusson, S.P., Aagaard, P., Rosager, S., Dyhre-Poulsen, P. & Kjær, M. (2001) Load-displacement properties of the human triceps surae aponeurosis in vivo. Journal of Physiology 531, 277–287.

Magnusson, S.P., Hansen, P., Aagaard, P., et al. (2003a) Differential strain pattern of the human triceps surae aponeurosis and free tendon. Acta Physiologica Scandinavica 177, 185–195.

Magnusson, S.P., Beyer, N., Abrahamsen, H., Aagaard, P., Neergaard, K. & Kjær, M. (2003b) Increased cross-sectional area and reduced tensile stress of the achilles tendon in elderly compared with young women. Journal of Gerontology 58, 123–127.

Marsolais, D., Cote, C.H. & Frenette, J. (2003) Nonsteroidal anti-inflammatory drug reduces neutrophil and macrophage accumulation but does not improve tendon regeneration. Laboratory Investigation 83, 991–999.

Miller, B.F., Olesen, J.L., Hansen, M., *et al.* (2005) Coordinated collagen and muscle protein synthesis in human patella tendon and quadriceps muscle after exercise. *Journal of Physiology* **567**, 1021–1033.

Petersen, W., Bobka, T., Stein, V. & Tillman, B. (2000) Blood supply of the peroneal tendons: injection and immunohistochemical studies of cadaver tendons. *Acta Orthopaedica Scandinavica* **71**, 168–174.

Rosager, S., Aagaard, P., Dyhre-Poulsen, P., Neergaard, K., Kjær, M. & Magnusson, S.P. (2002) Load-displacement properties of the human triceps surae aponeurosis and tendon in runners and non-runners. *Scandinavian Journal of Medicine and Science in Sports* **12**, 90–98.

Rosen, P., Eckel, J. & Reinauer, H. (1983) Influence of bradykinin on glucose uptake and metabolism studied in isolated cardic myocytes and isolated perfused heart. *Zeitchrift für Physiologische Chemie* **364**, 1431–1438.

Sommer, H.M. (1987) The biomechanical and metabolic effects of a running regimen on the Achilles tendon in the rat. *International Orthopaedics* **11**, 71–75.

Woo, S.L-Y., Gomez, M.A., Woo, Y.K. & Akeson, W.M. (1982) Mechanical properties of tendon and ligaments. The relationship of immobilization and exercise on tissue remodeling. *Biorheology* **19**, 397–408.

Chapter 6

Human Tendon Overuse Pathology: Histopathologic and Biochemical Findings

ALEXANDER SCOTT, KARIM M. KHAN, JILL L. COOK, AND VINCENT DURONIO

Overuse disorders remain one of the biggest challenges for sports medicine practitioners. This chapter provides a contemporary description of the major features of tendinopathies. Biopsies obtained in patients with chronic tendinopathy reveal no significant inflammation at the cellular or biochemical levels in the tendon proper. The major findings in tendon are an increase in ground substance and neovascularization, collagen disruption and disarray, increased matrix remodeling, and key tenocyte abnormalities that include altered phenotype as well as distinct areas of proliferation, death, and metaplasia. Taken together, these changes are not entirely consistent with a "failed healing response" model. The mechanisms of pain in tendinosis have yet to be established and may variously involve nociceptors in the paratenon, the tendon, and the tendon insertion, depending on the location of pathology. A major unanswered question is whether there are site-specific processes that lead to tendon pathology at various anatomic locations. It is hoped that the description of tendinosis presented here will improve clinicians' understanding of the nature of this pathology, provide them with the ability to give better explanations of the pathology underlying tendinipathy to their patients, and to set reasonable expectations about the time to recovery.

Introduction

Understanding of pathology provides a solid foundation for evidence-based prevention and treatment. In recent years, increasing recognition of the recalcitrant nature of overuse tendinopathies has led to an upsurge of research into all aspects of tendon, including pathologic investigations. The number of papers retrieved in PubMed with the search items "tendon" and "pathology" more than doubled between 1992 and 2002.

Human tendon pathology can be studied in various ways (Riley 2004). It can be defined according to its macroscopic features (gross pathology), or its microscopic features using the light and electron microscope (histopathology). More recently, human tendon pathology has also been examined using molecular biology techniques. The advent of DNA arrays and reverse transcriptase polymerase chain reaction (RT-PCR) means that gene expression can be measured in normal and pathologic tendons (Ireland *et al.* 2001; Alfredson *et al.* 2003a). The extent of tendon pathology can also be described or quantified according to functional outcomes or by mechanical testing (Sano *et al.* 1998).

This contemporary review of overuse tendon pathology demonstrates that the common chronic overuse pathology is tendinosis, not tendonitis. Tendinosis involves altered expression of matrix proteins, growth factors, and cytokines, pointing to a pathologic process involving the resident tenocytes, endothelium, perivascular cells, and neurons (Maffulli *et al.* 1998, 2003; Khan *et al.* 2002). Type I and III collagen synthesis is increased concomitantly with altered matrix metalloprotease (MMP) activity, leading to a pathologic state of remodeling that fails to restore normal tendon architecture and function (Maffulli *et al.* 2000; Ireland *et al.* 2001; Fu *et al.* 2002a, b; Riley *et al.* 2002; Tillander *et al.* 2002; Alfredson *et al.* 2003b). Glycosaminoglycans accumulate among collagen fibers or form frank regions of fibrocartilagenous metaplasia which develop as a response to compressive loading at the site of the lesion, or to a deregulation of cell phenotype, or both (Riley *et al.* 1994b; Tucci *et al.* 1997; Almekinders *et al.* 2003). Persistent neovessels (with accompanying sensory nerve fibers) are also a feature of the chronic stage of scar tissue remodeling in humans, and may be associated with the development of chronic symptoms (Cook *et al.* 2000; Khan & Cook 2000; Alfredson *et al.* 2003b). Many neovessels display intimal hyperplasia and narrowing of the lumen, and so although blood flow is increased overall, ischemia may still predominate at the site of the lesion (Kvist *et al.* 1988; Jósza & Kannus 1997; Pufe *et al.* 2001). Perhaps as a result of ischemia and ongoing mechanical loading, abnormally high local expression of cytokines (vascular endothelial growth factor, VEGF and transforming growth factor β, TGF-β) are seen, leading to modulation of proliferation and apoptosis among fibroblasts, and vascular cells (Pierce *et al.* 1991; Vogel & Hernandez 1992; Banes *et al.* 1995; Fenwick *et al.* 2001; Premdas *et al.* 2001; Pufe *et al.* 2001; Rolf *et al.* 2001; Sakai *et al.* 2001). Taken together, the changes result in a swollen, painful tendon in a chronic, degenerative state.

We hope that this summary of chronic tendon overuse pathology will: (i) highlight the necessity to avoid simplistic anti-inflammatory explanations and treatments when setting treatment goals with patients; and (ii) stimulate further debate and research into the efficacy and mechanism of action of current and emerging treatment options.

Methods

This chapter provides a detailed description of human tendon overuse pathology from a range of perspectives—macroscopic, microscopic, molecular, and functional. Before painting this contemporary picture of tendon pathology, we briefly describe normal tendon from the same perspectives for comparison.

Results—what do we know?

Normal tendon

Tendons are load-bearing structures that transmit the forces generated by muscle to their bony insertion, thereby making joint movement possible (Jósza & Kannus 1997). The basic elements of tendon are cells, collagen bundles, and ground substance, a viscous substance rich in proteoglycans and hyaluronan. Together, the collagen and ground substance comprise the extracellular matrix. Collagen is arranged in hierarchical levels of increasing complexity beginning with tropocollagen, a triple-helix polypeptide chain, which unites into fibrils, fibers (primary bundles), fascicles (secondary bundles), tertiary bundles, and finally the tendon itself (O'Brien 1997). Mature collagen and its associated proteoglycans provide tendon with its tensile strength and shield the intratendinous cells from injury.

MACROSCOPIC ANATOMY

The tendon is covered by the epitenon, a loose, fibrous sheath containing the vascular, lymphatic, and nerve supply. More superficially, the epitenon is surrounded by paratenon, a loose, fibrous, fatty tissue with an inner synovial lining. Together, the paratenon and epitenon are sometimes called the peritendon. The peritendon is continuous with the endotendon which houses the nerves and vessels, and divides the tendon proper into fascicles. A two-layered synovial sheath surrounds some tendons as they pass areas of increased friction. The outer layer is the fibrotic (ligamentous) sheath and the inner layer is the synovial sheath, consisting of thin visceral and parietal sheets. These tendon coverings can be affected by the pathology of paratenonitis, which is discussed in a subsequent section (see below).

The myotendinous and osseotendinous junctions are highly specialized regions where the tension generated by muscle fibers is transmitted to the tendon and bone, respectively. These regions are best explored using the transmission electron microscope and are discussed further below.

LIGHT MICROSCOPIC APPEARANCE

Under the light microscope, normal human tendon consists of dense, clearly defined, parallel, and slightly wavy collagen bundles. Collagen has a characteristic reflective appearance under polarized light known as birefringence. Between the collagen bundles are fibroblasts (tenocytes) with spindle-shaped nuclei and sparse cytoplasm. Tenocytes synthesize the ground substance and procollagen building blocks of the tendon matrix. Some authors also comment on the presence of tenoblasts—more rounded cells which sit atop collagen fibrils, are sparsely distributed throughout the matrix, are more abundant around vessels, and proliferate at sites of local remodeling. A network of capillaries runs parallel to the collagen fibers in the tendon (Jósza & Kannus 1997).

Ground substance (glycosaminoglycans or GAGs) can be stained for routine light microscopic evaluation. In normal tendon, GAGs provide structural support for the collagen fibers and also regulate the extracellular assembly of procollagen into mature collagen. Some GAGs are incorporated into collagen fibrils during the early, lateral assembly of fibrils (Canty & Kadler 2002). Other GAGS are interfibrillar, maintaining a hydrated viscoelastic structure, and allow sliding of fibers and fascicles relative to one another (lubrication). At the light microscopic level, using Alcian blue stain, normal ground substance is usually undetectable, although in some tendons seams of GAGs are visible between collagen bundles (Fallon et al. 2002). For example, histologic analysis of the rotator cuff tendon shows layers of loosely organized Alcian blue-stained material (GAGs) running between the longitudinal collagen fiber bundles, which may be necessary to allow transmission of inhomogeneous strains during glenohumeral stabilization (Berenson et al. 1996; Fallon et al. 2002).

NORMAL ULTRASTRUCTURAL APPEARANCE

Normal human tendon, when examined under the electron microscope (EM), displays prominent cross-striations of fibrils which are caused by the overlapping of laterally adjacent superhelices. The periodicity of the striations measures approximately 55 nm in longitudinal section (Evans et al. 1998) and arises as a result of the quarter-overlapped lateral packing of collagen fibrils.

Despite the apparently simple appearance of tendon on light microscopy, EM reveals that the three-dimensional ultrastructure of human tendons is complex (Józsa et al. 1991). EM demonstrates that the collagen fibrils are highly organized, not only longitudinally but also transversely and horizontally; the longitudinal fibrils run not only parallel, but also cross each other to form spirals (plaits) which may uncoil and recoil during loading and unloading. In transverse sections, the longitudinal fibrils vary in diameter from 50 to 300 nm, generally have a smooth profile, and appear homogenous in content (Evans et al. 1998). In longitudinal views, some GAGs appear randomly oriented whereas others are associated with collagen fibrils in a regular period corresponding to the banding pattern of collagen, indicating a highly ordered interaction between GAGs and collagen in the normal state (Scott 1996).

The ultrastructure of epitenon, peritendon, and endotendon reveals a woven network of longitudinal, oblique, and transverse collagen fibrils. This arrangement appears to serve as an effective buffer to resist longitudinal, transverse, horizontal, and also rotational forces during movement and activity (Enna & Dyer 1976).

When the myotendinous and osseotendinous junctions are viewed using EM, the structures hinted at by the light microscopic evidence can be better examined. At the myotendinous junction, the surface of the muscle cells form processes and have a highly indented sarcolemma into which the densely bundled actin filaments of the terminal sarcomeres insert. A network of collagen fibers that extend from tendon fills the recesses between the muscle cell's branching processes and joins with the basement membrane. At the osseotendinous junction, EM examination reveals densely packed, randomly oriented collagen fibers of various diameters which are continuous with those of the unmineralized and mineralized fibrocartilage. Fibrils insert between adjacent lamellae of cortical bone (Clark & Stechschulte 1998). Scanning electron microscopy

(SEM) and polarized light microscopy (PLM) show that, unlike tendon fibers elsewhere, those in the calcified fibrocartilage are not crimped. The tendon fibrils interdigitate among the separate bone lamellar systems (osteons), but do not merge with the collagen systems of the individual lamellae. The segment of calcified tendon that interdigitates with bone is less cellular than the more proximal zone of calcified fibrocartilage (Clark & Stechschulte 1998).

With respect to the ultrastructure of organelles, it appears that normal tenocytes contain sparse polyribosomes and rough endoplasmic reticulum, a Golgi complex, and secretory vesicles that serve to synthesize and transport matrix molecules to the cell surface. Tendon sheaths, when present at sites of increased friction, are populated by synoviocytes identical to those of synovial joint linings. These are characterized by numerous subplasmalemmal, pinocytic, and secretory vesicles (Schmidt & Mackay 1982). Macrophages with abundant lysosomes are occasionally seen. Adipocytes and granulecontaining mast cells are normally encountered only in the loose connective tissue (endotendon, peritendon) rather than the tendon proper.

NORMAL TENDON BIOCHEMISTRY: HUMAN DATA

There is an increasing recognition that tendon remodeling may have important roles in both healthy and pathologic tendon. Biochemist David Eyre is renowned for discovering the collagen cross-links now increasingly used in bone metabolism research (Eyre 1997). His earliest studies of cross-links were in tendon (Eyre et al. 1984). Hydroxypryridinium cross-links increase as tendon ages, and can be used to estimate turnover rates. The limiting factor at present is that cross-links are plentiful in all forms of cartilage, bone, dentin, ligament, tendon, fascia, intervertebral disc, lung, gut, cervix, aorta, and vitreous humor. Thus, changes in serum or urine levels of biomarkers are not specific for tendon.

The cross-links within and between mature collagen molecules provide mechanical stiffness. They also provide resistance to breakdown by proteases; this resistance contributes to the remarkably long half-life of collagen in tendon (greater than 100 days)

(Sell 1995). The patellar tendon has a significantly higher content of dihydroxylysinonorleucine than other tendons, suggesting that there are tendon-specific differences in cross-links (Fujii et al. 1994). In fact, when various biochemical factors are assessed, the patellar tendon collagen more closely resembles the collagen from the anterior cruciate ligament than that of periarticular tendons. This is of interest given that the patellar tendon is one of the commonly used graft tissues for ACL reconstruction. The functional role of these different specific cross-links, however, remains unclear and provides fruitful material for future investigations.

Whereas cross-linked collagen provides tensile strength and stiffness, ground substance is recognized as a vital, responsive gel that contributes to the viscoelastic properties of tendon and the lubrication and spacing that is essential for interfibrillar gliding and cross-tissue interactions. It also provides a medium for the diffusion of dissolved nutrients and gases. Although the proteoglycans and GAGs make up less than 1% of the dry weight of tendon, they contribute greatly to the volume and viscoelasticity of the tissue by maintaining water within the tissues. The water molecules are entrapped by the negatively charged GAGs with their preponderance of hydrophilic hydroxyl groups.

GAGs are linear polysaccharides that, with the exception of hyaluronic acid, are covalently bound to a protein core, forming a proteoglycan. The main GAGs of tendon are dermatan sulfate, chondroitin sulfate, keratin sulfate, and heparin sulfate. The proteoglycans in tendon include small (decorin, biglycan, lumican) and large (versican, aggrecan) molecules. Decorin, the best characterized, is so named because it appears to "decorate" the outside of fibrils. This dermatan sulfate-rich proteoglycan with its single GAG side-chain forms "shape modules" that form interfibrillar bridges, thereby maintaining the normal registry and alignment of tendon (Scott et al. 1998; Koob & Summers 2002). In human tendons, the major chondroitin sulfate proteoglycans appear to be versican and aggrecan (Waggett et al. 1998). Aggrecan is also linked to keratan sulfate and hyaluronan, and is present in both tensional and compressed regions of tendon, but is more abundant in compressed regions (Rees et al. 2000).

Versican is predominantly located in the perivascular matrix, as well as in the pericellular matrix around tenocyte arrays where it buffers the loads transmitted from the fibrillar matrix (Ritty *et al.* 2003). There is a rapid turnover of the small proteoglycan biglycan, indicating the existence of molecular pathways that, if deregulated, could compromise the integrity of the matrix and potentially contribute to tendon dysfunction.

The importance of GAGs in interfibrillar sliding is supported by studies of whole tendon. Synchrotron X-ray scattering, a novel method of examining tendon tissue (Puxkandl *et al.* 2002), allows simultaneous measurement of the elongation of fibrils inside the tendon and of tendon as a whole. In normal tendon, overall strain is greater than the strain in the individual fibrils, which demonstrates that some deformation occurs in the matrix between fibrils. Moreover, the ratio of fibril strain to tendon strain depends on the applied strain rate. When the speed of deformation is increased, this ratio increases. Thus, the mechanical behavior of whole tendon is consistent with a hierarchical model, where fibrils and interfibrillar matrix interact to form a coupled viscoelastic system.

TENDON IS NOT A "UNIFORM" STRUCTURE

Tendons are not all identical but vary in their anatomy, physiology, and thus, not surprisingly, their biochemistry. Tendons in compressed regions tend to express proteoglycans more typical of fibrocartilage (Waggett *et al.* 1998). The sulfated GAG content of the normal cadaver supraspinatus tendon is 3–10 times greater than in the common biceps tendon (Riley *et al.* 1994a). The major GAG of the supraspinatus is chondroitin sulfate with a smaller proportion of dermatan sulfate. In contrast, the common biceps tendon contains predominantly dermatan sulfate with less chondroitin sulfate (Riley *et al.* 1994a). The increased amount of GAG in the supraspinatus may serve to resist compression and to separate and lubricate collagen bundles as they move relative to each other (shear) during normal shoulder motion (Berenson *et al.* 1996).

In addition to the variation among different tendons, there are striking differences in the composition of tendons along their length. In the Achilles tendon and its insertion, type I, III, V, and VI collagens, decorin, biglycan, fibromodulin, and lumican have been reported in both the mid-tendon and the fibrocartilage, although their relative expression differed with site. The expression patterns of versican and aggrecan were complementary; versican mRNA was present in the mid-tendon and absent from the fibrocartilage, while aggrecan mRNA was present in the fibrocartilage and absent from the mid-tendon (Waggett *et al.* 1998). The range and distribution of ECM molecules detected in the Achilles tendon probably reflect the differing forces that act upon its various regions. The mid-tendon largely transmits tension and is characterized by molecules typical of fibrous tissues, whereas fibrocartilage must resist compression as well as tension and thus also contain molecules typical of cartilage.

Human tendon pathology—macroscopic and microscopic

There have been many advances in the description of overuse human tendon pathology in recent years. Thus, we review the macroscopic pathology, summarize histologic and immunohistologic changes, and describe insights from biochemistry and molecular biology into cell–matrix abnormalities of tendon that has suffered overuse injury.

MACROSCOPIC OVERUSE TENDINOPATHY—TENDINOSIS

Macroscopically, painful tendon affected by overuse (e.g. Achilles, patellar, lateral elbow, rotator cuff tendinopathy) loses its normal glistening white appearance and becomes gray or brown. It is hard to the feel and grates when the surgeon's scalpel cuts through it.

A second gross feature of tendinosis is a general proliferation of capillaries and arterioles. Alfredson and Öhberg suggested that this abnormal tendon vascularity (neovascularization, seen on color Doppler) is associated with tendon pain (Öhberg *et al.* 2001; Öhberg & Alfredson 2002).

A novel approach to evaluating tendon vasculature in tendinosis is called orthogonal polarization spectral imaging. This method has been applied to the rotator cuff tendon during arthroscopy of the shoulder. Biberthaler *et al.* (2003) visualized and quantified, *in vivo*, the microcirculation of the painful rotator cuff during arthroscopic surgery. They found that at the edge of the lesion, the functional capillary density was significantly reduced whereas the diameter of the vessels that were present did not differ. This finding was confirmed by histology (Biberthaler *et al.* 2003). This provides impetus for further research that aims to clarify the role of tendon vascularity in pathogenesis and pain production via accompanying nerve fibers. The relationship between pain and vascularity is discussed further Chapter 12.

LIGHT MICROSCOPIC FINDINGS IN TENDINOSIS

In tendinosis, light microscopy reveals abnormalities in collagen, in ground substance, and among tenocytes and endothelial cells (Jarvinen *et al.* 1997) (Figs 6.1 & 6.2). A characteristic feature is collagen disruption, disarray, and disorientation. Some collagen fibers appear to separate, giving the impression of loss of their parallel orientation. There is a decrease in fiber diameter, and a decrease in the overall density or packing of collagen. Collagen microtears can also occur and these may be surrounded by erythrocytes, fibrin, and fibronectin deposits. Within fascicles, there is unequal and irregular crimping, loosening and increased waviness, or complete loss of crimp structure, in contrast to the normal tight parallel bundled appearance. There is an increase in thinner, type III collagen and increased collagen solubility. These changes lead to decreased birefringence of the tendon under polarized light microscopy (Jarvinen *et al.* 1997). Special stains consistently demonstrate an increase in mucoid ground substance (GAGs) which can exist in association with vessels, with fibrocartilagenous metaplasia, or can be diffusely interspersed throughout the tendon (Figs 6.1–6.3) (Khan *et al.* 1996; Movin *et al.* 1997).

There is great variation in the cellular density and vascularity in tendinosis. In some areas, tenocytes are abnormally plentiful, have rounded nuclei giving them an ovoid or chondroid appearance, and may stain positively with nuclear proliferation

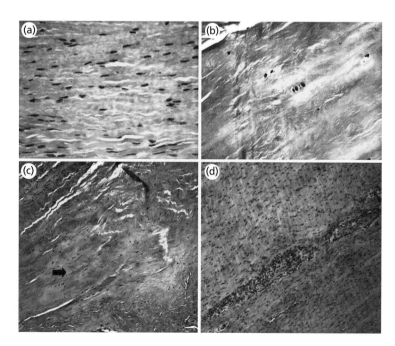

Fig. 6.1 (Hematoxylin and eosin (H&E)/Alcian blue) Early patellar tendinosis in asymptomatic athletes. (a) Increased numbers of metabolically active tenocytes. (b) Loss of cellularity, with clusters of chondroid tenocytes. (c) Increased amount of glycosaminoglycan (blue material). (d) Increased prominence of capilliaries.

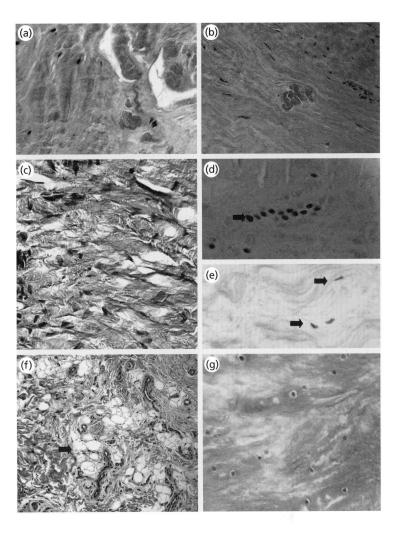

Fig. 6.2 Advanced patellar tendinosis in symptomatic athletes. (a–c; H&E) Collagen degeneration and variable tenocyte density. (d) Scattered tenocyte proliferation (arrow: Ki67) and (e) apoptosis (arrow: anti-ssDNA). (f) Fatty (arrow: H&E) and (g) cartilaginous (Alcian blue/Nuclear red) metaplasia at the patellar insertion in two different athletes.

markers (Fig. 6.2d). In contrast, other areas of the tendon may contain fewer tenocytes than normal, while those remaining occasionally demonstrate necrotic or apoptotic features (Jarvinen *et al.* 1997). A more frequent finding, however, is a simple absence of tenocytes caused presumably by an earlier episode of cell death. Regions of neovascularization are frequently observed. Rarely, there is infiltration of lymphocytes, macrophages, or neutrophils (Jarvinen *et al.* 1997).

Thus, the essence of tendinosis is apparent from its different appearance from normal tendon with respect to tendon cells, non-collagenous matrix, and collagen fibers and vasculature. (Jarvinen *et al.* 1997;

Khan *et al.* 1999) This is not a new discovery as Perugia *et al.* (1976) noted the "remarkable discrepancy between the terminology generally adopted for these conditions (which are obviously inflammatory because the ending 'itis' is used) and their histopathologic substratum."

RELATIONSHIP OF HISTOLOGIC
ABNORMALITIES AND MECHANICAL
PROPERTIES OF HUMAN TENDON

Few studies have measured the mechanical consequences of tendinosis. Sano *et al.* (1997, 1998) examined the relationship between the degrees of

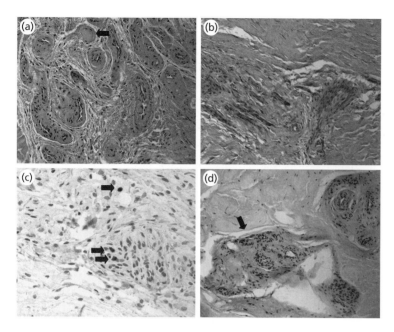

Fig. 6.3 Vascular abnormalities in symptomatic athletes. (a,b; H&E) Increased capillary density. (c) Proliferating endothelial cells (Ki67). (d) Increased glycosaminoglycans in association with vessels (Alcian blue/Nuclear red).

histologic abnormality at the supraspinatus insertion, the tensile strength, and the site of failure in cadaveric tendon (average age 62 years; range 39–83 years). Having applied a tensile load to tendon failure, he found that the histologic score of degeneration was negatively correlated with the ultimate tensile stress at the insertion. Disruptions of tendon fibers were located mostly in the articular half of the tendon and appeared to reduce the tensile strength of the tendon and thus, constitute a primary pathogenic factor promoting rotator cuff tear.

PARATENONITIS

Another type of overuse tendon pathology is paratenonitis. This term has been proposed as an umbrella term for the separate entities of peritendinitis, tenosynovitis (single layer of areolar tissue covering the tendon), and tenovaginitis (double-layer tendon sheath). A similar histologic picture may be present in the endotendon, which often becomes expanded after injury, but this is difficult to distinguish clinically. Examples include paratenonitis of the abductor pollicis longus and extensor pollicis longus (de Quervain disease), of the flexor hallucis longus as it passes the medial

malleolus of the tibia (Jósza & Kannus 1997), and (more recently recognized) of the flexor tendons at the wrist contributing to idiopathic carpal tunnel syndrome (Tsujii *et al.* 2006).

The acute histopathology of paratenonitis is edema and hyperemia of the paratenon with infiltration of inflammatory cells. After hours to a few days, fibrinous exudate fills the tendon sheath and causes the "crepitus" that can be felt on clinical examination. In chronic paratenonitis, fibroblasts proliferate in association with a perivascular lymphocytic infiltrate. Peritendinous tissue becomes macroscopically thickened and new connective tissue adhesions occur, populated by myofibroblasts (Jarvinen *et al.* 1997). Fibrocartilagenous metaplasia is sometimes seen on the visceral lining, suggesting a compressive force within the sheath (Clarke *et al.* 1998). Blood vessels proliferate, but often show narrowing of the lumen because of an expanded neointima. Marked inflammatory changes are seen in more than 20% of the arteries (Kvist & Jarvinen 1982).

ULTRASTRUCTURE CHANGES IN TENDINOSIS

EM studies of pathologic tendon have reported a wide variety of cellular and matrix abnormalities.

In some areas, abnormal tenocytes contain pronounced rough endoplasmic reticulum (RER), well-developed Golgi apparatus with cisternae dilated with electron-dense material implying increased proteoglycan and protein production, whereas in other areas tenocytes were few or absent. Necrotic and apoptotic tenocytes have both been reported (Galliani *et al.* 2002). In addition, there is also unequal and irregular crimping or loss of the normal crimping pattern, implying a loss of the normal stress–strain properties of tendon.

Józsa & Kannus (1997) have described: (i) hypoxic degeneration; (ii) hyaline degeneration; (iii) mucoid or myxoid degeneration; (iv) fibrinoid degeneration; (v) lipoid degeneration; (vi) calcification; and (vii) fibrocartilaginous and bony metaplasia. Although nomenclature is not systematized and there may be some overlap between Józsa & Kannus's descriptions and the historic pathologic labels, it may be that different pathologies can coexist and may depend on the anatomic site and the nature of the insult that caused them (e.g. hypoxia versus mechanical loading, acute versus chronic injury). Thus, tendinosis may be the end result of a number of etiologic processes.

Evidence of abnormal tendon cells in tendinopathy came in an elegant study of patients with tennis elbow where the common extensor tendon showed a pronounced reactive change consisting of mesenchymal cell proliferation along with aggregates of newly formed vascular channels, underscoring the importance of neovascularization in tendon overuse injury. The origins of differentiating endothelial cells, mesenchymal cells, and tenocytes remain controversial (Sarkar & Uhthoff 1980).

TENDINOSIS—INSIGHTS FROM MOLECULAR BIOLOGY

The abovementioned histologic findings indicate that tendinosis does not simply result from mechanical fatigue of collagen. The abundance of GAGs, neurovascular ingrowth, and tenocyte morphology suggest several distinct pathologic processes.

Contemporary molecular biology techniques provide an exciting, comprehensive picture of tendinosis. Although many questions remain, we can now propose a general model where tendon cells are continuously remodeling and responding to their extracellular milieu and matrix in an ongoing feedback loop. This cell–matrix feedback loop could conceivably go awry at several key points, leading to cell transformation, accumulation or breakdown of particular matrix components, and altered tendon function (Table 6.1). Some important areas for future research are now beginning to be defined.

A central question in the molecular biology of tendon is to identify the chain of events leading to pain in tendinosis (Khan *et al.* 2000). Fu *et al.* (2002b) reported an increased basal expression of cyclo-oxygenase 2 in tendinosis biopsies, as well as an increase in the production, *in vitro*, of prostaglandin E_2 (PGE_2) by tendinosis cultures. In contrast, Alfredson *et al.* (2000), using *in vivo* microdialysis, failed to find an elevation of PGE_2 in patients with Achilles tendinosis and lateral elbow tendinopathy. While the first group of researchers concluded that PGE_2 may have a role in the chronic phase of tendinosis, the second concluded the opposite. In attempting to resolve this discrepancy, it should be noted that the increase in PGE_2 production by cultured tendinosis cells was rather small (less than 50%) and this may be undetectable *in vivo*. In contrast to Fu *et al.* (2002b), Graham Riley's laboratory has reported that cultured Achilles tendinosis specimens did not generate any substantial baseline PGE_2 (Corps *et al.* 2003). PGE_2 production was strongly induced by interleukin-1(IL-1), however, which is reported to be present in surrounding peritendinous tissues but absent from the tendon itself in the chronic stages (Table 6.1). Thus, the role of inflammatory mediators, if any, in tendon and peritendon pain remains unclear.

In support of the hypothesis that PGE_2 does not offer a complete explanation of tendinosis pain, Alfredson *et al.* (2000, 2002) reported increased lactate (twofold greater than controls) and glutamate in the tendinosis lesion. Both of these substances have been associated with nociception. In addition, substance P-containing neural ingrowth was identified. It seems likely that there may be different molecular mechanisms of pain at different points in the development of tendinosis.

The finding of increased lactate by *in vivo*

Table 6.1 Molecular findings in chronic, non-ruptured tendinopathies.

Molecule	Likely significance of change	Reference
Tendon		
↑ Collagen I mRNA	Healing/remodeling response	(Ireland *et al.* 2001; Corps *et al.* 2004)
↑ MMP-2 mRNA	↑ Matrix breakdown	(Ireland *et al.* 2001; Alfredson *et al.* 2003a)
↑ MMP-1, ↓ TIMP-1	↑ Matrix breakdown	(Fu *et al.* 2002b)
↑ Collagen III	↑ Presence of smaller fibrils	(Jarvinen *et al.* 1997)
	↓ fibril strength	
↑ Fibronectin mRNA	Altered cell–matrix interaction	(Alfredson *et al.* 2003a)
↑ GAG, ↑ chondroitin sulfate	↑ Tendon swelling	(Corps *et al.* 2004)
↓ MMP-3 mRNA	GAG accumulation	(Ireland *et al.* 2001)
↓ Dermatan sulfate, ↓ decorin mRNA	Abnormal fibril size regulation	(Benazzo *et al.* 1996)
		(Alfredson *et al.* 2003a)
↑ Lactate	↑ Anaerobic metabolism	(Alfredson *et al.* 2001; Alfredson *et al.* 2002)
↑ COX-2	↑ Collagen synthesis vasodilation	(Fu *et al.* 2002b)
↑ TGF-β	↑ GAG and collagen synthesis	(Fu *et al.* 2002b)
	↓ GAG degradation	
↑ VEGF-R mRNA	↑ Angiogenesis	(Alfredson *et al.* 2003a)
	↑ Permeability of vessels	
↑ PDGF-R, ↑ PCNA, NMDAR	↑ Tenocyte proliferation	(Rolf *et al.* 2001; Alfredson *et al.* 2003a)
↑ IGF-I	↑ Tenocyte survival	
	↑ Tenocyte proliferation	(Hansson *et al.* 1989)
↑ CD30	Endothelial proliferation	(Biberthaler *et al.* 2003)
↑ PGP 9.5, ↑ SP	Neural ingrowth	(Alfredson *et al.* 2001)
	Pain, vasodilation	
Tendon linings and bursae		
↑ Fibronectin, ↑ Fibronogen	Inflammation, scarring	(Kvist *et al.* 1988)
↑ SP	Pain, edema	(Gotoh *et al.* 1988)
↑ IL-1 mRNA	Inflammation, pain	(Gotoh *et al.* 2001)
↑ IL-6	Inflammation, repair	(Freeland *et al.* 2002)
↑ PGE$_2$	Pain, inflammation	(Freeland *et al.* 2002)
↑ VEGF mRNA	Neovascularization	(Yanagisawa *et al.* 2001)
↑ Tenascin-C	Altered cell–matrix interactions	(Hyvonen *et al.* 2003)

CD, cellular differentiation marker; COX, cyclo-oxygenase; GAG, glycosaminoglycan; IGF, insulin-like growth factor; IL, interleukin; MMP, matrix metalloprotease; PCNA, proliferating cell nuclear antigen; PDGF, platelet-derived growth factor; PGE$_2$, prostaglandin E$_2$; PGP, protein gene product; SP, substance P; TGF, transforming growth factor; TIMP, tissue inhibitor of MMP; VEGF, vascular endothelial growth factor.

microdialysis in the patellar, Achilles, and extensor carpi radialis brevis tendons implies the presence of anaerobic conditions in the tendinosis lesion. Clarifying the relationship between anaerobic or hypoxic conditions, pain, and the other cellular and matrix abnormalities described below requires further research. For example, Achilles tendinosis and tendon rupture are associated with increased expression of VEGF (Pufe *et al.* 2001; Alfredson *et al.* 2003a). Immunohistochemical, biochemical, molecular, and cell biology techniques showed that VEGF could be immunostained in tenocytes of ruptured and fetal Achilles tendons, but not in those of normal adults (Pufe *et al.* 2001). In microvessels, the VEGF receptor VEGFR-1 (flt-1) was also seen. High VEGF levels were measured in homogenates from ruptured adult tendons whereas levels were lower in fetal tendon and negligible in normal adult Achilles tendons. These results prove the presence of an angiogenic peptide and neovascularization in ruptured and tendinopathic tendons. Whether such observed variations in growth factor expression and neovascularization are a cause or an effect of anaerobic conditions will also need to be examined.

TGF-β and platelet-derived growth factor (PDGF) have both been implicated in patellar tendinosis, and may have a role both in the abnormal cellularity and in the altered matrix production and remodeling (Rolf *et al.* 2001; Fu *et al.* 2002a,b). Rolf *et al.* (2001) assessed cellularity with respect to cell proliferation and the expression of PDGF receptor β (PDGFRβ). Tendinosis tissue had increased cellularity ($P < 0.001$) compared with controls, and also a higher proliferative index, based on proliferating cell nuclear antigen (PCNA) staining ($P < 0.001$). The conditions that alter expression of proliferative cytokines and their receptors in tendinosis have not yet been identified. However, the mechanisms that underpin local growth factor upregulation and ongoing cellular proliferation in tendinosis need to be established.

The abnormal extracellular matrix in tendinopathies has been characterized in detail for some tendons, although the underlying cause of the alterations has not been identified. Supraspinatus tendons from patients with a chronic rotator cuff rupture have significantly increased concentrations of hyaluronan, chondroitin, and dermatan sulfate compared with "normal," cadaveric, supraspinatus tendons. The authors suggested this finding may represent an adaptation to an alteration in the types of loading (tension vs. compression vs. shear) which act on the rotator cuff tendons in the shoulder (Riley *et al.* 1994b). Conversely, pathologic factors such as low oxygen tension or the autocrine and paracrine influence of growth factors may also be important in the altered matrix following rupture.

The injured supraspinatus tendon appears to possess an intrinsic healing capability characterized by long-term upregulation of procollagen production. Riley *et al.* (1994a,b) reported that the GAG composition of tendon specimens from patients with chronic tendon rupture was consistent with that of newly synthesized matrix, even in chronically ruptured tendon from older individuals. Hamada *et al.* (1997) used *in situ* hybridization localize cells containing alpha 1 type I procollagen mRNA in chronically and more recently torn rotator cuff tendon. In biopsies from complete-thickness tears, actively synthesizing cells were significantly more abundant at the proximal tendon stumps in the specimens that were obtained less than 4 months after trauma, compared with those obtained 4 months or more after trauma. In the less substantial tears (partial thickness), the number of active cells was maintained even in long-standing tears. The labeled cells at the margins of concomitant intra-tendinous extensions of the tears were detected even in the long-standing tears.

In addition to altered collagen and proteoglycan synthesis, altered matrix remodeling is a feature of tendinosis. Riley *et al.* (2002) reported an increased expression of MMP enzymes including MMP-1, MMP-2, MMP-9, and MMP-13 in human rotator cuff pathology. Higher rates of turnover in the non-ruptured supraspinatus may be part of an adaptive response to the mechanical demands on the tendon and to an imbalance in matrix synthesis and degradation. Fu *et al.* (2002a) reported similar results when studying the expression of procollagen type I, MMP-1, and tissue inhibitor of metalloproteinase 1 (TIMP-1) by immunohistochemistry in human patellar tendinosis tissues and healthy patellar tendons. *In situ* gelatin zymography was used to detect collagenolytic activities. The production of MMP-1, TIMP-1, and collagenolytic activities was also compared in cell cultures from tendinosis samples and controls. Tendinosis tissues and cultures showed an increase in the expression level of MMP-1 and a decrease in that of TIMP-1, a condition favoring collagen degradation. However, not all results on MMP-1 have been consistent (Tillander *et al.* 2002).

The complexity of cell–matrix interactions makes the study of tendinosis challenging. In pathologic tendons, an abnormally hydrated matrix could promote altered local binding of factors. This altered binding may, in turn, modulate cytokine and growth factor activity, and thus cellular activity. It will be a challenge to untangle the chain of events leading to altered matrix and altered cellular activities characteristic of tendinosis.

The role of TGF-β has been scrutinized with respect to tendon overuse injury because it is a cytokine strongly associated with matrix remodeling. TGF-β isoforms (β1, β2, and β3) and their signaling receptors (TGF-βRI and TGF-βRII) are present at sites of blood vessels both in normal and in injured Achilles tendons (Fenwick *et al.* 2001). Pathologic tendon showed an increase in cell numbers and in the percentage of TGF-β2 expression as well as an increase in the number of cells expressing TGF-βRII. TGF-βRI was restricted to blood vessels and was absent from cells in the fibrillar matrix. The authors concluded that despite the presence and upregulation of TGF-β2, TGF-β signaling may be dependent on TGF-βRI. If this were the case, it would explain why chronic tendon lesions fail to resolve and suggests that the addition of exogenous TGF-β may have little effect on chronic tendinopathy. This important finding remains to be explored further.

Another member of the TGF-β superfamily that is implicated in tendon injury and repair is cartilage-derived morphogenetic protein-1 (CDMP-1). CDMP-1 appears to be activated in the torn rotator cuff (Nakase *et al.* 2002). The localization and expression of CDMP-1 was examined by *in situ* hybridization and immunohistochemistry. Active cells synthesizing the alpha-1 chain of collagen type I mRNA were localized predominantly in the torn edge and in the bursal side rather than in the joint side, and minimally evident in tissue that was more distant from the torn edge. CDMP-1 had a similar distribution as the alpha-1 chain of collagen type I. These data provide the first observational evidence that CDMP-1 was activated specifically at the site of the torn rotator cuff tendon.

The different cellular environment of tendon insertions, as opposed to the tendon proper, might influence the process of matrix remodeling at the tendon–bone insertion. Gotoh *et al.* (1997) examined the contribution of IL-β, cathepsin D, and MMP-1 to osteochondral destruction at the osseotendinous junction. Strong immunoreactivity was found in torn supraspinatus insertions, but not in the insertions of intact tendons. Macrophages and multinucleated giant cells showed immunoreactivity for all three mediators and were often found at the interface between the osteochondral margin of the enthesis and the granulation tissue, suggesting that they may be involved in osteochondral destruction. The authors concluded that granulation tissue may contribute to the development of rotator cuff tears by weakening the insertion. Specific studies of the osseotendinous junction are required, as many instances of tendon pathology occur specifically at these insertion points.

GENETICS

Atlas cDNA arrays (CLONTECH) have recently been used to examine tissue from four patients with Achilles tendon disorders, to identify changes in the expression of genes that regulate cell–cell and cell–matrix interactions. The greatest difference between the normal (postmortem) and tendinosis tissue samples was the downregulation of MMP-3 (stromelysin) in all the tendinosis samples. The expression levels of type I and III collagen were significantly higher in the degenerate compared to the "normal" samples (Ireland *et al.* 2001). The downregulation of MMP-3 has also been identified in a cDNA array and confirmed by real-time PCR by Alfredson *et al.* (2003a). MMP-3 is a broad-spectrum degradative enzyme which can cleave collagens and proteoglycans. Ireland *et al.* (2001) speculated that the downregulation of MMP-3 may contribute to the increased levels of GAGs that are characteristic of tendinosis.

cDNA arrays have also been used to confirm the absence of inflammatory cells and cytokines in Achilles tendinosis. There was no increase in the mRNA for typical markers of lymphocytes, monocytes, and granulocytes (CD70, CD27, and CD33) (Alfredson *et al.* 2003a). In addition, the RNAs for IL-1 and TNF-α, important cytokine mediators of inflammation, were not detected. The authors noted that surgical biopsy studies represent the end-stage of tendon pathology so there remains a need to examine tissue from earlier stages of the disease process. These authors also noted that "failed healing" (insufficient cell activity, or cell senescence) has often been proposed as an etiological factor in tendinosis, but that the finding of increased expression of genes for type I and III collagen and probably for proteoglycans and other non-collagen proteins did not support that model.

WHAT ROLE DOES APOPTOSIS HAVE IN TENDINOPATHIES?

Because areas of hypocellularity are a prominent feature in advanced tendinosis lesions, the question arises as to the cause and mode of cell death, and its overall importance in the pathologic process. There are two forms of cell death: apoptosis and necrosis. Necrosis, or "accidental" cell death, generally results from conditions where the integrity of the cell membrane is lost (e.g. direct trauma, toxins, ischemia) and is characterized by spillage of the cellular contents into the extracellular space. In contrast, apoptosis or "programmed" cell death is unleashed by dedicated enzymes (caspases) in response to various cellular stresses including DNA damage, hypoxia, oxidative stress, or loss of cell–matrix contact. Apoptotic and necrotic tenocytes are both observed in tendinosis of the elbow (Galliani *et al.* 2002) and shoulder (Tuoheti *et al.* 2005). In patellar tendinosis (Fig. 6.2d), apoptosis is not as prominent as has been reported for the other tendons (< 1% of the total cellularity), but nevertheless patients display about twice as many apoptotic cells compared to controls. Conversely, following tendon rupture, a high percentage of apoptotic fibroblast-like cells has been reported for the supraspinatus (Yuan *et al.* 2002). Remarkably, ongoing apoptosis was observed even months after rupture, particularly in older patients; because the tissue remains hypercellular, this suggests that proliferation and apoptosis were occurring simultaneously. Treatment with growth factors, anabolic levels of mechanical loading, or stem cell implantation might have the potential to prevent ongoing apoptosis and stimulate remaining cells to proliferate and align, thereby restoring and organizing the lost tendon cells.

Clinical relevance

There remains a substantial lack of understanding about the chain of events leading to tendinosis. However, armed with a detailed basic science description of the cellular and matrix abnormalities of tendinosis, clinicians are in a better position than they were previously to describe the nature of tendinosis and paratenonitis pathology to patients. Although the relationship between structural and biochemical abnormalities and pain is not yet clear, the fact that collagen remodeling takes place over months rather than days requires the time frame of recovery to be adjusted according. It is unlikely in the near future that any single pharmacotherapy

will be able to normalize the cellular and matrix abnormalities of the chronic stage of tendinosis.

Future directions

A number of important questions about the histopathologic nature of tendinosis remain outstanding. First, what is the time course of tendinosis (including the first steps in the tendinosis cascade) and the relationship between observed features such as cell death and proliferation, matrix damage, remodeling and metaplasia, neurovascular ingrowth and symptoms? This will require a combination of cell biology tools and animal models of tendinopathy, with particular attention to early time points.

Second, better attempts to draw associations between tendinosis in humans and experimental models are needed. Even basic questions such as the origin of hypercellularity in patellar or Achilles tendinosis remain essentially unexamined in both animal and human tendon. A comprehensive model of the tendinosis cascade with proposed triggers needs to be developed, as has been carried out for osteoarthritis, to allow us to identify and prevent the most upstream point in the process, to synthesize findings on various aspects of the pathology, and to draw correspondences with symptoms on the one hand and mechanistic laboratory studies on the other.

Third, we need to further explore the relationship between histopathology and clinically meaningful outcomes. There is an emerging relationship between the presence of nerves and vessels, and chronic pain, as detailed above. However, to answer the question which athletes are most at risk for developing painful tendon conditions, and which ones will benefit most from the various treatment options (exercise, sclerotherapy, nitric oxide), a baseline risk assessment including imaging findings, genetic testing, biomechanical assessment, and tendon biopsy analysis needs to be prospectively evaluated. If validated, these measures could be subjected to a randomized trial to examine their ability, alone or in combination, to predict injury and response to treatment.

With respect to treatment, there is an urgent need to describe the histopathologic changes that occur with various physical, pharmacologic, and surgical treatments. The challenge has been to obtain tissue *in vivo* from such therapeutic interventions.

Once such descriptive studies have been performed, researchers will strive to understand the mechanisms that underpin the described changes.

There are a large number of treatments that need to be understood; the range of possible mechanisms explaining even those that are supported by randomized trial evidence is very large. Thus, the field of tendon histopathology research provides great opportunity for new investigators.

References

Alfredson, H., Bjur, D., Thorsen, K., Lorentzon, R. & Sandstrom, P. (2002) High intratendinous lactate levels in painful chronic Achilles tendinosis. An investigation using microdialysis technique. *Journal of Orthopedic Research* **20**, 934–938.

Alfredson, H., Forsgren, S., Thorsen, K. & Lorentzon, R. (2001) *In vivo* microdialysis and immunohistochemical analyses of tendon tissue demonstrated high amounts of free glutamate and glutamate NMDAR1 receptors, but no signs of inflammation, in Jumper's knee. *Journal of Orthopedic Research* **19**, 881–886.

Alfredson, H., Ljung, B.O., Thorsen, K. & Lorentzon, R. (2000) *In vivo* investigation of ECRB tendons with microdialysis technique: no signs of inflammation but high amounts of glutamate in tennis elbow. *Acta Orthopaedica Scandinavica* **71**, 475–479.

Alfredson, H., Lorentzon, M., Backman, S., Backman, A. & Lerner, U.H. (2003) cDNA-arrays and real-time quantitative PCR techniques in the investigation of chronic Achilles tendinosis. *Journal of Orthopedic Research* **21**, 970–975.

Alfredson, H., Öhberg, L. & Forsgren, S. (2003) Is vasculo-neural ingrowth the cause of pain in chronic Achilles tendinosis? An investigation using ultrasonography and colour Doppler, immunohistochemistry, and diagnostic injections. *Knee Surgery, Sports Traumatology, Arthroscopy* **11**, 334–338.

Almekinders, L.C., Weinhold, P.S. & Maffulli, N. (2003) Compression etiology in tendinopathy. *Clinics in Sports Medicine* **22**, 703–710.

Banes, A.J., Tsuzaki, M., Hu, P., *et al.* (1995) PDGF-BB, IGF-I and mechanical load stimulate DNA synthesis in avian tendon fibroblasts *in vitro*. *Journal of Biomechanics* **28**, 1505–1513.

Benazzo, F., Stennardo, G. & Valli, M. (1996) Achilles and patellar tendinopathies in athletes: pathogenesis and surgical treatment. *Bulletin—Hospital for Joint Diseases* **54**, 236–240.

Berenson, M.C., Blevins, F.T., Plaas, A.H. & Vogel, K.G. (1996) Proteoglycans of human rotator cuff tendons. *Journal of Orthopedic Research* **14**, 518–525.

Biberthaler, P., Wiedemann, E. Nerlich, A., *et al.* (2003) Microcirculation associated with degenerative rotator cuff lesions. *In vivo* assessment with orthogonal polarization spectral imaging during arthroscopy of the shoulder. *Journal of Bone and Joint Surgery. American volume* **85**, 475–480.

Canty, E.G. & Kadler, K.E. (2002) Collagen fibril biosynthesis in tendon: a review and recent insights. *Comparative Biochemistry and Physiology. Part A—Molecular and Integrative Physiology* **133**, 979–985.

Clark, J.D. & Stechschulte, J. Jr. (1998) The interface between bone and tendon at an insertion site: a study of the quadriceps tendon insertion. *Journal of Anatomy* **192** (Part 4), 605–616.

Clarke, M.T., Lyall, H.A., Grant, J.W. & Matthewson, M.H. (1998) The histopathology of de Quervain's disease. *Journal of Hand Surgery. British volume* **23**, 732–734.

Cook, J.L., Khan, K.M., Kiss, Z.S., Purdam, C.R. & Griffiths. L. (2000) Prospective imaging study of asymptomatic patellar tendinopathy in elite junior basketball players. *Journal of Ultrasound Medicine* **19**, 473–479.

Corps, A.N., Curry, V.A., Harrall, R.L., Dutt, D., Hazelman, B.L. & Riley, G.P. (2003) Ciproflaxicin reduces the stimulation of prostaglandin E$_2$ output by interleukin-1β in human tendon-derived cells. *Rheumatology* **42**, 1306–1310.

Corps, A.N., Robinson, A.H.N., Movin, T., *et al.* (2004) Versican splice variant messenger RNA expression in normal human Achilles tendon and tendinopathies. *Rheumatology* **43**, 969–972.

Enna, C.D. & Dyer, R.F. (1976) Tendon plasticity: a property applicable to reconstructive surgery of the hand. *Hand* **8**, 118–124.

Evans, N.A., Bowrey, D.J. & Newman, G.R. (1998) Ultrastructural analysis of ruptured tendon from anabolic steroid users. *Injury* **29**, 769–773.

Eyre, D.R. (1997) Bone biomarkers as tools in osteoporosis management. *Spine* **22**, 17S–24S.

Eyre, D.R., Koob, T.J. & Van Ness, K.P. (1984) Quantitation of hydroxypyridinium crosslinks in collagen by high-performance liquid chromatography. *Analytical Biochemistry* **137**, 380–388.

Fallon, J., Blevins, F.T., Vogel, K. & Trotter, J. (2002) Functional morphology of the supraspinatus tendon. *Journal of Orthopedic Research* **20**, 920–926.

Fenwick, S.A., Curry, V., Harrall, R.L., Hazleman, B.L., Hackney, R. & Riley, G.P. (2001) Expression of transforming growth factor-beta isoforms and their receptors in chronic tendinosis. *Journal of Anatomy* **199**, 231–240.

Freeland, A.E., Tucci, M.A., Barbieri, R.A., Angel, M.F. & Nick, T.G. (2002) Biochemical evaluation of serum and flexor tenosynovium in carpal tunnel syndrome. *Microsurgery* **22**, 378–385.

Fu, S.C., Chan, B.P., Wang, W., Pau, H.M., Chan, K.M. & Rolf, C.G. (2002) Increased expression of matrix metalloproteinase 1 (MMP-1) in 11 patients with patellar tendinosis. *Acta Orthopaedica Scandinavica* **73**, 658–662.

Fu, S.C., Wang, W., Pau, H.M., Wong, Y.P., Chan, K.M. & Rolf, C.G. (2002) Increased expression of transforming growth factor-β1 in patellar tendinosis. *Clinical Orthopaedics and Related Research* **73**, 174–183.

Fujii, K., Yamagishi, T., Nagafuchi, T., Tsuji, M. & Kuboki, Y. (1994) Biochemical properties of collagen from ligaments and periarticular tendons of the human knee. *Knee Surgery, Sports Traumatology, Arthroscopy* **2**, 229–233.

Galliani, I., Burattini, S., Mariani, A.R., Riccio, M., Cassiani, G. & Falcieri, E. (2002) Morpho-functional changes in human tendon tissue. *European Journal of Histochemistry* **46**, 3–12.

Gotoh, M., Hamada, K., Yamakawa, H., Inoue, A. & Fukuda, H. (1988) Increased substance P in subacromial bursa and shoulder pain in rotator cuff diseases. *Journal of Orthopedic Research* **16**, 618–621.

Gotoh, M., Hamada, K., Yamakawa, H., Tomonaga, A., Inoue, A. & Fukuda, H. (1997) Significance of granulation tissue in torn supraspinatus insertions: an immunohistochemical study with antibodies against interleukin-1β, cathepsin D, and matrix metalloprotease-1. *Journal of Orthopedic Research* **15**, 33–39.

Gotoh, M., Hamada, K., Yamakawa, H., *et al.* (2001) Interleukin-1-induced subacromial synovitis and shoulder pain in rotator cuff diseases. *Rheumatology* **40**, 995–1001.

Hamada, K., Tomonaga, A., Gotoh, M., Yamakawa, H. & Fukuda, H. (1997) Intrinsic healing capacity and tearing process of torn supraspinatus tendons: *in situ* hybridization study of alpha 1 (I) procollagen mRNA. *Journal of Orthopedic Research* **15**, 24–32.

Hansson, H.A., Brandsten, C., Lossing, C. & Petruson, K. (1989) Transient expression of insulin-like growth factor I immunoreactivity by vascular cells during angiogenesis. *Expermental and Molecular Pathology* **50**, 125–138.

Hyvonen, P., Melkko, J., Lehto, V.P. & Jalovaara, P. (2003) Involvement of the subacromial bursa in impingement syndrome as judged by expression of tenascin-C and histopathology. *Journal of Bone and Joint Surgery. British volume* **85**, 299–305.

Ireland, D., Harrall, R., Curry, V., *et al.* (2001) Multiple changes in gene expression in chronic human Achilles tendinopathy. *Matrix Biology* **20**, 159–169.

Jarvinen, M., Jozsa, L., Kannus, P., Jarvinen, T.L., Kvist, M. & Leadbetter, W. (1997) Histopathological findings in chronic tendon disorders. *Scandinavian Journal of Medicine and Science in Sports* **7**, 86–95.

Jósza, L. & Kannus, P. (1997) *Human Tendons*. Human Kinetics, Champaign, IL.

Józsa, L., Kannus, P., Balint, J.B. & Reffy, A. (1991) Three-dimensional ultrastructure of human tendons. *Acta Anatomica* **142**, 306–312.

Khan, K.M., Bonar, F., Desmond, P.M., *et al.* (1996) Patellar tendinosis (jumper's knee): findings at histopathologic examination, US, and MR imaging. Victorian Institute of Sport Tendon Study Group. *Radiology* **200**, 821–827.

Khan, K. & Cook, M.J. (2000) Overuse tendon injuries: Where does the pain come from? *Sports Medicine and Arthroscopy Reviews* **8**, 17–31.

Khan, K.M., Cook, J.L., Bonar, F., Harcourt, P. & Astrom, M. (1999) Histopathology of common tendinopathies. Update and implications for clinical management. *Sports Medicine* **27**, 393–408.

Khan, K.M., Cook, J.L., Kannus, P., Maffulli, N. & Bonar, S.F. (2002) Time to abandon the "tendinitis" myth. *British Medical Journal* **324**, 626–627.

Khan, K.M., Cook, J.L. & Taunton, J.E. (2000) Overuse tendinosis, not tendinitis. Part 1: A new paradigm for a difficult clinical problem. *Physican and Sports Medicine* **28**, 38–48.

Koob, T.J. & Summers, A.P. (2002) Tendon—bridging the gap. *Comparative Biochemestry and Physiology. Part A, Molecular and Integrative Physiology* **133**, 905–909.

Kvist, M. & Jarvinen, M. (1982) Clinical, histochemical and biomechanical features in repair of muscle and tendon injuries. *International Journal of Sports Medicine* **3** (Suppl. 1), 12–14.

Kvist, M.H., Lehto, M.U., Józsa, L., Jarvinen, M.H. & Kvist, T. (1988) Chronic achilles paratenonitis. An immunohistologic study of fibronectin and fibrinogen. *American Journal of Sports Medicine* **16**, 616–623.

Maffulli, N., Ewen, S.W., Waterston, S.W., Reaper, J. & Barrass, V. (2000) Tenocytes from ruptured and tendinopathic achilles tendons produce greater quantities of type III collagen than tenocytes from normal achilles tendons. An *in vitro* model of human tendon healing. *American Journal of Sports Medicine* **28**, 499–505.

Maffulli, N., Khan, K.M. & Puddu, G. (1998) Overuse tendon conditions: time to change a confusing terminology. *Arthroscopy* **14**, 840–843.

Maffulli, N., Wong, J. & Almekinders, L.C. (2003) Types and epidemiology of tendinopathy. *Clinics in Sports Medicine* **22**, 675–692.

Movin, T., Gad, A., Reinholt, F.P. & Rolf, C. (1997) Tendon pathology in long-standing achillodynia. Biopsy findings in 40 patients. *Acta Orthopaedica Scandinavica* **68**, 170–175.

Nakase, T., Sugamoto, K., Miyamoto, T., *et al.* (2002) Activation of cartilage-derived morphogenetic protein-1 in torn rotator cuff. *Clinical Orthopedics and Related Research* 140–145.

O'Brien, M. (1997) Structure and metabolism of tendons. *Scandinavian Journal of Medicine and Science in Sports* **7**, 55–61.

Ohberg, L. & Alfredson, H. (2002) Ultrasound guided sclerosis of neovessels in painful chronic Achilles tendinosis: pilot study of a new treatment. *British Journal of Sports Medicine* **36**, 173–175.

Ohberg, L., Lorentzon, R. & Alfredson, H. (2001) Neovascularisation in Achilles tendons with painful tendinosis but not in normal tendons: an ultrasonographic investigation. *Knee Surgery, Sports Traumatology, Arthroscopy* **9**, 233–238.

Perugia, L., Ippolitio, E., Postachinni, F. (1976) A new approach to the pathology, clinical features and treatment of stress tendinopathy of the Achilles tendon. *Italian Journal Orthopaedics and Traumatology* **2** (1), 5–21.

Pierce, G.F., Vande Berg, J., Rudolph, R., Tarpley, J.T. & Mustoe, A. (1991) Platelet-derived growth factor-BB and transforming growth factor beta 1 selectively modulate glycosaminoglycans, collagen, and myofibroblasts in excisional wounds. *American Journal of Pathology* **138**, 629–646.

Premdas, J., Tang, J.B., Warner, J.P., Murray, M.M. & Spector, M. (2001) The presence of smooth muscle actin in fibroblasts in the torn human rotator cuff. *Journal of Orthopedic Research* **19**, 221–228.

Pufe, T., Petersen, W., Tillmann, B. & Mentlein, R. (2001) The angiogenic peptide vascular endothelial growth factor is expressed in foetal and ruptured tendons. *Virchows Archiv* **439**, 579–585.

Puxkandl, R., Zizak, I., Paris, O., *et al.* (2002) Viscoelastic properties of collagen: synchrotron radiation investigations and structural model. *Philosophical Transactions of the Royal Society of London. Series B, Biological Sciences* **357**, 191–197.

Rees, S.G., Flannery, C.R., Little, C.B., Hughes, C.E., Caterson, B. & Dent, C.M. (2000) Catabolism of aggrecan, decorin and biglycan in tendon. *Biochemical Journal* **350** (Part 1), 181–188.

Riley, G. (2004) The pathogenesis of tendinopathy. A molecular perspective. *Rheumatology* **43**, 131–142.

Riley, G.P., Curry, V., DeGroot, J., *et al.* (2002) Matrix metalloproteinase activities and their relationship with collagen remodelling in tendon pathology. *Matrix Biology* **21**, 185–195.

Riley, G.P., Harrall, R.L., Constant, C.R., Chard, M.D., Cawston, T.E. & Hazleman, B.L. (1994) Glycosaminoglycans of human rotator cuff tendons: changes with age and in chronic rotator cuff tendinitis. *Annals of the Rheumatic Diseases* **53**, 367–376.

Riley, G.P., Harrall, R.L., Constant, C.R., Chard, M.D., Cawston, T.E. & Hazleman, B.L. (1994) Tendon degeneration and chronic shoulder pain: changes in the collagen composition of the human rotator cuff tendons in rotator cuff tendinitis. *Annals of the Rheumatic Diseases* **53**, 359–366.

Ritty, T.M., Roth, R. & Heuser, J.E. (2003) Tendon cell array isolation reveals a previously unknown fibrillin-2-containing macromolecular assembly. *Structure* **11**, 1179–1188.

Rolf, C.G., Fu, B.S., Pau, A., Wang, W. & Chan, B. (2001) Increased cell proliferation and associated expression of PDGFRβ causing hypercellularity in patellar tendinosis. *Rheumatology* **40**, 256–261.

Sakai, H., Fujita, K., Sakai, Y. & Mizuno, K. (2001) Immunolocalization of cytokines and growth factors in subacromial bursa of rotator cuff tear patients. *Kobe Journal of Medical Sciences* **47**, 25–34.

Sano, H., Ishii, H., Yeadon, A., Backman, D.S., Brunet, J.A. & Uhthoff, H.K. (1997) Degeneration at the insertion weakens the tensile strength of the supraspinatus tendon: a comparative mechanical and histologic study of the bone-tendon complex. *Journal of Orthopedic Research* **15**, 719–726.

Sano, H., Uhthoff, H.K., Backman, D.S., *et al.* (1998) Structural disorders at the insertion of the supraspinatus tendon. Relation to tensile strength. *Journal of Bone and Joint Surgery. British volume* **80**, 720–725.

Sarkar, K. & Uhthoff, H.K. (1980) Ultrastructure of the common extensor tendon in tennis elbow. *Virchows Archiv A, Pathological Anatomy and Histology* **386**, 317–330.

Schmidt, D. & Mackay, B. (1982) Ultrastructure of human tendon sheath and synovium: implications for tumor histogenesis. *Ultrastructural Pathology* **3**, 269–283.

Scott, J.E. (1996) Proteodermatan and proteokeratan sulfate (decorin, lumican/fibromodulin) proteins are horseshoe shaped. Implications for their interactions with collagen. *Biochemistry* **35**, 8795–8799.

Scott, J.E., Dyne, K.M., Thomlinson, A.M., *et al.* (1998) Human cells unable to express decoron produced disorganized extracellular matrix lacking "shape modules" (interfibrillar proteoglycan bridges). *Experimental Cell Research* **243**, 59–66.

Sell (1995) Aging of long-lived proteins: extracellular matrix (collagens, elastins, proteoglycans) and lens crystallins. In: *Handbook of Physiology. 11 Aging* (Masaro, E., ed.). Oxford University Press, New York.

Tillander, B., Franzen, L. & Norlin, R. (2002) Fibronectin, MMP-1 and histologic changes in rotator cuff disease. *Journal of Orthopedic Research* **20**, 1358–1364.

Tsujii, M., Hirata, H., Yoshida, T., Imanaka-Yoshida, K., Morita, A. & Uchida, A. (2006) Involvement of tenascin-C and PG-M/versican in flexor tenosynovial pathology of idiopathic carpal tunnel syndrome. *Histology and Histopathology* **21**, 511–518.

Tucci, M.A., Barbieri, R.A. & Freeland, A.E. (1997) Biochemical and histological analysis of the flexor tenosynovium in patients with carpal tunnel syndrome. *Biomedical Sciences Instrumentation* **33**, 246–251.

Tuoheti, Y., Itoi, E., Pradhan, R.L., *et al.* (2005) Apoptosis in the supraspinatus tendon with stage II subacromial impingement. *Journal of Shoulder and Elbow Surgery* **14**, 535–541.

Vogel, K.G. & Hernandez, D.J. (1992) The effects of transforming growth factor-beta and serum on proteoglycan synthesis by tendon fibrocartilage. *European Journal of Cell Biology* **59**, 304–313.

Waggett, A.D., Ralphs, J.R., Kwan, A.P., Woodnutt, D. & Benjamin, M. (1998) Characterization of collagens and proteoglycans at the insertion of the human Achilles tendon. *Matrix Biology* **16**, 457–470.

Yanagisawa, K., Hamada, K., Gotoh, M., *et al.* (2001) Vascular endothelial growth factor (VEGF) expression in the subacromial bursa is increased in patients with impingement syndrome. *Journal of Orthopedic Research* **19**, 448–455.

Yuan, J., Murrell, G.A., Wei, A.Q. & Wang, M.X. (2002) Apoptosis in rotator cuff tendonopathy. *Journal of Orthopedic Research* **20**, 1372–1379.

Chapter 7

Mechanobiologic Studies of Cellular and Molecular Mechanisms of Tendinopathy

JAMES H-C. WANG, SAVIO L-Y. WOO, WEI-HSIU HSU, AND DAVID A. STONE

It is well recognized that mechanical forces regulate the form and function of connective tissues. However, abnormal mechanical loading conditions result in connective tissue disorders such as tendinopathy, which is a prevalent tendon disorder in both athletic and occupational settings. Although there are numerous publications that discuss the etiology, diagnosis, and treatment of various forms of tendinopathy, the precise pathogenesis of tendinopathy remains unclear. Previous *in vitro* model studies showed that the cyclic stretching of tendon fibroblasts subjected to various stretching magnitudes, frequencies, and durations upregulates the expression of lipid inflammatory mediator, including $cPLA_2$, $sPLA_2$, and COX. Both *in vitro* and *in vivo* studies have shown that mechanical loading of tendons or tendon fibroblasts increases the production of prostaglandin E_2 (PGE_2). Animal model studies also showed that injection of PGE_1 or PGE_2 results in inflammation and degeneration around and within the tendon, as well as the disorganization of collagen matrix and decreased collagen fibril diameter, typical of tendinopathy-associated pathologic conditions.

In future tendinopathy research, several lines of research directions should be pursued. These include: (i) to elucidate the role of phospholipase A_2 (PLA_2) in the development of tendinopathy; (ii) to determine the role of leukotrienes (e.g. LTB_4) and their interaction with PGE_2 in tendon homeostasis as well as pathogenesis of tendinopathy; (iii) to study the role of proinflammatory cytokines (e.g. interleukins IL-1β and IL-6) and degradative enzymes, including matrix metalloproteinases MMP-1, MMP-3, and MMP-13, in tendon degeneration; (iv) to investigate the interactive effects of inflammatory mediators with various mechanical loading conditions on tendons; and (v) to create refined animal models of tendinopathy so that effective protocols for treatment and prevention of tendinopathy can be developed. The ultimate goal in tendinopathy research is to devise scientifically based treatment and preventive strategies to reduce the incidence of tendinopathy in athletic settings and in the workplace.

Introduction

Mechanical forces have a profound effect on connective tissue cells. For example, it is well known that gravity, tension and compression, and shear stresses influence cellular functions (e.g. gene expression and protein synthesis). As a result, these mechanical forces have a crucial role in maintaining tendon homeostasis as well as in repairing and remodeling after tendon injuries. While mechanical forces are beneficial in the ways described, excessive, repetitive mechanical loading of tendons has detrimental effects which can result in pathophysiologic changes in tendons, including tendinopathy (Leadbetter 1992). Therefore, it is essential to understand how mechanical forces induce pathophysiologic changes in tendons at the cellular and molecular levels. Cell mechanobiology, an interdisciplinary field that studies biologic responses of cells to mechanical forces and the mechanotransduction mechanisms, may help elucidate the molecular mechanisms of tendinopathy. In general, cells may be viewed as sensors and transducers of mechanical forces. The sensing and transduction of forces take place in two steps:

1 Mechanical coupling, which enables the transformation of applied forces into detectable physical stimuli (e.g. matrix deformations); followed by

2 Mechanotransduction, which transduces the stimuli into a cascade of molecular events, including gene expression, production of autocrine or paracrine factors, and expression of specific receptors.

In this chapter, the mechanisms of tendinopathy at the molecular, cellular, and tissue levels are discussed. First, the cascade of inflammatory events that result from lipid metabolism in response to stimuli such as mechanical forces are briefly reviewed. Then, the effect of cyclic mechanical stretching on the expression and production of inflammatory mediators (e.g. PGE_2) by human tendon fibroblasts are described. This is followed by studies where the effect of these mediators on tendon fibroblasts *in vitro* and tendons *in vivo* are presented. Finally, directions for future research on tendinopathy using mechanobiologic approaches as well as new strategies for the prevention and treatment of tendinopathy are suggested.

Inflammatory mediators from lipid metabolism

Although the etiology of tendinopathy remains elusive, it is generally believed that excessive, repetitive mechanical loading on the tendon is the initial event, which leads to tendon inflammation, degeneration, and, in some cases, rupture (Archambault *et al.* 1995; Almekinders & Temple 1998). *In vivo* studies with rabbits show that after ankle joints were passively flexed and extended for 2 hours per day, three times a week over a total of 6 weeks, their Achilles tendons were found to be grossly inflamed and fibrillated (Backman *et al.* 1990). Histologic examination revealed the presence of inflammatory cell infiltrates, edema, fibroblast proliferation, and increased vascularity. Repetitive mechanical loading by treadmill running has also been shown to induce tendinosis (or tendon degeneration) in rats (Soslowsky *et al.* 2000). Moreover, elevated PGE_2 levels were found in the human tendon after

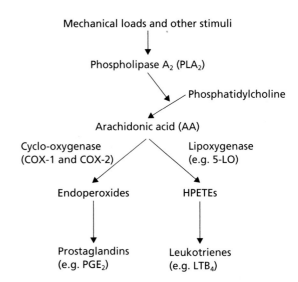

Fig. 7.1 A simplified illustration of the production of arachidonic acid metabolites. (After Fantone, J.C. (1990) Basic concepts in inflammation. In: *Sports-induced Inflammation: Clinical and Basic Science Concepts* Leadbetter W.B., Buckwalter J.B., Gordon S.L., eds. American Academy of Orthopaedic Surgeons, Park Ridge, IL.)

repetitive dynamic loading (Langberg *et al.* 1999). In addition, it is known that mechanical trauma to tissues increases the production of leukotrienes, which induce tissue edema (Denzlinger *et al.* 1985). *In vitro* studies also showed that repetitive mechanical loading of human tendon fibroblasts increases the production of both PGE_2 and LTB_4 (Almekinders *et al.* 1993; Wang *et al.* 2003, 2004; Li *et al.* 2004). Thus, these findings suggest that excessive, repetitive mechanical loading of tendons cause tendon inflammation and degeneration by the generation of inflammatory mediators from arachidonic acid (AA) metabolites. Figure 7.1 illustrates the production of AA metabolites, which are further described in detail below.

Phospholipase A_2

The PLA_2 family of enzymes consists of several isotypes, including cytosolic PLA_2 ($cPLA_2$) and secretary PLA_2 ($sPLA_2$). The $cPLA_2$ is expressed ubiquitously and upregulated by inflammatory stimuli (Vadas & Pruzanski 1990; Samad *et al.* 2001).

Secretory PLA_2 is implicated in the regulation of regional blood flow to inflamed sites (Vadas *et al.* 1981). Previous studies have shown that cyclic stretching of human flexor tendon fibroblasts increases levels of PGE_2 (Almekinders *et al.* 1993; Wang *et al.* 2003). PLA_2 catalyzes the hydrolysis of fatty acids at the sn-2 position of glycerophospholipids and, as a result, yields AA (Kaiser 1999). PLA_2 activation is thought to be important in the synthesis of prostaglandins including PGE_2, because it is the first step in the cell's production of AA, which is converted to prostaglandins and leukotrienes via the cyclo-oxygenase (COX) and 5-lipoxygenase (5-LO) pathways, respectively (Smith *et al.* 1996). Moreover, PLA_2 itself has an important role in initiating tissue inflammation. For example, intratracheal, intradermal, and intra-articular injection of PLA_2 in rabbits induces profound inflammatory lesions (Gonzalez-Buritica *et al.* 1989). Similar to biochemical stimuli, mechanical forces applied to cells can also activate PLA_2 and result in the increased production of PGE_2 by: (i) activation of PLA_2; (ii) release of AA; and (iii) increased production of PGE_2 (Binderman *et al.* 1988). In human endothelial cells, for example, flow shear stresses increase $cPLA_2$ activity in an apparently stress magnitude-dependent manner (Pearce *et al.* 1996).

Cyclo-oxygenase

The production of prostaglandins requires COX to convert AA to prostaglandin H_2, the committed step in prostanoid synthesis. Two COX isoforms, COX-1 and COX-2, have been identified (Smith *et al.* 1996), and both catalyze the same reaction. The two enzymes, however, are variably expressed in different tissues. COX-1 is expressed constitutively in many types of cells, and COX-2 is induced mainly at inflammatory sites, although it is also constitutively expressed in the kidney and parts of the central nervous system (Geis 1999). It is generally believed that in response to inflammatory stimuli, such as cytokines and bacterial products, COX-2 but not COX-1 is upregulated (Cryer & Feldman 1998). Nevertheless, it is reported that in addition to COX-2, COX-1 expression can also be induced, which contributes to high levels of prostaglandin production

when stimulated by lipopolysaccharide, a potent inflammatory agent (McAdam *et al.* 2000).

Prostaglandin E_2 and leukotriene B_4

Prostaglandins belong to a class of lipids that are distinguished by their potent physiologic properties and rapid metabolic turnover. PGE_2, one of the most abundant prostaglandins in many tissues, is synthesized from AA and mediates tendon and ligament inflammation (Almekinders & Temple 1998). It is believed that non-steroidal anti-inflammatory drugs (NSAIDs) decrease tissue inflammation through inhibition of prostaglandin synthesis. Fibroblasts can produce high levels of PGE_2 in response to mechanical loading in many human tissues (Baracos *et al.* 1983; Yamaguchi *et al.* 1994). For example, in human periodontal ligament fibroblasts and human finger flexor tendon fibroblasts, cyclic stretching of these cells increased PGE_2 production in a stretching frequency-dependent manner (Almekinders *et al.* 1993, 1995; Yamaguchi *et al.* 1994). These studies revealed that human tendon or ligament fibroblasts can produce high levels of PGE_2 when subjected to repetitive mechanical loading *in vitro*. It has also been established that PGE_2 modulates various cellular functions, including the suppression of the transforming growth factor-β (TGF-β) stimulated expression of total protein, collagen, and fibronectin in human lung fibroblasts (Diaz *et al.* 1989). In addition, exogenous addition of PGE_2 to culture decreases proliferation and collagen synthesis of human tendon fibroblasts in a dosage-dependent manner (Cilli *et al.* 2004). Thus, high levels of PGE_2 produced by tendon fibroblasts in response to repetitive mechanical loading are likely involved in the development of tendinopathy by the induction of tendon inflammation that eventually leads to degeneration.

In addition to PGE_2, leukotrienes, such as LTB_4, are also produced via the 5-LO pathway. An abundance of LTB_4 is present in damaged tissues. For example, mechanical trauma in an anesthetized rat induced a large increase in the production of leukotrienes (Denzlinger *et al.* 1985), which is sufficient to induce tissue edema often seen in degenerative tendons. *In vitro* studies have shown that repetitive mechanical loading of human tendon fibroblasts increases the production of LTB_4 levels (Almekinders *et al.* 1993; Li *et al.* 2004). It is known that LTB_4 is a potent chemoattractant for neutrophils, and injection of LTB_4 into tissues results in the accumulation of neutrophils at the injection site (Casale *et al.* 1992). Therefore, the excessive accumulation and activation of neutrophils by LTB_4 causes tissue damage as a result of their release of proteases and reactive oxygen species (Crooks & Stockley 1998). Thus, high levels of LTB_4 production by tendon fibroblasts in response to excessive mechanical loading will result in inflammation leading to the development of tendinopathy (Dahlen *et al.* 1981).

Effect of mechanical stretching on the production of inflammatory mediators

Because the tendon transmits force from muscles to bone, the tendon is usually subjected to different levels of repetitive mechanical stretching, which subjects tendon fibroblasts to tensile strains. Therefore, *in vitro* models that can stretch cells at known stretching magnitudes and frequencies will enable one to examine the mechanobiologic responses of tendon fibroblasts to repetitive mechanical stretching.

For this purpose, we have developed a novel model system to study the cellular and molecular mechanisms of tendinopathy (Fig. 7.2). The system consists of a stretching apparatus and silicone dishes with microgrooved culture surfaces. Silicone, a transparent, elastic, and non-toxic material to cells

(Wang 2000), was used to make deformable dishes for growing and stretching human tendon fibroblasts. The silicone dishes have microgrooves on their culture surfaces, which are aligned along the long axis of the dish, that is, the direction along which the membrane is stretched (the stretching direction) (Wang *et al.* 2003). The advantage of this system is that one can control the alignment, shape, and mechanical stretching conditions of human tendon fibroblasts to mimic *in vivo* conditions (Fig. 7.3). Therefore, the corresponding biologic responses of human tendon fibroblasts *in vivo* can be modeled more closely, so that one may elucidate the cellular and molecular mechanisms of tendinopathy.

Using this system, we have investigated the inflammatory response of human patellar tendon fibroblasts (HPTFs) to repetitive mechanical stretching conditions. HPTFs were obtained from tendon pieces trimmed from patellar tendon autografts that were used for reconstruction of the anterior cruciate

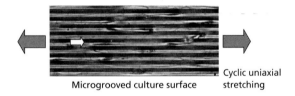

Microgrooved culture surface   Cyclic uniaxial stretching

Fig. 7.3 Human patellar tendon fibroblasts were grown on microgrooved silicone surface. These cells were elongated in shape and aligned with the direction of uniaxial stretching. (Reproduced from Li, Z. *et al.* (2004) *American Journal of Sports Medicine* **32**, 435–440 with permission.)

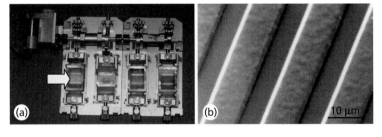

Fig. 7.2 (a) A novel *in vitro* system for studying mechanobiology of tendon fibroblasts. The system consists of silicone dishes (arrow) mounted on the custom-made stretching apparatus. (b) The culture surface of the silicone dish contains microgrooves oriented along the dish's long axis, that is, the stretching direction. The profile of the microgroove is close to a rectangle, with the width of the ridges and grooves being 10 μm, and the depth being about 3 μm. (Reproduced from Wang, J.H. *et al.* (2003) *Connective Tissue Research* **44**, 128–133 with permission.)

ligament of young, healthy donors. These fibroblasts were grown in microgrooved silicone dishes and subjected to cyclic mechanical stretching with various stretching magnitudes and frequencies.

PLA$_2$ expression and activation

PLA$_2$ activation is the first step for a stimulated cell to produce AA, which is then converted into prostaglandins and leukotrienes by COX and 5-LO, respectively. We have found that tendon fibroblasts subjected to 8% stretching for 4 hours followed by 4 hours of rest increased cPLA$_2$ expression by 88% compared to non-stretched cells. Moreover, the sPLA$_2$ activity level increased by 190% (Fig. 7.4).

It should be noted that 8% stretch, as well as 4% and 12% stretches, is the nominal strain imposed on the silicone dish in which the cells are grown. Because of the incomplete transfer of dish deformation to dish culture surface as well as the dish substrate strains to the individual cells, the actual strains on the cells on the dish surface are smaller than the applied nominal strain (Wang 2000). In endothelial cells, for example, it has been shown that cell strain was about 77.2% of the substrate strain (Wang *et al.* 2001).

COX expression

To further define the effect of mechanical stretching on the expression of COX, we performed another study and found a large increase in both COX-1 and COX-2 expression levels after 8% and 12% stretch for 4 hours, followed by 4 hours of rest. With 4% stretching, COX-2 levels markedly increased while COX-1 levels did not (Fig. 7.5).

The effect of stretching frequency on COX expression levels was also investigated. After 8% stretching at 0.1 Hz, the COX-1 level did not significantly increase, whereas the COX-2 level increased compared to the non-stretched control group. On the other hand, both COX-1 and COX-2 levels increased significantly after 8% stretching at 0.5 Hz. Similarly, 8% stretching at 1.0 Hz significantly increased both COX-1 and COX-2 levels. However, the increase in the COX-2 level was more pronounced than that of COX-1 (Fig. 7.6).

Because there was a concurrent increase in PGE$_2$ production and COX expression following cyclic stretching, an additional experiment was performed to verify that the increase in COX expression contributed to the increase in PGE$_2$ production. It was found that when indometacin, a specific COX

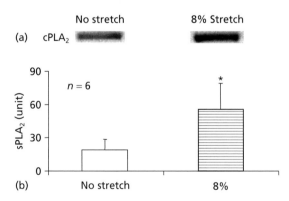

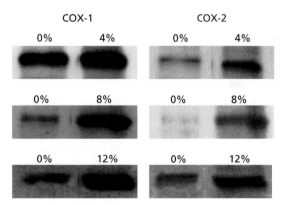

Fig. 7.4 The effect of cyclic stretching on the expression levels of cPLA$_2$ and sPLA$_2$. Cyclic stretching (8%) of human patellar tendon fibroblasts markedly increased cPLA$_2$ protein expression compared with that of non-stretched fibroblasts (a). The level of sPLA$_2$ secretion by stretched fibroblasts was also markedly increased (b) (*P <0.05). (Reproduced from Wang, J.H., Li, Z., Yang, G. & Khan, M. (2004) *Clinical Orthopaedics and Related Research* 243–250 with permission.)

Fig. 7.5 The effect of cyclic stretching on COX expression. At 4% stretching, COX-1 expression levels of human patellar tendon fibroblasts slightly increased compared with non-stretched controls, but COX-2 levels markedly increased. However, at 8% and 12% stretching, both COX-1 and COX-2 levels markedly increased. Note that the cells were cyclically stretched at 0.5 Hz for 4 hours, followed by 4 hours of rest. (Reproduced from Wang, J.H. *et al.* (2003) *Connective Tissue Research* **44**, 128–133 with permission.)

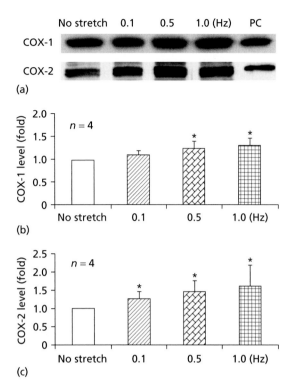

(a)

(b)

(c)

Fig. 7.6 The effect of cyclic stretching frequency on COX expression. With increased stretching frequency from 0.1, 0.5, to 1.0 Hz, both COX-1 and COX-2 expression levels increased, but the level of the increase in COX-2 expression was markedly larger than that of COX-1 (*P <0.05; PC, positive control). (From Wang, J.H., Li, Z., Yang, G. & Khan, M. (2004) *Clinical Orthopaedics and Related Research* 243–250 with permission.)

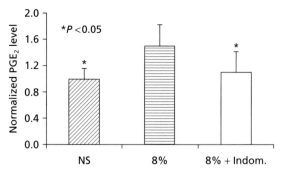

Fig. 7.7 Addition of indometacin (25–50 μmol) decreased stretching-induced PGE_2 production by human patellar tendon fibroblasts. Note that PGE_2 measurements for the stretched cells were normalized with respect to that of non-stretched cells and cell numbers for proper comparisons among the three experimental conditions. NS, no stretching; 8%, 8% stretching; 8% + Indom., 8% stretching in the presence of indometacin. (The bar represents ± SD; $5 \leq n \leq 10$ for each condition; and *P <0.05, compared to 8% stretching.) (Reproduced from Wang, J.H. *et al.* (2003) *Connective Tissue Research* **44**, 128–133 with permission.)

inhibitor, was present in cell cultures, PGE_2 levels after 8% stretching were found to be significantly decreased compared to those without indometacin treatment (Fig. 7.7). Moreover, PGE_2 levels from the cyclically stretched cells with indometacin treatment were not significantly different from those cells without stretching and without indometacin treatment. These findings indicate that the increased expression and/or activation of COX because of cyclic stretching is responsible for the increased PGE_2 production.

PGE_2 and LTB_4 production

In human periodontal ligament fibroblasts, cyclic mechanical stretching has been shown to increase

PGE_2 production, with the level of increase dependent on stretching magnitude (Yamaguchi *et al.* 1994). Similarly, in human finger flexor tendon fibroblasts, cyclic biaxial stretching also increased PGE_2 production in a stretching frequency-dependent manner (Almekinders *et al.* 1993, 1995). In addition, we recently found that compared to cells without stretching, 8% and 12% cyclic stretching of the tendon fibroblasts at 0.5 Hz for 24 hours significantly increased the levels of PGE_2 1.7-fold and 2.2-fold, respectively, whereas 4% cyclic stretching did not significantly increase levels of PGE_2. Furthermore, PGE_2 levels were increased 1.6-fold with 8% versus 4% cyclic stretching and 1.9-fold with 12% versus 4% cyclic stretching (Fig. 7.8), which demonstrates that the increase in PGE_2 levels are stretching magnitude dependent. The results also suggest that PGE_2 production by tendon fibroblasts in response to repetitive mechanical loading may be involved in tendon inflammation.

The effect of stretching frequency on human tendon fibroblasts was then investigated. It was found that immediately after cyclic stretching, there were no significant differences in PGE_2 production

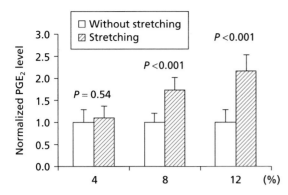

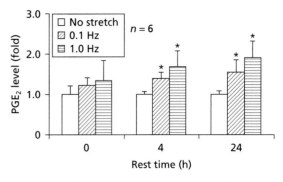

Fig. 7.8 The effect of cyclic stretching on PGE_2 production in human patellar tendon fibroblasts. Fibroblasts significantly increased the production of PGE_2 at 8% and 12% but not at 4%. The cells were cyclically stretched at 0.5 Hz for 24 hours, followed by incubation for an additional 20 hours in the presence of exogenous AA (20 μmol). (Reproduced from Wang, J.H. *et al.* (2003) *Connective Tissue Research* **44**, 128–133 with permission.)

Fig. 7.9 The effect of stretching frequency on PGE_2 production in human patellar tendon fibroblasts. The cells were stretched at 8% for 4 hours, followed by rest for 0, 4, and 24 hours. It is shown that PGE_2 production by stretched fibroblasts increased with increased stretching frequency and with increased rest time, the stretching frequency effect was more pronounced (*P <0.05). (Reproduced from Wang, J.H., Li, Z., Yang, G. & Khan, M. (2004). *Clinical Orthopaedics and Related Research* 243–250 with permission.)

between the high-frequency stretching group and the low-frequency stretching group. However, the levels of PGE_2 increased more in the high-frequency group compared with the low-frequency group as rest time increased. Specifically, immediately after 4 hours of stretching, the stretched fibroblasts produced consistently higher levels of PGE_2 compared with non-stretched fibroblasts. However, after 4 hours of rest, PGE_2 levels increased on average by 40% and 69% for the 0.1-Hz group and the 1.0-Hz group, respectively, compared to the non-stretched control group. After 24 hours of rest, PGE_2 levels were increased by 55% and 90% for the 0.1-Hz group and the 1.0-Hz group, respectively, compared to the non-stretched control group (Fig. 7.9). These results reveal that the cellular response to mechanical stretching persists even after the mechanical stimulus is removed.

In addition, it was found that cyclic stretching of HPTFs increased LTB_4 levels significantly compared to unstretched controls in a stretching magnitude-dependent fashion (Fig. 7.10). Specifically, with both 8% and 12% stretching but not 4%, LTB_4 production increased significantly compared to the control without stretching. Furthermore, LTB_4 levels at 8% or 12% stretching were significantly increased compared to 4%, but there was no significance

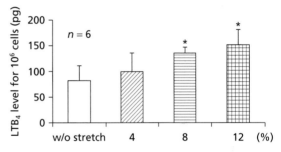

Fig. 7.10 The effect of cyclic mechanical stretching on LTB_4 production by human patellar tendon fibroblasts. Cyclic stretching at 8% and 12% but not 4% significantly increased LTB_4 production compared with the cells without stretching. In addition, LTB_4 levels at 8% were significantly increased compared with 4%, but not so compared with 12% stretching. (Reproduced from Li, Z., Yang, G., Khan, M., Stone, D., Woo, S.L. & Wang, J.H. (2004) *Journal of Sports Medicine* **32**, 435–440 with permission.)

difference in the LTB_4 level between 8% and 12% stretching.

Interestingly, blocking the production of PGE_2 with indometacin increased the level of LTB_4 produced by the tendon fibroblasts, which had been stretched for 4 hours and rested for an additional

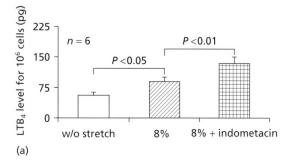

(a)

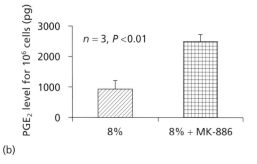

(b)

Fig. 7.11 (a) The relationship between COX and 5-LO pathways in human patellar tendon fibroblasts under cyclic mechanical stretching. Inhibiting COX with indometacin (25 μmol) decreased PGE_2 production but increased LTB_4 production by tendon fibroblasts. (b) Similarly, decreasing LTB_4 production by tendon fibroblasts with MK-886 (10 μmol) markedly increased PGE_2 production compared with the untreated stretched cells. (Reproduced from Li, Z., Yang, G., Khan, M., Stone, D., Woo, S.L. & Wang, J.H. (2004) *American Journal of Sports Medicine* **32**, 435–440 with permission.)

4 hours. Similarly, decreasing the LTB_4 production with MK-886 increased PGE_2 production levels (Fig. 7.11).

It should be noted that although we have focused on the role of inflammatory products (e.g. PGE_2 and LTB_4) from AA metabolism in the development of tendinopathy, other inflammatory mediators such as IL-1 may also be involved. IL-1 is a known potent inducer of MMPs, which induce degradation of the extracellular matrix (Unemori *et al.* 1994). It has been shown that IL-1β treated tendon fibroblasts increased the expression of COX-2, IL-6, MMP-1, and MMP-3 (Tsuzaki *et al.* 2003) and that mechanical loading of tendon fibroblasts also increased the gene expression of MMP-1 and MMP-3 (Archambault *et al.* 2002). There was also a synergistic effect of IL-

1β and stretching. Therefore, both IL-1β and MMPs induced by repetitive mechanical loading could cause extracellular matrix degradation, which is often observed in patients with tendinopathy (Jarvinen *et al.* 1997). In addition, repetitive mechanical stretching of tendon fibroblasts increased the expression of stress-activated protein kinases (SAPK/JNK) in a stretching magnitude-dependent manner. The persistent SAPK/JNK activation has been linked to the initiation of the apoptotic cascade (Arnoczky *et al.* 2002) and therefore may be involved in the development of tendinopathy.

Mechanisms of tendinopathy—going from *in vitro* to *in vivo* studies

It has been established that prostaglandins mediate diverse biologic processes in many types of cells. These include cell proliferation (Elias *et al.* 1985a,b), inflammatory and immune responses (Harada *et al.* 1982; Betz & Fox 1991), and the production of extracellular matrix proteins (Barile *et al.* 1988; Diaz *et al.* 1993). In human lung fibroblasts, for example, prostaglandins suppress the production of total protein, collagen, and fibronectin when the cells were stimulated with TGF-β (Diaz *et al.* 1989). Thus, high levels of PGE_2 resulting from repetitive mechanical stretching will likely affect the proliferation and protein synthesis of human tendon fibroblasts. We will explore this mechanism from *in vitro* to *in vivo* studies.

In vitro studies

HPTFs were derived from the tendon samples of young, healthy donors (21 and 38 years old) using explant tissue culture techniques (Wang *et al.* 2003). The cells were plated in 6-well plates at 6×10^4 cells per well. After culturing for 24 hours, PGE_2 (Sigma, St. Louis, MO) was added to the wells of the plates. Three concentrations of PGE_2 (1, 10, and 100 ng/mL) were used for the experimental groups, and fibroblasts without PGE_2 treatment were used as the control group. All the cells in the experimental and control groups were incubated for an additional 48 hours. To determine the number of viable cells in cultures, an MTT assay was used (Yang *et al.* 2004).

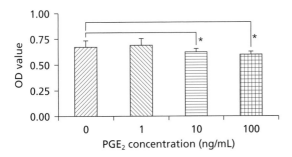

Fig. 7.12 The effect of PGE$_2$ on the proliferation of human patellar tendon fibroblasts. Higher dosages of PGE$_2$ (10 and 100 ng·mL) significantly decreased the fibroblast proliferation (*P <0.05). Note that OD values represent the number of viable cells in culture. (Reproduced from Cilli, F., Khan, M., Fu, F. & Wang, J.H. (2004) *Clinical Journal of Sport Medicine* **14**, 232–236 with permission.)

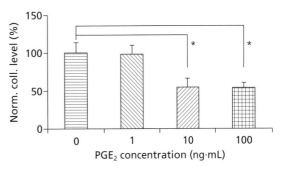

Fig. 7.13 The effect of exogenous PGE$_2$ on the collagen production of human patellar tendon fibroblasts. The addition of PGE$_2$ to cell cultures at a dosage of 10 or 100 ng·mL significantly decreased collagen production by the fibroblasts (*P <0.0001). Note that collagen levels were normalized by cell numbers and represented by percentage changes with respect to that of fibroblasts without PGE$_2$ treatment. (Reproduced from Cilli, F., Khan, M., Fu, F. & Wang, J.H. (2004) *Clinical Journal of Sport Medicine* **14**, 232–236 with permission.)

It was found that cell proliferation at 1 ng/mL PGE$_2$ was not significantly different from that of the control group. At concentrations of 10 and 100 ng/mL PGE$_2$, however, fibroblast proliferation decreased significantly by 7.3% and 10.8%, respectively, compared to cells without PGE$_2$ treatment. Also, fibroblast proliferation at 100 ng/mL PGE$_2$ was not significantly different from that at 10 ng/mL PGE$_2$ (Fig. 7.12). These results suggest that tendon fibroblast proliferation may be regulated by the secretion of PGE$_2$ by tendon fibroblasts in response to repetitive mechanical stretching *in vivo*.

We further examined the effect of PGE$_2$ on collagen secretion. Human patellar tendon fibroblasts were plated in each well of four separate 6-well plates, with 10^5 fibroblasts in each well. This high cell density was used to ensure that the cells were confluent so that cell proliferation was minimized and collagen synthesis was maximized. In addition, 25 μg/mL ascorbic acid was added to the growth medium in the wells at the time of plating to promote collagen synthesis. The cells were then incubated in this medium for 48 hours. After 48 hours, PGE$_2$, with dosages of 0 (control), 1, 10, and 100 ng/mL, were then added to individual wells of the plates. The cells were incubated in this medium for an additional 72 hours.

Using a Sircol collagen assay (Biocolor Assays, Ireland) to measure total collagen levels in the medium, it was found that there was no significant difference in collagen production at 1 ng/mL PGE$_2$ compared to the control group. However, at higher PGE$_2$ concentrations (10 and 100 ng/mL), collagen production significantly decreased by 45.2% and 45.7%, respectively. There was no statistical difference, however, in collagen production between PGE$_2$ concentrations of 10 and 100 ng/mL (Fig. 7.13). Taken together, these results show that high levels of PGE$_2$ decrease collagen production by tendon fibroblasts and suggest that high levels of PGE$_2$ present in the tendon matrix *in vivo* could not only participate in tendon inflammation but also decrease fibroblast proliferation and collagen production that could lead to tendon matrix degeneration.

In vivo studies

Many studies have pointed to the fact that repetitive mechanical loading leads to the microscopic failure of collagen fibrils or bundles with concomitant inflammatory responses in these symptomatic tendons. The understanding of tendinopathy, however, is primarily based on tissue samples taken at the time of surgery, histologic analysis of biopsy materials, and biomechanical measurement of human specimens. Therefore, they do not address the developmental mechanisms of tendinopathy (Almekinders & Temple 1998). Therefore, efforts have been made to develop injection animal models for studying tendinopathy at the cellular and molecular levels. These studies are briefly reviewed below.

Collagenase injection

In this model, bacterial collagenase was injected into the Achilles tendon of the horse or rabbit (Silver *et al.* 1983; Backman *et al.* 1990) and into the rat's supraspinatus tendon (Soslowsky *et al.* 1996). It was found that collagenase injection caused tendon degeneration at an early time but the tendon appeared to heal at a later time (Soslowsky *et al.* 1996; Stone *et al.* 1999). This model appears to represent a normal tendon healing response resulting from a "traumatic insult" to the tendon. However, the development of tendinopathy is an insidious process and in many cases, healing does not occur (Sharma & Maffulli 2005). Thus, the questions of what factors are responsible for initiating tendinopathy and how the tendon thereafter develops into pathophysiologic conditions (e.g. tendon degeneration) cannot be addressed by the collagenase injection model.

Cytokine injection

A rabbit model for the study of tendinitis was developed at the Musculoskeletal Research Center (Stone *et al.* 1999). In this model, species-matched cell activating factor (CAF), which is composed of inflammatory cytokines, was injected into rabbit patellar tendons. During the first 4 weeks, the CAF injection affected neither the cross-sectional area nor the structural properties of the tendon. By 16 weeks, however, the tendons treated with CAF failed at significantly lower loads than controls (Fig. 7.14). In contrast, collagenase injections in the study increased the cross-sectional area of the patellar tendons, indicating that healing occurred and scar tissue was produced. Collagenase injections also slightly decreased the stiffness of the patella–whole patellar tendon–tibia complex, but increased the

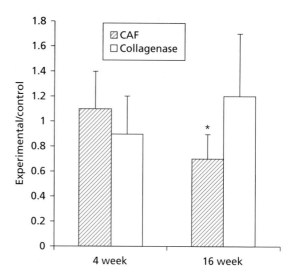

Fig. 7.14 Ultimate load of the rabbit patellar tendons injected with cytokine preparation (CAF) or collagenase after 4 and 16 weeks (*$P < 0.05$). (Reproduced from Stone, D., Green, C., Rao, U., *et al.* (1999) *Journal of Orthopaedic Research* **17**, 168–177 with permission.)

collagen cross-link density by a factor of four at 16 weeks. Tendons injected with CAF were not significantly different from their controls. Furthermore, collagen content was significantly decreased at 4 weeks compared with the control tendons that received the collagenase injection but not for those that received the CAF injection. It should be noted that this CAF model could be further improved because the CAF was produced by synovial fibroblasts treated with phorbol myristate, an inflammatory agent, instead of repetitive mechanical loading.

PGE injection

The important role of prostaglandins in the development of tendinopathy has been recognized. Peritendinous injection of PGE_1 around the rat Achilles' tendon leads to degeneration as well as inflammation around and within the tendon (Sullo *et al.* 2001). We have shown that cyclic stretching of HPTFs *in vitro* could markedly increase PGE_2 production. Also, treatment of tendon fibroblasts with PGE_2 decreases cell proliferation and collagen production *in vitro*. In addition, elevated PGE_2 levels were found in the human tendon after repetitive

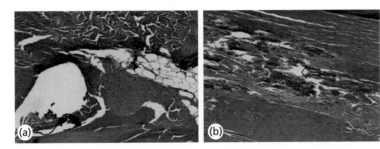

Fig. 7.15 The effect of intratendinous injection of PGE$_2$ into the rabbit patellar tendon by H&E staining. (a) With injection of 50 ng PGE$_2$, there were some fatty infiltration and areas of disorganized tissue can also be seen (arrow). (b) With injection of 500 ng PGE$_2$, more extensive degeneration and loss of parallel collagen fibrils were evident (blank arrow). (Original magnification ×10) (Reproduced from Khan, M.H., Li, Z. & Wang, J.H. (2005) *Clinical Journal of Sport Medicine* **15**, 27–33 with permission.)

mechanical loading (Langberg *et al.* 1999). Therefore, PGE$_2$ is likely to be involved in the development of tendinopathy.

To test this possibility *in vivo*, we injected PGE$_2$ into rabbit patellar tendons and examined its effect on the tendon matrix (Khan *et al.* 2005). Light microscopy of hematoxylin and eosin (H&E) stained tendon samples showed that tendons injected with 50 ng PGE$_2$ contained focal areas of degeneration. Fatty infiltration was also noted in the tendon surrounded by highly disorganized tissue (Fig. 7.15a). There was a focal area of cellular hyperproliferation, but the matrix appeared to be regular in appearance. Overall, tendons injected with 500 ng PGE$_2$ appeared much more degenerated than those injected with 50 ng PGE$_2$. The loss of parallel collagen fiber organization in the PGE$_2$-treated tendons was evident, and the presence of a large number of cells of unknown origin was noted within the tendons (Fig. 7.15b). In contrast, tendons from the three different control groups (no injection, normal saline injection, and needle-stick only) had a uniform appearance with fibroblasts arranged in parallel. In addition, fibroblasts had thin, flattened nuclei. The extracellular matrix was regular without obvious degenerative changes, and there were no inflammatory cells present. Overall, the control tendons appeared to be tightly packed and highly organized.

Transmission electron microscopy (TEM) analysis of tendons injected with 50 ng PGE$_2$ showed that the diameter of collagen fibrils appeared smaller than those of controls, and the space between fibrils was

larger and more irregular (Fig. 7.16a). Tendons injected with 500 ng PGE$_2$ appeared to show more loosely packed collagen fibrils than those injected with 50 ng PGE$_2$ (Fig. 7.16b). For control tendons that were given a needle-stick only, TEM revealed tightly packed collagen fibrils with both thick and thin fibrils organized in such a way that there was little unfilled space between them (Fig. 7.16c). Tendons injected with normal saline showed a similar tightly packed appearance (Fig. 7.16d). Quantitative analysis of the diameters of collagen fibrils showed that those treated with either 50 or 500 ng PGE$_2$ were significantly smaller than that of the saline control (Fig. 7.17); however, there was no significant difference in the collagen fibril diameter between 50 and 500 ng PGE$_2$ groups, which suggests that a low dosage of PGE$_2$ (50 ng) may have saturated the PGE$_2$ receptors (Yu *et al.* 2002) in a way that a higher dosage of PGE$_2$ (500 ng) had no further effects.

Taken together, these studies demonstrate that the "injection animal model" is a reliable, cost-effective approach to studying the molecular mechanisms of tendinopathy. The use of the "injection animal model" can be further improved by using multiple inflammatory mediators that are produced by tendon fibroblasts in response to various mechanical loading conditions.

Conclusions and future directions

Tendinopathy remains a common problem for both professional and recreational athletes. There is also

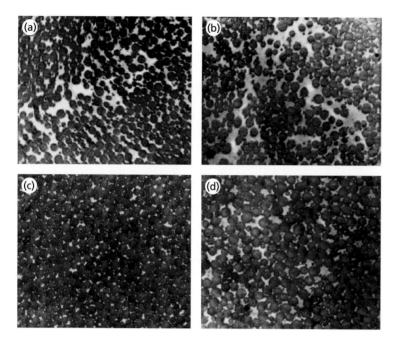

Fig. 7.16 The effect of intratendinous injection of PGE_2 on collagen fibril organization by transmission electron microscopy (TEM). It is apparent that collagen fibrils of tendons injected with 50 ng PGE_2 (a) or 500 ng PGE_2 (b) were more disorganized compared with tendons that received needle-stick only (c) or saline injection (d). (Original magnification ×8000.) (Reproduced from Khan, M.H., Li, Z. & Wang, J.H. (2005) *Clinical Journal of Sport Medicine* **15**, 27–33 with permission.)

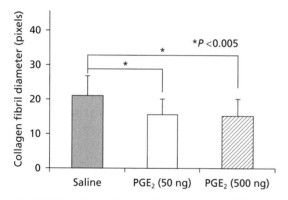

Fig. 7.17 The effect of intratendinous injection of PGE_2 on collagen fibril diameter. The diameter of collagen fibrils of tendons with injection of PGE_2 was smaller than those without PGE_2 injection. Specifically, for the 50 and 500 ng injection groups, the collagen fibril diameter (mean $\pm$ SD) was 16.1 ± 4.8 (pixels) and 15.7 ± 5.3 (pixels), respectively, compared with 21.6 ± 5.5 (pixels) in the saline injected group. (Reproduced from Khan, M.H., Li, Z. & Wang, J.H. (2005) *Clinical Journal of Sport Medicine* **15**, 27–33 with permission.)

an increased incidence of tendinopathy in occupational settings (Statistics 2001; Maffulli & Kader 2002). Although sports medicine physicians pay much attention to acute, traumatic conditions, such as frank tendon tears, chronic tendinopathy may result in a much longer delay from training and competition, or return to the workplace (Kujala *et al.* 1986). In addition, because of the limited understanding of the molecular and cellular mechanisms of tendinopathy, its treatments are largely empirical and the clinical outcome of these treatments remains unpredictable.

Therefore, to understand the mechanisms of tendinopathy better, we have developed a novel model system, which can simulate the alignment, shape, and mechanical loading conditions of human tendon fibroblasts *in vivo*. Using such a system, we have identified that repetitive mechanical stretching of human tendon fibroblasts will increase the expression and activity levels of PLA_2, enabling the cells to produce abundant AA. The repetitively stretched tendon fibroblasts also markedly increase COX expression. The elevation of COX expression is dependent upon stretching magnitude, frequency, and duration. Cyclic stretching also induced high levels of PGE_2 and LTB_4 production. Further, our data suggest that the COX and 5-LO pathways are inversely related, such that decreasing PGE_2 production increases LTB_4 levels and vice versa. Finally, *in vivo* animal studies using the rabbit patellar tendon as a model revealed that repeated exposure to PGE_2 could cause degenerative changes in the tissue. Therefore, we believe that both the COX and 5-LO pathways are responsive to repetitive mechanical loading, and their inflammatory products, including PGE_2 and LTB_4, are likely involved in the onset and/or progression of tendinopathy.

To understand further the mechanisms of tendinopathy at the molecular and cellular levels, several lines of future research are suggested. First, the role of PLA_2 in tendinopathy development needs to be investigated more closely. PLA_2 catalyzes the hydrolysis of fatty acids at the sn-2 position of glycerophospholipids and, as a result, yields AA, which has been shown to convert into two categories of inflammatory mediators: prostaglandins and leukotrienes, both of which cause tissue inflammation (Gonzalez-Buritica *et al.* 1989). We have shown that cyclic stretching of human tendon fibroblasts increases PLA_2 expression levels and its activity. This raises the possibility that stretching-induced PLA_2 may not only be responsible for initiating the production of inflammatory mediators by tendon fibroblasts, but may be also involved in the onset of tendinopathy.

Second, we need to understand more completely how prostaglandins and leukotrienes together influence tendon homeostasis. It is known that prostaglandins mediate diverse biologic processes in many types of cells, including cell proliferation (Elias *et al.* 1985a,b), inflammatory and immune responses (Harada *et al.* 1982; Betz & Fox 1991), and the production of extracellular matrix proteins (Barile *et al.* 1988; Diaz *et al.* 1993). Thus, high levels of PGE_2 production by tendon fibroblasts under repetitive, excessive mechanical loading conditions may downregulate the proliferation and protein synthesis of human tendon fibroblasts *in vivo*. On the other hand, leukotrienes such as LTB_4 are known to be a potent chemotactic agent for infiltration of neutrophils and monocytes/macrophages, which can damage tissue by releasing proteases and

reactive oxygen species. This is supported by evidence that elevated concentrations of LTB_4 were found in inflammatory disorders such as cystic fibrosis, psoriasis, chronic bronchitis, and asthma, as well as rheumatoid arthritis. Our *in vitro* studies have shown that human tendon fibroblasts produce both PGE_2 and LTB_4 following repetitive mechanical stretching conditions. However, the expression of PGE_2 and LTB_4 receptors on cell surfaces in response to repetitive mechanical stretching should also be investigated. Once this knowledge is available, therapy with PGE_2 and LTB_4 receptor antagonists may be developed to treat tendinopathy.

Third, with the advent of microarray technologies, it is now possible to determine the differential expression of a large number of genes in tendon fibroblasts subjected to various repetitive mechanical loading conditions. This approach has the potential to identify specific genes and their proteins that are involved in the onset and progression of tendinopathy. In this regard, a number of candidate genes (e.g. IL-1β, IL-6, MMP-1, MMP-3, and MMP-13) may be of special interest. These known genes and proteins as well as others could serve as "biomarkers" for the clinical diagnosis of tendinopathy in its early stages.

In addition, the interaction between the expression of cytokines, which are released at the site of tissue injury by infiltrated inflammatory cells such as neutrophils and macrophages, and various mechanical loading conditions (e.g. various stretching magnitudes) should be investigated further. Once the mechanisms of tendinopathy are better understood, the creation of animal models of tendinopathy should be pursued, which would then become more rational and more useful. With refined animal models, new and more effective protocols can be developed to minimize the occurrence of tendinopathy and treat tendinopathy in athletic settings as well as in the workplace.

What we know

- Repetitive mechanical loading of the tendon is one of the major etiologic factors that cause tendinopathy.
- Repetitive mechanical loading of human tendon

fibroblasts induces high levels of expression and production of inflammatory mediators (e.g. PLA_2, COX, PGE_2, and LTB_4).

• Repetitive mechanical loading regulates inflammatory gene expression of human tendon fibroblasts.

What we need to know

• The "biomarkers" of tendinopathy at different developmental stages.
• The effect of stretching-induced PLA_2 (e.g. $cPLA_2$ and $sPLA_2$) on tendon fibroblasts *in vitro* and on tendons *in vivo*.
• The effect of stretching-induced PGE_2 and LTB_4 and other isoforms of prostaglandins and leukotrienes on tendon fibroblasts *in vitro* and on tendons *in vivo*.
• The expression of the extracellular matrix proteins as well as MMPs under various mechanical loading conditions.
• The interaction between the production of inflammatory mediators and various mechanical loading conditions in tendon fibroblasts subjected to the treatment of inflammatory cytokines (e.g. IL-1β).

How we get there

• Refine *in vitro* models to determine inflammatory responses of human tendon fibroblasts to various repetitive mechanical loading conditions.
• Use microarray and proteomics technologies to determine the gene expression and protein production of multiple inflammatory mediators under various mechanical loading conditions.
• Use molecular techniques to determine the effects of increasing or suppressing inflammatory gene expression on human tendon fibroblasts *in vitro* and on tendons *in vivo* under mechanical loading conditions.
• Develop new technologies to accurately measure inflammatory mediators present in animal tendons under repetitive mechanical loading conditions.

Clinical revelance and significance of cell mechanobiology

Tendons consist of a complex, fibroblast-embedded matrix composed of collagen fibers, adhesion proteins, and proteoglycans. The primary function of the tendon is to transmit muscular forces to the bone. As a result of this dynamic environment, tendon fibroblasts are subjected to mechanical loading and respond by altering metabolic functions, including increasing DNA synthesis as well as production of extracellular matrix proteins (e.g. type I collagen) as part of the normal physiologic cellular responses. Pathophysiologic conditions, however, could occur under excessive, abnormal mechanical loading conditions. The consequence of pathophysiologic cellular responses is the development of tendinopathy, which includes a group of highly prevalent tendon disorders that involve tendon inflammation and degeneration. Despite its prevalence, the molecular mechanisms of tendinopathy remain poorly understood.

Cell mechanobiology, an interdisciplinary study that is concerned with the biologic responses of cells to mechanical forces and the mechanotransduction mechanisms, may aid in understanding the mechanisms of tendinopathy at the cellular and molecular levels. Because tendon fibroblasts are responsible for maintaining as well as repairing and remodeling the extracellular matrix, it is particularly important to understand how tendon fibroblasts respond to mechanical loading conditions with different magnitudes, frequencies, and durations. Therefore, *in vitro* studies that determine the response of tendon fibroblasts to various mechanical loading conditions have enhanced our understanding of tendon homeostasis as well as the pathogenesis of tendinopathy.

Nowadays, the conservative treatment of tendinopathy consists of rest, therapeutic exercise, and anti-inflammatory drugs. These clinical treatments, however, are largely empirical. Moreover, the efficacy of these treatments is relatively low and recurrences are common. The study of tendon fibroblast mechanobiology will shed new light on the pathogenesis of tendinopathy at the molecular and cellular levels. With new scientific findings, additional *in vitro* and *in vivo* models can be developed and used to optimize protocols for clinical management of tendinopathy as well as training regimens to reduce or prevent tendinopathy.

References

Almekinders, L.C. & Temple, J.D. (1998) Etiology, diagnosis, and treatment of tendonitis: an analysis of the literature [see comments]. *Medicine and Science in Sports & Exercise* **30**, 1183–1190.

Almekinders, L.C., Banes, A.J. & Ballenger, C.A. (1993) Effects of repetitive motion on human fibroblasts. *Medicine & Science in Sports & Exercise* **25**, 603–607.

Almekinders, L.C., Baynes, A.J. & Bracey, L.W. (1995) An *in vitro* investigation into the effects of repetitive motion and nonsteroidal antiinflammatory medication on human tendon fibroblasts. *American Journal of Sports Medicine* **23**, 119–123.

Archambault, J., Tsuzaki, M., Herzog, W. & Banes, A.J. (2002) Stretch and interleukin-1β induce matrix metalloproteinases in rabbit tendon cells *in vitro*. *Journal of Orthopaedic Research* **20**, 36–39.

Archambault, J.M., Wiley, J.P. & Bray, R.C. (1995) Exercise loading of tendons and the development of overuse injuries. A review of current literature. *Sports Medicine* **20**, 77–89.

Arnoczky, S.P., Tian, T., Lavagnino, M., Gardner, K., Schuler, P. & Morse, P. (2002) Activation of stress-activated protein kinases (SAPK) in tendon cells following cyclic strain: the effects of strain frequency, strain magnitude, and cytosolic calcium. *Journal of Orthopaedic Research* **20**, 947–952.

Backman, C., Boquist, L., Friden, J., Lorentzon, R. & Toolanen, G. (1990) Chronic Achilles paratenonitis with tendinosis: an experimental model in the rabbit. *Journal of Orthopaedic Research* **8**, 541–547.

Baracos, V., Rodemann, H.P., Dinarello, C.A. & Goldberg, A.L. (1983) Stimulation of muscle protein degradation and prostaglandin E_2 release by leukocytic pyrogen (interleukin-1). A mechanism for the increased degradation of muscle proteins during fever. *New England Journal of Medicine* **308**, 553–558.

Barile, F.A., Ripley-Rouzier, C., Siddiqi, Z.E. & Bienkowski, R.S. (1988) Effects of prostaglandin E_1 on collagen production and degradation in human fetal lung fibroblasts. *Archives of Biochemistry and Biophysics* **265**, 441–446.

Betz, M. & Fox, B.S. (1991) Prostaglandin E_2 inhibits production of Th1 lymphokines but not of Th2 lymphokines. *Journal of Immunology* **146**, 108–113.

Binderman, I., Zor, U., Kaye, A., Shimshoni, Z., Harell, A. & Somjen, D. (1988) The transduction of mechanical force into biochemical events in bone cells may involve activation of phospholipase A_2. *Calcified Tissue International* **42**, 261–266.

Casale, T.B., Abbas, M.K. & Carolan, E.J. (1992) Degree of neutrophil chemotaxis is dependent upon the chemoattractant and barrier. *American Journal of Respiratory Cell and Molecular Biology* **7**, 112–117.

Cilli, F., Khan, M., Fu, F. & Wang, J.H. (2004) Prostaglandin E_2 affects proliferation and collagen synthesis by human patellar tendon fibroblasts. *Clinical Journal of Sport Medicine* **14**, 232–236.

Crooks, S.W. & Stockley, R.A. (1998) Leukotriene B_4. *International Journal of Biochemistry and Cell Biology* **30**, 173–178.

Cryer, B. & Feldman, M. (1998) Cyclooxygenase-1 and cyclooxygenase-2 selectivity of widely used nonsteroidal anti-inflammatory drugs. *American Journal of Medicine* **104**, 413–421.

Dahlen, S.E., Bjork, J., Hedqvist, P., *et al.* (1981) Leukotrienes promote plasma leakage and leukocyte adhesion in postcapillary venules: *in vivo* effects with relevance to the acute inflammatory response. *Proceedings of the National Academy of Sciences (USA)* **78**, 3887–3891.

Denzlinger, C., Rapp, S., Hagmann, W. & Keppler, D. (1985) Leukotrienes as mediators in tissue trauma. *Science* **230**, 330–332.

Diaz, A., Munoz, E., Johnston, R., Korn, J.H. & Jimenez, S.A. (1993) Regulation of human lung fibroblast alpha 1(I) procollagen gene expression by tumor necrosis factor alpha, interleukin-1 beta, and prostaglandin E_2. *Journal of Biological Chemistry* **268**, 10364–10371.

Diaz, A., Varga, J. & Jimenez, S.A. (1989) Transforming growth factor-beta stimulation of lung fibroblast prostaglandin E_2 production. *Journal of Biological Chemistry* **264**, 11554–11557.

Elias, J.A., Rossman, M.D., Zurier, R.B. & Daniele, R.P. (1985a) Human alveolar macrophage inhibition of lung fibroblast growth. A prostaglandin-dependent process. *American Review of Respiratory Disease* **131**, 94–99.

Elias, J.A., Zurier, R.B., Schreiber, A.D., Leff, J.A. & Daniele, R.P. (1985b) Monocyte inhibition of lung fibroblast growth: relationship to fibroblast

prostaglandin production and density-defined monocyte subpopulations. *Journal of Leukocyte Biology* **37**, 15–28.

Geis, G.S. (1999) Update on clinical developments with celecoxib, a new specific COX-2 inhibitor: what can we expect? *Scandinavian Journal of Rheumatology Supplement* **109**, 31–37.

Gonzalez-Buritica, H., Khamashita, M.A. & Hughes, G.R. (1989) Synovial fluid phospholipase A_2s and inflammation. *Annals of the Rheumatic Diseases* **48**, 267–269.

Harada, Y., Tanaka, K., Uchida, Y., *et al.* (1982) Changes in the levels of prostaglandins and thromboxane and their roles in the accumulation of exudate in rat carrageenin-induced pleurisy: a profile analysis using gas chromatography-mass spectrometry. *Prostaglandins* **23**, 881–895.

Jarvinen, M., Józsa, L., Kannus, P., Jarvinen, T.L., Kvist, M. & Leadbetter, W. (1997) Histopathological findings in chronic tendon disorders. *Scandinavian Journal of Medicine and Science in Sports* **7**, 86–95.

Kaiser, E. (1999) Phospholipase A_2: its usefulness in laboratory diagnostics. *Critical Reviews in Clinical Laboratory Sciences* **36**, 65–163.

Khan, M.H., Li, Z. & Wang, J.H. (2005) Repeated exposure of tendon to prostaglandin-E_2 leads to localized tendon degeneration. *Clinical Journal of Sport Medicine* **15**, 27–33.

Kujala, U.M., Kvist, M. & Osterman, K. (1986) Knee injuries in athletes. Review of exertion injuries and retrospective study of outpatient sports clinic material. *Sports Medicine* **3**, 447–460.

Langberg, H., Skovgaard, D., Karamouzis, M., Bulow, J. & Kjær, M. (1999) Metabolism and inflammatory mediators in the peritendinous space measured by microdialysis during intermittent isometric exercise in humans. *Journal of Physiology* **515** (Part 3), 919–927.

Leadbetter, W.B. (1992) Cell–matrix response in tendon injury. *Clinics in Sports Medicine* **11**, 533–578.

Li, Z., Yang, G., Khan, M., Stone, D., Woo, S.L-Y. & Wang, J.H. (2004) Inflammatory response of human tendon fibroblasts to cyclic mechanical stretching. *American Journal of Sports Medicine* **32**, 435–440.

Maffulli, N. & Kader, D. (2002) Tendinopathy of tendo achillis. *Journal*

of Bone and Joint Surgery. British volume
84, 1–8.

McAdam, B.F., Mardini, I.A., Habib, A., *et al.* (2000) Effect of regulated expression of human cyclooxygenase isoforms on eicosanoid and isoeicosanoid production in inflammation. *Journal of Clinical Investigation* **105**, 1473–1482.

Pearce, M., McIntyre, T., Prescott, S., Zimmerman, G. & Whatley, R. (1996) Shear stress activates cytosolic phospholipase A_2 ($cPLA_2$) and MAP kinase in human endothelial cells. *Biochemical and Biophysical Research Communications* **218**, 500–504.

Samad, T.A., Moore, K.A., Sapirstein, A., *et al.* (2001) Interleukin-1beta-mediated induction of Cox-2 in the CNS contributes to inflammatory pain hypersensitivity. *Nature* **410**, 471–475.

Sharma, P. & Maffulli, N. (2005) Tendon injury and tendinopathy: healing and repair. *Journal of Bone and Joint Surgery. American volume* **87**, 187–202.

Silver, I.A., Brown, P.N., Goodship, A.E., *et al.* (1983) A clinical and experimental study of tendon injury, healing and treatment in the horse. *Equine Veterinary Journal Supplement* **1**, 1–43.

Smith, W.L., Garavito, R.M. & DeWitt, D.L. (1996) Prostaglandin endoperoxide H synthases (cyclooxygenases)-1 and -2. *Journal of Biological Chemistry* **271**, 33157–33160.

Soslowsky, L.J., Carpenter, J.E., DeBano, C.M., Banerji, I. & Moalli, M.R. (1996) Development and use of an animal model for investigations on rotator cuff disease. *Journal of Shoulder and Elbow Surgery* **5**, 383–392.

Soslowsky, L.J., Thomopoulos, S., Tun, S., *et al.* (2000) Neer Award 1999. Overuse activity injures the supraspinatus tendon in an animal model: a histologic and biomechanical study. *Journal of Shoulder and Elbow Surgery* **9**, 79–84.

Statistics, B.O.L. (2001) *Survey of Occupational Injuries and Illnesses in 1994.* United States Department of Labor, Washington, DC.

Stone, D., Green, C., Rao, U., *et al.* (1999) Cytokine-induced tendinitis: a preliminary study in rabbits. *Journal of Orthopaedic Research* **17**, 168–177.

Sullo, A., Maffulli, N., Capasso, G. & Testa, V. (2001) The effects of prolonged peritendinous administration of PGE_1 to the rat Achilles tendon: a possible animal model of chronic Achilles tendinopathy. *Journal of Orthopaedic Science* **6**, 349–357.

Tsuzaki, M., Guyton, G., Garrett, W., *et al.* (2003) IL-1β induces COX2, MMP-1, -3 and -13, ADAMTS-4, IL-1β and IL-6 in human tendon cells. *Journal of Orthopaedic Research* **21**, 256–264.

Unemori, E.N., Ehsani, N., Wang, M., Lee, S., McGuire, J. & Amento, E.P. (1994) Interleukin-1 and transforming growth factor-alpha: synergistic stimulation of metalloproteinases, PGE_2, and proliferation in human fibroblasts. *Experimental Cell Research* **210**, 166–171.

Vadas, P. & Pruzanski, W. (1990) Phospholipase A_2 activation is the pivotal step in the effector pathway of inflammation. *Advances in Experimental Medicine and Biology* **275**, 83–101.

Vadas, P., Wasi, S., Movat, H.Z. & Hay, J.B. (1981). Extracellular phospholipase A_2 mediates inflammatory hyperaemia. *Nature* **293**, 583–585.

Wang, J.H. (2000) Substrate deformation determines actin cytoskeleton reorganization: a mathematical modeling and experimental study. *Journal of Theoretical Biology* **202**, 33–41.

Wang, J.H., Goldschmidt-Clermont, P., Wille, J. & Yin, F.C. (2001) Specificity of endothelial cell reorientation in response to cyclic mechanical stretching. *Journal of Biomechanics* **34**, 1563–1572.

Wang, J.H., Jia, F., Yang, G., *et al.* (2003) Cyclic mechanical stretching of human tendon fibroblasts increases the production of prostaglandin E_2 and levels of cyclooxygenase expression: a novel *in vitro* model study. *Connective Tissue Research* **44**, 128–133.

Wang, J.H., Li, Z., Yang, G. & Khan, M. (2004) Repetitively stretched tendon fibroblasts produce inflammatory mediators. *Clinical Orthopaedics and Related Research* 243–250.

Yamaguchi, M., Shimizu, N., Goseki, T., *et al.* (1994) Effect of different magnitudes of tension force on prostaglandin E_2 production by human periodontal ligament cells. *Archives of Oral Biology* **39**, 877–884.

Yang, G., Crawford, R.C. & Wang, J.H. (2004) Proliferation and collagen production of human patellar tendon fibroblasts in response to cyclic uniaxial stretching in serum-free conditions. *Journal of Biomechanics* **37**, 1543–1550.

Yu, J., Prado, G.N., Schreiber, B., Polgar, P. & Taylor, L. (2002) Role of prostaglandin E_2 EP receptors and cAMP in the expression of connective tissue growth factor. *Archives of Biochemistry and Biophysics* **404**, 302–308.

Chapter 8

In Vivo Function of Human Achilles and Patella Tendons During Normal Locomotion

PAAVO V. KOMI AND MASAKI ISHIKAWA

Knowledge on the function and mechanical loading of human tendons has increased considerably when direct *in vivo* measurement techniques have been applied in natural movement situations. Two basic techniques have been used in these measurements: buckle transducer and optic fiber techniques. Both techniques have been applied in measurements of several activities, ranging from low speed walking to maximal hopping, jumping, and running. A wide range of tensile forces (1.4–9.5 kN) has been recorded under these conditions. Achilles tendon (AT) and patella tendon have been explored more extensively. AT can sustain very high forces, which in some individuals can reach as high values as 9.5 kN, corresponding to 12.5 times body weight. More important, however, is the observation that, especially during the early contact phase of running, the rate of AT force development increases linearly with the increase in running speed. This suggests that this parameter, instead of the peak force levels, should be used to characterize the loading of the tensile tissue. These direct force measurements can be complemented with simultaneous ultrasonographic recordings of the length changes in the fascicle and tendinous structures. The available information emphasizes that each muscle–tendon unit behaves individually, depending on the specific movement and intensity of effort. This basic knowledge and research of tensile/ligament loading has considerable clinical relevance, especially for treatment modalities and the design of artificial structures.

Introduction

It has been a long time wish and challenge among researchers to be able to capture exactly and continuously the loading of the various musculoskeletal structures in the human body. Especially relevant in this regard has been a need to record continuously the loading of an individual tissue (e.g. tendon or ligament) in its natural environment, i.e. when it is functioning together with other similar or different (e.g. muscle) tissues. It is very likely that the loading (and function) of a tissue may be very different when one compares the "natural" setting with that of an isolated tissue loading. The natural setting involves not only different structural elements, but also interference from the nervous system (e.g. sensory input with various connections, variable central command to the muscles). Tendons are of particular interest because, besides being an important part of the muscle–tendon complex (MTC; or muscle–tendon unit), their chief function is to transfer force produced by the contractile component to the joint and/or bone connected in series.

The human AT represents an important part of lower extremity function. It is a common tendon for the triceps surae muscle group, and it possesses considerable elastic potential. This elastic potential combined with the activities of the muscular components gives the MTC efficient possibilities for force production during locomotion. Because of their anatomic position, the AT and its muscles (soleus and gastrocnemius) are the first structures to take up the impact loads in many activities. They are therefore also accessible to either chronic or sudden injuries. To evaluate both performance potential and possible injury mechanism, it is useful to know the loads (forces) imposed on the AT or other tendons in real activity conditions. The methods used to determinate these forces have been both direct and indirect.

An indirect approach can refer to such methods as the mathematic solution of the muscle force in the indeterminate musculosketal system. This requires the grouping of muscles to reduce the number of unknowns for the appropriate equations of motion. An example of this type of approach can be taken from the study of Scott and Winter (1990) who described an AT model and its use to estimate AT loading during the stance phase of running. Electromyography (EMG) has been used to estimate loading of individual human skeletal muscles. The method may sound promising, especially because a linear or slightly curvilinear relationship can be established between EMG activity and muscular force (Komi & Buskirk 1972; Bouisset 1973), but unfortunately EMG is a very poor predictor of continuous force record, because it is very sensitive to different types of muscle action (isometric, eccentric, concentric) and to the velocity action in dynamic situations (Komi 1983). The list of problems increases when one considers that EMG is very adaptable to training and detraining (Häkkinen & Komi 1983) as well as to fatigue (Komi 1983). In certain dynamic situations such as hopping, EMG may be momentarily silent while considerable force can be recorded from the AT during the same time period (Moritani *et al*. 1990).

Considering that indirect estimates are often also time consuming, it is understandable that researchers became interested in developing methods to directly record *in vivo* human tendon and ligament forces during dynamic activities. As is often the case in technologic developments of measuring devices, tendon transducers were first developed and used in animal experiments. Salmons (1969) was the first to introduce the design of the buckle-type transducer for directly recording *in vivo* tendon forces in animals. Since then a number of experiments have

been performed to measure individual forces during cat and monkey locomotion. These buckle-type transducers are surgically implanted on selected tendons, and after an appropriate healing and recovery period, *in vivo* recording can be performed under a range of movement conditions, such as walking, running, jumping, hopping, and bicycling.

Further technical developments for direct tendon force measurements resulted in a new approach, the optic fiber technique (Komi *et al*. 1996). The present report deals with studies performed with these two methods. The material is complemented with another type of approach: *in vivo* ultrasonography, which can be used successfully for describing the behavior of human tendon during normal activities. Available information is expected to be important for understanding the mechanics of individual muscles, tendons, and ligaments *in vivo*, and consequently of relevance to biomechanists, muscle physiologists, neurophysiologists, and to those working in the delicate area of motor control.

Methods to study *in vivo* tendon loading

Implantable transducers

BUCKLE TRANSDUCER

The application of an *in vivo* measurement technique required several stages of development and trials with animals (for details see Komi *et al*. 1987). These stages included such technical questions as transducer designs, details of surgical operation, and duration of implantation. They were then followed by an experiment with a human subject in which the E-form transducer was implanted around the AT and kept *in situ* for 7 days before measurements were performed during slow walking (Komi *et al*. 1984). This type of transducer did not, however, satisfy the requirements of pain-free, natural locomotion, and the transducer design was changed to Salmons' original buckle type (Salmons 1969).

The design of the transducer has previously been presented in detail (Komi 1990; Komi *et al*. 1987, 1992). The transducer consists of a main buckle frame, two

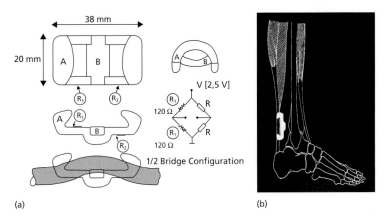

Fig. 8.1 (a) Schematic presentation of the "buckle"-type transducer designed for experiments in which human subjects could perform even maximal activities (e.g. in running and jumping). (A) Main buckle frame; (B) cross-bar. R_1 and R_2, resistors of the $1/2$ Wheatstone bridge configuration. The lower part demonstrates schematically (and with slight exaggeration) the bending of the Achilles tendon when the transducer is *in situ*. (b) Schematic presentation of the buckle transducer implanted around the Achilles tendon. (Komi *et al*. *In vivo* registration of Achilles tendon forces in man. *International Journal of Sports Medicine* **8**, 3–8, 1987. Copyright © 1987. Used with permission.)

strain gauges, and a center bar placed across the frame (Fig. 8.1). The frame and the center bar are molded from stainless steel. Three different kinds of frames are available, and each frame has three different kinds of cross-bars. The differences in frame size and in cross-bar bending ensure that a suitable transducer is available for almost any size of adult human AT. To assist in the selection of the best possible transducer size, a roentgenogram of the ankle of the subject (lateral view) is obtained before surgery. The final selection is performed during the operation, when the tendon is visible and can be easily palpated and the thickness measured again. To avoid possible sideways movement of the buckle, the width of the tendon must match the interior width of the buckle frame as closely as possible. The cross-bar is selected to allow a slight bend in the tendon. If the bending is excessive, the tendon structures may suffer damage. The transducer shown in Fig. 8.1 has a frame of middle size (38 mm in length, 20 mm in width, and 13.5 mm in height).

The transducer is implanted under local anesthesia. During the surgery, which lasts 15–20 min, the subject is in a prone position on the operating table. Fifteen to 20 mL of 1% lidocaine with adrenaline ($4\ g{\cdot}mL^{-1}$) is injected around the calcaneal tendon.

To provide normal proprioception during movements, lidocaine is not injected into the tendon or muscle tissue. Evidence has been presented that when local anesthesia is injected directly into the muscle, the myoelectric response of the muscle could be affected (Inoue & Frank 1962; Sabbahi *et al.* 1979). An incision of approximately 50 mm in length is made on the lateral side just anterior to the tendon to avoid damage to small saphenous vein and the sural nerve. The size of the buckle is matched with that of the tendon. The correct-sized cross-bar is then placed under the tendon into the slots of the frame. This causes a small bend in the tendon, as demonstrated schematically in Fig. 8.1. The cable containing the wires from the strain gauges is threaded under the skin and brought outside approximately 10 cm above the transducer. After the cut is sutured and carefully covered with sterile tapes, the cable of the transducer is connected to an amplifying unit for immediate check-up. Figure 8.1 demonstrates a lateral radiographic view of the transducer *in situ*.

Calibration of the transducer is performed immediately prior to the experiments. In contrast to animal experiments, an indirect method must be applied to calibrate the AT transducer placed on human subjects. It is performed on a special calibration table where both static and dynamic loads can be applied. The details of the calibration procedure have been explained (Komi *et al.* 1987), and some critical aspects of the procedure were subsequently discussed (Komi 1990).

Use of the buckle transducer in the study of AT force (ATF) measurements produces important parameters such as peak-to-peak force and rate of force development that can then be used to describe the loading characteristics of the tendon under normal locomotion. When these parameters are combined with other external measurements, such as cinematography for calculation of MTC length changes, the important concepts of muscle mechanics, such as instantaneous length–tension and force–velocity relationships can be examined in natural situations such as stretch–shortening cycle (SSC) activities (Fukashiro & Komi 1987; Komi 1990)

(Table 8.1). Simultaneous recording of EMG activities can add to the understanding of the force potentiation mechanism during SSC-type movement.

The major advantage of direct *in vivo* measurement is the possibility of continuous recording of ATF, which is also immediately available for inspection. The second important feature in this measurement approach is that several experiments can be performed in one session and the movements are truly natural.

The buckle transducer method is quite invasive, and may receive objections for use by the ethical committee in question. Because of the relatively large size of the buckle, there are not many tendons that can be selected for measurements. However, The AT is an ideal one because of the large space between the tendon and bony structures within the Karger triangle. Other restrictions in the use of this method are difficulties in the calibration procedure,

Table 8.1 *In vivo* tensile force measurements during natural human locomotion.

Reference	Year	Tendon	Transducer type	Movement(s)
Komi *et al.*	1984	Achilles	E-form (invasive)	Slow walking
Gregor *et al.*	1984	Achilles	Buckle (invasive)	Cycling
Komi *et al.*	1985	Achilles	Buckle (invasive)	Walking (1.2–1.8 ms^{-1}), running (3–9 ms^{-1})
Komi	1990	Achilles	Buckle (invasive)	Walking (1.2–1.8 ms^{-1}), running (3–9 ms^{-1}) and jumping
Gregor *et al.*	1991	Achilles	Buckle (invasive)	Cycling
Komi *et al.*	1992	Achilles	Buckle (invasive)	SJ, CMJ, hopping
Fukashiro *et al.*	1993	Achilles	Buckle (invasive)	SJ, CMJ
Fukashiro *et al.*	1995b	Achilles	Buckle (invasive)	SJ, CMJ, hopping
Nicol *et al.*	1995	Achilles	Optic (invasive)	Ankle dorsiflexion reflex
Gollhofer *et al.*	1995	Achilles	Optic (invasive)	Ankle dorsiflexion reflex
Komi *et al.*	1995	Achilles, Patella, Biceps brachii	Optic (invasive)	Isometric plantar flexion, Isometric knee extension, Isometric elbow flexion
Finni *et al.*	1998	Achilles	Optic (invasive)	Wasking (1.1–1.8 ms^{-1})
Arndt *et al.*	1998	Achilles	Optic (invasive)	Isometric plantarflexions
Nicol & Komi	1998	Achilles	Optic (invasive)	Passive dorsiflexion stretches
Finni *et al.*	2000	Achilles, patella	Optic (invasive)	Submaximal SJ and CMJ
Finni *et al.*	2001a	Achilles, patella	Optic (invasive)	Hopping
Finni *et al.*	2001b	Patella	Optic (invasive)	Submaximal SJ, CMJ and DJ
Finni *et al.*	2001c	Patella	Optic (invasive)	Maximal knee extension (SSC), CMJ and rebound jump
Finni & Komi	2002	Patella	Optic (invasive)	Submaximal SJ and DJ
Finni *et al.*	2003a	Patella	Optic (invasive)	Knee extension (eccentric and concentric)
Kyrolainen *et al.*	2003	Achilles	Buckle (invasive)	Running (3–5 ms^{-1}), long jump
Ishikawa *et al.*	2003	Patella	Optic (invasive)	DJ, SJ
Ishikawa *et al.*	2005b	Achilles	Optic (invasive)	Walking (1.4 ms^{-1})

CMJ, countermovement jump; DJ, drop jump; SJ, squat jump; SSC, stretch–shortening cycle.

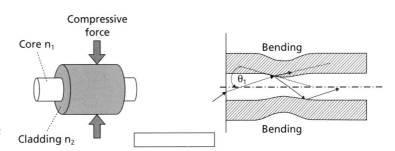

Fig. 8.2 Basic principle demonstrating how the compression on the optic fiber (left) causes microbending (right) and loss of light through the core–cladding interface.

and problems in the application of the technique when long-term and repeated implantation may be of interest. As is the case in animal experiments, the buckle transducer method cannot isolate the forces of the contractile tissue from the tendon tissues. The method can therefore be used to demonstrate the loading characteristics of the entire MTC only.

OPTIC FIBER TECHNIQUE

In order to overcome some of the disadvantages of the buckle transducer technique, an alternative method has recently been developed. As was the case for the buckle method, this new optic fiber technique was also first applied to animal tendon (Komi *et al.* 1996). However, it had already been applied with success as a pressure transducer in sensitive skin applications (Bocquet & Noel 1987) and for measurement of foot pressure in different phases of cross-country skiing (Candau *et al.* 1993). The measurement is based on light intensity modulation by mechanical modification of the geometric properties of the plastic fiber. The structures of optical fibers used in animal and human experiments (Komi *et al.* 1996; Arndt *et al.* 1998; Finni *et al.* 1998, 2000) consist of two-layered cylinders of polymers with small diameters. When the fiber is bent or compressed, the light can be reduced linearly with pressure. The sensitivity is dependent on fiber index, fiber stiffness, and bending radius characteristics. Figure 8.2 characterizes the principle of the light modulation in the two-layer (cladding and core) fiber when the fiber diameter is compressed by an external force. The core and cladding will be deformed and a certain amount of light is transferred through the core–cladding interface. In order

to avoid the pure effect of bending of the fiber, the fiber must have a loop large enough to exceed the critical bending radius when inserted through the tendon (Fig. 8.3).

Figure 8.3 demonstrates how the optic fiber is inserted through the tendon. A hollow 19-gauge needle is first passed through the tendon (Fig. 8.3a). The sterile optic fiber is then passed through the needle; the needle is removed and the fiber remains *in situ* (Fig. 8.3b). Both ends of the fiber are then attached to the transmitter receiver unit and the system is ready for measurement (Fig. 8.3c). The calibration procedure usually produces a good linear relationship between external force and optic fiber signal. Figure 8.4 shows a representative example of such a relationship for the patella tendon measurements. The optic fiber technique has recently been applied to study mechanical behavior of AT and patella tendons in several experiments. Table 8.1 includes the most important references.

Although the optic fiber method may not be more accurate than the buckle transducer method, it has several unique advantages. First of all, it is much less invasive and can be reapplied to the same tendon after a few days' rest. In addition, almost any tendon can be studied, provided the critical bending radius is not exceeded. The optic fiber technique can also be applied to measure the loading of various ligaments. In the hands of an experienced surgeon, the optic fiber can be inserted even through deeper ligaments such as the anterior talofibular ligament. In such a case, however, special care must be taken to ensure that the optic fiber is in contact with the ligament only and that it is preserved from interaction with other soft tissue structures by catheters.

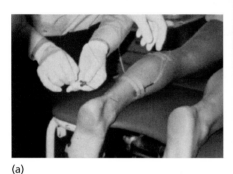

(a)

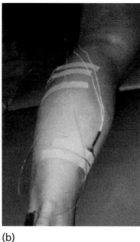

(b)

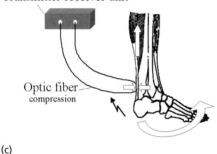

(c)

Fig. 8.3 Demonstration of the insertion of the optic fiber into the tendon. (a) After the 19-gauge needle has been inserted through the tendon, the 0.5-mm thick optic fiber is threaded through the needle. The needle is then removed and the optic fiber remains *in situ* inside the tendon (b), and both ends of the fiber are connected to the transmitter receiver unit (c). In real measurement situations this unit is much smaller and can be fastened on skin of the calf muscles. (Komi. Stretch–shortening cycle. *Journal of Biomechanics* **33**, 1197–1206, 2000. Copyright © 2000. Used with permission.)

Non-invasive scanning of fascicle–tendinous tissues

ULTRASONOGRAPHY

Since Howry (1965) demonstrated an ultrasonic echo interface between tissues such as that between fat and muscle, the B-mode ultrasonographic scanning of the non-invasive technique was used primarily to characterize the skeletal muscle gross architecture *in vivo* (Ikai & Fukunaga 1968, Yeh & Wolf 1978). High-quality imaging techniques, such as X-ray photography, magnetic resonance imaging (MRI), and ultrasonography have then been made available to non-invasively and directly estimate skeletal muscle architecture during static move-

ment conditions (Fellows & Rack 1987; Rugg *et al.* 1990; Fukunaga *et al.* 1992, 1996; Henriksson-Larsen *et al.* 1992, Rutherford & Jones 1992; Kawakami *et al.* 1993; Finni *et al.* 2003b). These techniques have now been extended to natural locomotion, and the instantaneous length changes in the fascicles and tendinous tissues (TT) can be estimated during human dynamic movements (Table 8.2).

Skeletal muscles consist of the juxtaposed bundles of parallel muscle fibers with ensheathing connective tissues. Each fascicle is comprised of several muscle fibers arranged in parallel and in series (Hijikata *et al.* 1993). In real-time ultrasonography, longitudinal sectional images over the mid-belly of the muscle are usually obtained with B-mode ultrasonic scanning on a linear array probe (electronic

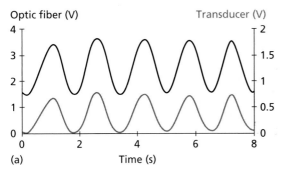

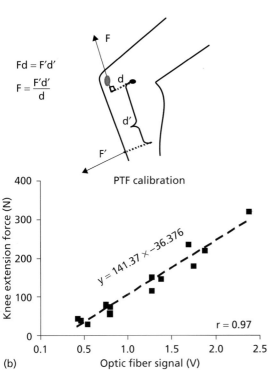

Fig. 8.4 (a) Records of an optic fiber and an external force transducer during quick dynamic loading and unloading of the knee extension movement. Please note how the two records follow each other. (b) Measured forces and moment arms for the calibration of patellar tendon force (PTF). The optic fiber output was related to the muscle force (F) that had been converted from the external force output (F') using equation Fd = Fd', where d is the moment arm of tendon force and d' the moment arm of the foot or leg. (Finni *et al. In vivo* triceps surae and quadriceps femoris muscle function in a squat jump and counter movement jump. *European Journal of Applied Physiology* **83**, 416–426, 2000. Copyright © 2000. Used with permission.)

transducer). In this scanning, muscle fascicles can appear as dark (hypoechogenic) lines lying between light (echogenic) striations of fat or connective tissue (Fig. 8.5) and run from the superficial to the deep aponeurosis. The precision, linearity, and reproducibility of this method have been confirmed (Henriksson-Larsen *et al.* 1992; Rutherford & Jones 1992; Kawakami *et al.* 1993, 2000). During human dynamic movements, the fascicles can be monitored directly by ultrasonic echoes from interfascicle connective tissues and aponeurosis.

IDENTIFICATION OF THE TENSILE STRUCTURES

According to Hill's classic model (Hill 1938), the MTC consists of contractile and series elastic components (CC and SEC, respectively). The major part of the SEC is located in the TT of a muscle. Some fundamental characteristics of SEC with regard to tendon have been documented (e.g. Huijing 1992). Generally, TT consists of the outer tendon and internal tendinous sheet, which is referred to as aponeurosis. For example, in measuring elasticity of TT in medial gastrocnemius (MG) during isometric plantarflexion contraction, the traveling distance on the cross-point of one certain fascicle on the deeper aponeurosis during the contraction can be measured from the series of ultrasonographic images (Fig. 8.5a). This distance can indicate the lengthening of deep aponeurosis and distal tendon because the cross-point between superficial aponeurosis and fascicles do not usually move during isometric contraction (Fukashiro *et al.* 1995b; Ito *et al.* 1998; Kubo *et al.* 1999). Another approach is to scan the end-point echo of MG tendon in the myotendinous junction (Fig. 8.5b). The traveling displacement of the reference point (the arrow point in Fig. 8.5b) during contraction is considered to represent the tendon elongation upon the loading (Maganaris & Paul 2000). In isometric conditions, the properties of TT and outer tendon are expressed by stress–strain and force–length relations, respectively. Stress indicates the force applied per unit area of outer tendon (cross-sectional area). Strain represents the length changes in TT relative to its initial length. The change in force can be obtained from the direct

Reference	Year	Muscle(s)	Movement(s)
Kubo *et al.*	2000	MG	Plantar flexion (SSC)
Fukunaga *et al.*	2001	MG	Walking (0.8 ms⁻¹)
Muraoka *et al.*	2001	VL	Cycling (pedaling)
Kurokawa *et al.*	2001	MG	SJ
Fukunaga *et al.*	2002a	Review (MG, VL)	
Fukunaga *et al.*	2002b	MG	Plantar flexion (SSC)
Kawakami *et al.*	2002	MG	Plantar flexion (SSC)
Finni & Komi	2002	VL	Submaximal SJ and DJ
Ishikawa *et al.*	2003	VL, MG	SJ, DJ
Kurokawa *et al.*	2003	MG	Countermovement jump

Table 8.2 Studies, which have applied the real-time fascicle and tendon length measurement during dynamic human movements.

DJ, drop jump; MG, medial gastrocnemius; SJ, squat jump; SSC, stretch–shortening cycle; VL, vastus lateralis.

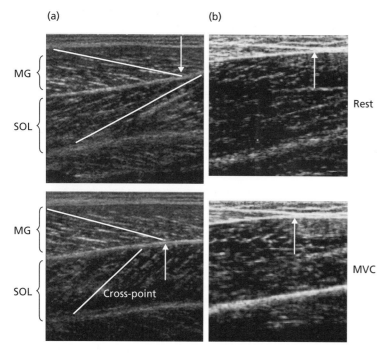

(a)   (b)

MG

SOL

Rest

MG

SOL

Cross-point

MVC

Fig. 8.5 Ultrasonographic images of the medial gastrocnemius (MG) and soleus (SOL) muscles during rest (top) and maximal voluntary isometric contraction (MVC; bottom). (a) The lines represent the selected fascicles of the two muscles. Please note the change in the length of the fascicles and in their pennation angles of each muscle. The cross-points are also shifted from rest to MVC. (b) The arrows show the end-point of MG tendon in the myotendinous junction.

in vivo tendon force measurements in the manner shown in the previous paragraphs. The distance traveled by a certain measured point in the ultrasonic echo can then be synchronized with the force record. The slope of the stress–strain and force–length relation is defined as stiffness of TT.

It must be pointed out, however, that this approach cannot yet be applied to dynamic movements because both the cross-points of the fascicle insertion and the origin can move during muscle activity. Also, the changes of the moment arm during the joint angle changes can affect the whole MTC length. Figure 8.6 uses a schematic model to illustrate how the length changes of TT can be estimated during dynamic movement conditions. In this model, the instantaneous length changes of TT are obtained by subtracting the horizontal part of the fascicle from MTC length. Muscle fascicle

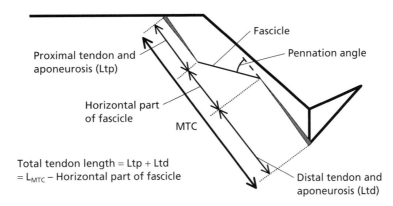

Total tendon length = Ltp + Ltd
= L$_{MTC}$ – Horizontal part of fascicle

Fig. 8.6 Schematic model illustrating how the tensile structures of the medial gastrocnemius muscle can be identified and their changes measured during dynamic movement conditions. The method requires that the total muscle–tendon complex (MTC) length is recorded continuously (e.g. cinematically during locomotion). The rest of the measurements are based on the continuous ultrasound records, such as shown in Fig. 8.5. The kinematics and ultrasononic records need to be time synchronized naturally. (After Zajac 1989; Kubo *et al.* 2000; Fukunaga *et al.* 2001; Kurokawa *et al.* 2001.)

lengths are then measured by taking the line distance between origin and insertion of the most clearly visualized muscle fascicles (Fukunaga *et al.* 2001; Kurokawa *et al.* 2001, 2003; Ishikawa *et al.* 2003, 2005a).

METHODOLOGIC PROBLEMS AND POSSIBLE ERRORS

To apply ultrasonography in dynamic movements, the appropriate probe frequency should be selected according to the width of the muscle region of interest. While probes producing higher frequencies have less penetrating ability, probes producing lower frequencies will provide greater depth of penetration but with less well-defined images. In most cases with human muscles, scanning is usually performed using the 5.0–7.5 MHz probes, although the evaluation of superficial muscle and tendons requires the use of the 7.5–10 MHz probes (Fornage 1986a,b). In addition, dynamic movements require an appropriately selected time resolution of ultrasonographic scan sampling (Kaya *et al.* 2002; Ishikawa *et al.* 2005a,b). After the probe has been selected, it is then placed over the mid-belly of the selected muscle. The soundhead is tipped slightly and medially or laterally to find the best images, which coincides with the plane of the muscle

fascicle (Herbert & Gandevia 1995; Narici *et al.* 1996). The investigator visually confirms the echoes reflected from aponeuroses and interspaces in order to avoid echoes of the reverberation artifacts and pitfalls of vascular origin. It must be noted, however, that in many cases with adult human superficial muscles, the probe length (e.g. 60 mm) does not cover the entire length of the fascicle. For this reason, appropriate approximations have been adapted for obtaining correct estimates of changes in the tensile structure lengths (Finni & Komi 2002; Muraoka *et al.* 2001; Ishikawa *et al.* 2003).

Tensile loading and locomotion

Achilles tendon loading during normal activities

As walking is a typical activity in humans, the first AT *in vivo* loadings were applied to normal walking (Komi *et al.* 1985; Komi 1990). Figure 8.7 is a representative example of what the buckle transducer records when the subjects walked on the long force platform at various constant speeds ranging from 1.2 to 1.8 m·s^{-1}. Each individual curve represents an averaged curve of a minimum of four ipsilanteral contacts. Figure 8.7 also demonstrates the occurrence of the slack in ATF upon the heel contact. The heel contact occurs at the instant of increase in the

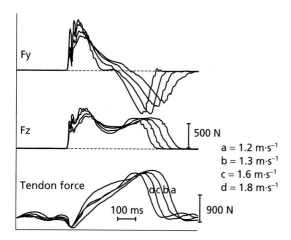

Fig. 8.7 Achilles tendon force curves during walking at different speeds. The beginning of the upward reflection of the ground reaction force curves (Fz and Fy) shows the heel contact (Komi *et al.* Biomechanical loading of Achilles tendon during normal locomotion (Komi *et al.* Biomechanical loading of Achilles tendon during normal locomotion. *Clinics in Sport Medicine* **11**, 521–531, 1992. Copyright © 1992. Used with permission).

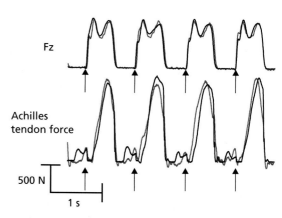

Fig. 8.8 Achilles tendon (optic fiber) and Fz ground reaction forces measured for one subject while walking at the same speed at after a 4-month interval. Black line: 1st measurement, gray line: 2nd measurement. The arrows represent the first point of heel contact with the ground.

vertical (Fz) and horizontal (Fy) curves of the force platform reaction forces. The peak-to-peak amplitude of ATF reached the value of 2.6 kN corresponding to 5.9 kN·$(cm^2)^{-1}$ when the cross-sectional area of the AT was 0.44 cm^2 in this particular subject. This peak value seems to be similar across all speeds, whereas the rate of ATF development is sensitive to speed so that it increases at faster walking.

Similar ATF records have been obtained recently with the optic fiber technique (Finni *et al.* 1998). It is also worth noting that the optic fiber recording can be very reproducible provided the research team has enough experiences in its application. Figure 8.8 is an excellent example of the similarity of ATF patterns when the subject walked at the same speed during a 4-month interval.

Sudden release of ATF upon heal contact on the ground (Figs 8.7 & 8.8) demonstrates that ATF loading is indeed very dynamic and variable. A similar pattern also occurs in running, where the sudden release of ATF is very clear in heel running (Fig. 8.9). This sudden release usually coincides with the release of electromyographic activation of the tibialis anterior muscle, resulting in a reduction

in stretch of the AT. Consequently, the velocity of plantar flexion is momentarily greater than the shortening velocity of the active soleus and gastrocnemius muscles. On the other hand, running with the ball contact (Fig. 8.9) results in a slightly different ATF response. The quick release of the force is almost absent in these curves.

The loading of AT has been usually characterized by the magnitude of the peak ATF. Figure 8.10(a) gives an example of one subject, who ran at different constant speeds. The highest maximum ATF was already attained at a speed of 6 m·s^{-1}, in which case the value was 9 kN corresponding to 12.5 body weight. When the cross-sectional area of the tendon was 0.81 cm^2, the peak force for this subject was 11 kN·$(cm^2)^{-1}$. This value is well above the range of the single load ultimate tensile strength (Butler *et al.* 1984) and also higher than those observed by Scott and Winter (1990) from their AT model calculations. It must be noted, however, that at the same speed of running, the different subjects seemed to obtain different ATFs. Thus, no representative average ATF values can be presented at this time. The Scott and Winter model (1990) provided similar observations as those in Fig. 8.10 in that the greatest tendon force was not obtained at the highest speeds. Thus, the plateauing of ATF after 6 m·s^{-1} in Fig. 8.10 may suggest re-examining the importance of the force

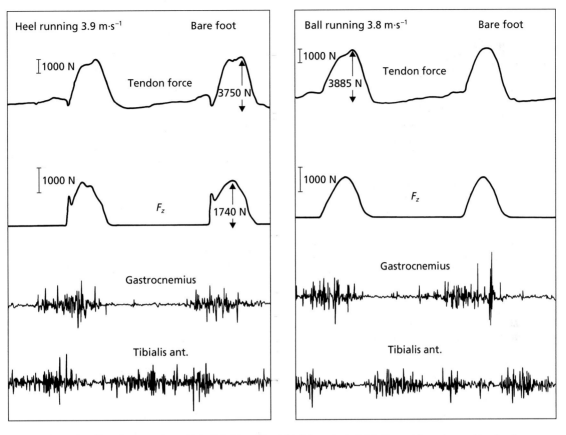

Fig. 8.9 Example of barefoot running with ball (left) and heel (right) contacts. Note the sudden release of tendon force upon heel contact on the force plate plate. (Komi P.V. Relevance of *in vivo* force measurements to human biomechanics. *Journal of Biomechanics* **23** (Suppl. 1), 23–34, 1990. Copyright © 1990. Used with permission.)

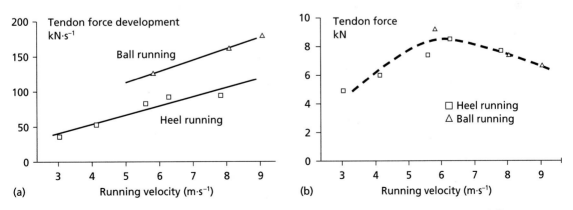

Fig. 8.10 Peak tendon forces (a) and peak rate of tendon force development (b) for one subject running at different velocities. (Komi P.V. Relevance of *in vivo* force measurements to human biomechanics. *Journal of Biomechanics* **23** (Suppl. 1), 23–34, 1990. Copyright © 1990. Used with permission.)

magnitude to characterize the loads imposed on the AT during various conditions. Figure 8.10(b) demonstrates that the highest rate of ATF development linearly increased in both running conditions with the increase in running speeds. Consequently, instead of emphasizing the magnitude of forces only, it may be more relevant for future discussions of tissue loading in living organisms to look at the rates at which the forces are developing at particular loading phases.

HOPPING AND JUMPING

Loading of individual MTC is naturally dependent on how specifically the movement influences the respective joints. For example, a vertical jump on a force platform can be performed in different ways, and one could expect the AT to become also correspondingly differently loaded. There are three examples of jumps and hops on the force platform that have been used in connection with ATF measurements:

1 Maximal vertical jump from a squat position without countermovement. This condition is performed as a pure concentric action and is called a squatting jump (SJ) (Komi & Bosco 1978);

2 Maximal vertical jump from an erect standing position with a preliminary countermovement. This jump is called a countermovement jump (CMJ) (Komi & Bosco 1978); and

3 Repetitive submaximal hopping in place with preferred frequency.

Figure 8.11 presents the results from a representative subject who performed these jumps while keeping his hands on his hips. It is noteworthy from this figure that although the peak ATFs in maximal SJ and maximal CMJ were 2.2 and 1.9 kN, the respective value in the very submaximal hopping was much higher, 4.0 kN. Hopping is characterized by the large mechanical work of the ankle joint and quite small work of the hip joint (Fukashiro & Komi 1987). It can further be suggested that the submaximal hopping with preferred frequency demonstrates great use of the elastic potential of the plantar flexor muscles.

The long jump is expected to be an activity where the joints, muscles, and tendons are highly loaded.

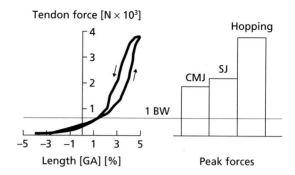

Fig. 8.11 Peak Achilles tendon forces in maximal countermovement (CMJ) and squatting (SJ) jumps as well as in submaximal hopping. The left side of the figure gives the force–length relationship during hopping for the contact phase on the ground. The length axis refers to the gastrocnemius muscle. (Komi *et al.* Biomechanical loading of Achilles tendon during normal locomotion. *Clinics in Sport Medicine* **11**, 521–531, 1992. Copyright © 1992. Used with permission).

Much to our surprise, the peak-to-peak ATF values were relatively low (approximately 2000 N) at the end of the braking of the long jump take-off motion (Fig. 8.12). The subject was an experienced former long jumper. More importantly, however, the sudden release of ATF upon heal contact was very dramatic, especially in the near maximal effort condition.

Comparison between patella and Achilles tendon loading in different activities

Compared with AT, patella tendon has not been as frequently examined for *in vivo* direct measurements during human movement. However, there are some efforts that are worth introducing here. Ishikawa *et al.* (2003) instructed their subjects to make maximal SJ, CMJ, and submaximal drop jumps (DJ) (the rebound jump height was equal to SJ) on a sledge apparatus. In these conditions, patella tendon force (PTF), as measured with the optic fiber technique, reached its highest values (approximately 7 kN) in DJ (Fig. 8.13). The respective values in maximal SJ and CMJ conditions were 3 and 6.5 kN, respectively. These movements also demonstrated another important feature of

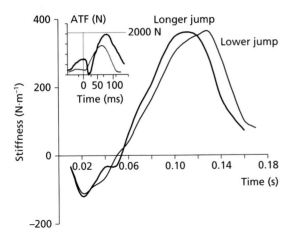

Fig. 8.12 The tendomuscular stiffness–time curves of the Achilles tendon–triceps surae muscle complex during the take-off contact phases of two different long jumps, good and low performances. Please note the dramatic Achilles tendon force (ATF) reduction immediately after heel contact during the long jump. ATF–time curves are shown in the insert for the longer jump (thick line) and for running at 5 m·s⁻¹ (gray line). (Kyrolainen *et al.* Neuromuscular behaviour of the triceps surae muscle–tendon complex during running and jumping. *International Journal of Sports Medicine* **24**, 153–155, 2003. Copyright © 2003. Used with permission.)

intramuscular behavior. The length change in MTC did not necessarily coincide with the length changes experienced by the fascicle and TT during SSC (see also Finni *et al.* 2001b; Fukunaga *et al.* 2001;

Kurokawa *et al.* 2001). They also suggest that TT is lengthened and subsequently shortened during the contact phase in all conditions; energy storage and its release from TT only occur in SJ performance (Kurokawa *et al.* 2001).

Another important observation from the work of Ishikawa *et al.* (2003) is that during high intensity DJs, the entire MTC showed dramatic shortening during the last movements of the push-off. This was entirely due to the quick recoil (shortening) of TT, as the fascicles changed its length only slightly during this phase. The clinical and performance-related significance of this phenomenon needs further exploration.

Fukashiro and Komi (1987) demonstrated with indirect estimation that the mechanical work of knee extension and plantar flexion may be considerably different depending on the type of activity. For example, knee extension produces greater work in CMJ, whereas the plantar flexors do the same in hopping. On the tendon level, this would imply that the patella tendon is more loaded in CMJ and the AT more in hopping. Our recent measurements with the optic fiber technique confirmed this suggestion. Figure 8.14 is from the work of Finni *et al.* (2000) and shows that in CMJ, PTF is greater than ATF and that in hopping the situation is the opposite. Secondly, when increasing the intensity of activity PTF increased more in CMJ and ATF more in hopping.

Fig. 8.13 Examples of length changes in the fascicle and tendinous tissues in the vastus lateralis (VL) during squat-jumps (SJ; left), countermovement jumps (CMJ; middle) and drop-jumps (DJ; right). The figures show respective electromyograph (EMG) activities as well as the patella tendon force (optic fiber technique) and the sledge force plate force. Dashed lines refer to the first contact (DJ) or the beginning of movements (SJ, CMJ), end of braking phase and the take-off moment, respectively.

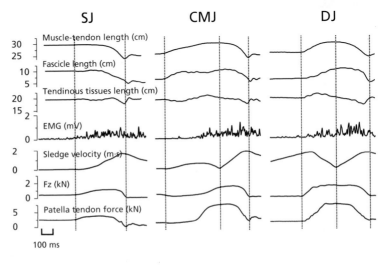

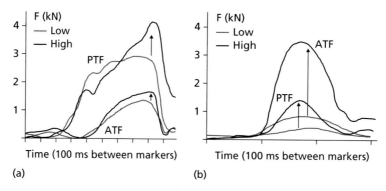

Fig. 8.14 Effect of intensity on tendon loading. During the large amplitude movements such as CMJ (a) or hopping with 56° knee joint displacement the patellar tendon was primarily loaded. In small amplitude hopping with knee flexion of 23° during the ground contact phase the Achilles tendon produced greatest forces (b). Increase in jumping intensity (upward arrows) did not alter the loading patterns but the peak forces were increased (Finni *et al. In vivo* triceps surae and quadriceps femoris muscle function in a squat jump and counter movement jump. *European Journal of Applied Physiology* **83**, 416–426, 2000. Copyright © 2000. Used with permission.)

Muscle mechanics and tendon loading during normal locomotion

WHOLE MUSCLE–TENDON COMPLEX

Hopping and running are typical examples of SSC activities where force and/or performance of MTC is potentiated (see e.g. Komi 2000). However, it is not the purpose of this article to go into the details of different possibilities in the potentiation mechanisms but, in order to characterize the loading (and role) of the tendinous structures in this phenomenon, it is important to first describe how the entire MTC behaves during SSC. The nature of force potentiation can be explored by looking first at the analog signals of AT (e.g. in running) (Fig. 8.15). The instantaneous force–length and force–velocity curves can then be computed from the parameters shown in Fig. 8.15. Figure 8.16 presents results of such an analysis from fast running, and it covers the functional ground contact phase only. It is important to note from this figure that the force–length curve demonstrates a very sharp increase in force during the stretching phase, which is characterized by a very small change in muscle length. Figure 8.16(b) shows the computed instantaneous force–velocity comparison suggesting high potentiation during the shortening phase (concentric

action). Figure 8.17 represents examples of EMG–length and EMG–velocity plots for moderate running. It clearly demonstrates that muscle activation levels are variable and primarily concentrated for the eccentric part of the cycle. This is important to consider when comparing the naturally occurring SSC actions with those obtained with isolated muscle preparations and constant activation levels throughout the cycle.

The classic force–velocity (F–V) relationship (Hill 1938) describes the fundamental mechanical properties of skeletal muscle. Its direct application to natural locomotion, such as SSC, may be difficult because of the necessity of *in situ* preparations to utilize constant maximal activation. When measured *in vivo* during SSC, the obtained F–V curve (Fig. 8.16) is a dramatic demonstration that the curves are very dissimilar to the classic curve obtained for the pure concentric action with isolated muscle preparations (e.g. Hill 1938) or with human forearm flexors (e.g. Wilkie 1950; Komi 1973). Although Fig. 8.16 does not present directly the comparison of the F–V curve for the final concentric (push-off) phase with the classic curve, it certainly suggests considerable force potentiation. Unfortunately, the human experiment as shown in Fig. 8.16 did not include comparative records obtained in a classic way. However, our recent

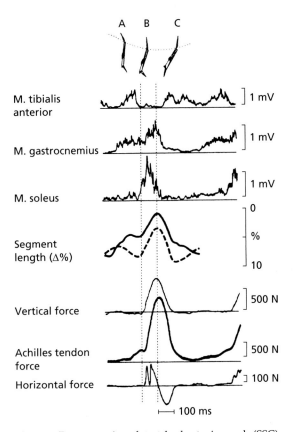

A   B   C

M. tibialis
anterior   ] 1 mV

M. gastrocnemius   ] 1 mV

M. soleus   ] 1 mV

                                                            0

Segment   %
length (Δ%)
                                                            10

Vertical force   ] 500 N

Achilles tendon
force   ] 500 N

Horizontal force   ] 100 N

⊢——⊣ 100 ms

Fig. 8.15 Demonstration of stretch–shortening cycle (SSC)
for the triceps surae muscle during the (functional)
ground contact phase of human running. Top: Schematic
position representing the three phases of SSC presented in
Fig. 8.1. The rest of the curves represent parameters in the
following order (from top to bottom): Rectified surface
EMG records of the tibialis anterior, gastrocnemius and
soleus muscles, segmental length changes of the two
plantar flexor muscles, vertical ground reaction force,
directly recorded Achilles tendon force, and the
horizontal ground reaction force. The vertical line
signifies the beginning of the foot (ball) contact on the
force plate. The subject was running at moderate speed
(Komi P.V. Relevance of *in vivo* force measurements to
human biomechanics. *Journal of Biomechanics* **23** (Suppl. 1),
23–34, 1990. Copyright © 1990. Used with permission.)

in vivo measurements with an optic fiber technique
were performed to obtain these comparisons (Finni
et al. 1998) (Fig. 8.17).

Although not yet performed at high running
speeds, these recent experiments with the optic fiber

technique suggest similar potentiation. Figure 8.18(a)
shows simultaneous plots for both PTF and ATF
during hopping. The records signify that in short
contact hopping the triceps surae muscle behaves in
a bouncing ball-type action (see also Fukashiro &
Komi 1987; Fukashiro *et al.* 1993, 1995b). When the
hopping intensity is increased or changed to CMJ,
the patella tendon force increases and the ATF may
decrease (Finni *et al.* 1998). The classic type of curve
obtained with constant maximal activation for an
isolated concentric action is also superimposed in
the same graph with the ATF (Fig. 8.18a). The
shaded area between the two AT curves suggests a
remarkable force potentiation for this submaximal
effort. It must be emphasized that the performance
potentiation in these comparisons has been made
between submaximal SSC and maximal isolated
concentric action.

Many of the *in vivo* measurement techniques
for humans have been developed following reports
on animal experiments (Sherif *et al.* 1983). Some of
these animal studies have included similar parameters to those used in our human studies, such as
muscle length, force, and EMG. The most relevant
report for comparison with our human experiments is that by Gregor *et al.* (1988); they measured
mechanical outputs of the cat soleus muscle during
treadmill locomotion. In that study, the results indicated that the force generated at a given shortening
velocity during the late stance phase was greater,
especially at higher speeds of locomotion, than the
output generated at the same shortening velocity
in situ. Thus, both animal and human *in vivo* experiments seem to give similar results with regard to the
F–V relationships during SSC.

The difference between the F–V curve and the
classic curve in isolated muscle preparations (Hill
1938) or in human experiments (Wilkie 1950; Komi
1973) may be partly brought about by natural differences in muscle activation levels between the two
types of activities. While the *in situ* preparations
may primarily measure the shortening properties
of the contractile elements in the muscle, natural
locomotion, primarily utilizing SSC action, involves
controlled release of high forces, caused primarily
by the eccentric action. This high force favors storage of elastic strain energy in the MTC. A portion of

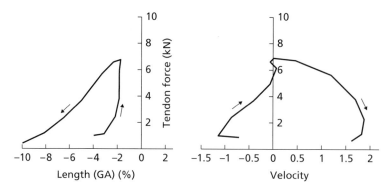

Fig. 8.16 Instantaneous force–length and force–velocity curves of the gastrocnemius muscle for stretch–shortening cycle (SSC) when the subject ran at fast speed (9 m·s⁻¹). The upward deflection signifies stretching (eccentric action) while the downward deflection signifies shortening (concentric action) of the muscle during ground contact. The horizontal axes have been derived from segmental length changes according to Grieve *et al.* (1978). (Komi P.V. Relevance of *in vivo* force measurements to human biomechanics. *Journal of Biomechanics* **23** (Suppl. 1), 23–34, 1990. Copyright © 1990. Used with permission.)

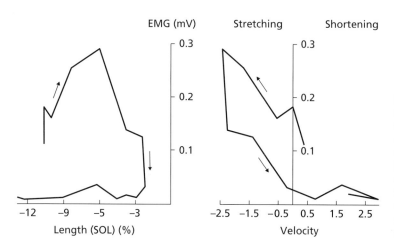

Fig. 8.17 Instantaneous EMG–length and EMG–velocity curves of the soleus muscle for stretch–shortening cycle (SSC) when the subject ran at moderate speed. The arrows indicate how the events changed from stretching to shortening during the contact phase. Please note that the EMG activity is primarily concentrated for the eccentric part of the cycle.

this stored energy can be recovered during the subsequent shortening phase and used for performance potentiation. Both animal and human experiments seem therefore to agree that natural locomotion with primarily SSC muscle action may produce muscle outputs that can be very different to the conditions of isolated preparations, where activation levels are held constant and storage of strain energy is limited. The SSC enables the triceps surae muscle to perform very efficiently in activities such as walking, running, and hopping. Recent evidence has demonstrated that the gastrocnemius and soleus muscles also function in bicycling in SSC, although

the active stretching phases are not so apparent as in running or jumping (Gregor *et al.* 1988, 1991).

Important additional features can be seen in Fig. 8.18. The patterns between ATF and PTF records differ considerably when the movement is changed from a CMJ to hopping. On CMJ—characterized by a smaller eccentric phase—the patella tendon is much more loaded than the AT, which is more strongly loaded in hopping. Thus, the muscle mechanics are not similar in all SSC activities, and generalizations should not be made from one condition and from one specific muscle only. In contrast to hopping, for example, the elastic recoil

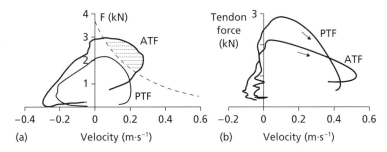

Fig. 8.18 Examples of instantaneous force–velocity curves measured in human hopping and countermovement jumps. The records in (a) (submaximal hopping) present greater loading of the Achilles tendon (ATF) compared to the patella tendon (PTF). The situation is reversed in the case of countermovement jumps (b). The records signify the functional phases of the ground contact. The left side of both figures represent eccentric action and the right side concentric action. The dashed line signifies the force–velocity curve for plantar flexors measured in the classic way. (After Finni *et al.* 2000, 2001a.)

of the triceps surae muscle plays a much smaller role in CMJ (Fukashiro *et al.* 1993, 1995b; Finni *et al.* 1998). This is expected because in CMJ the stretch phase is slow and the reflex contribution to SSC potentiation is likely to be much less than in hopping.

One important note of caution is necessary when interpreting the muscle mechanics based on the methods shown above. Both in animal and human experiments—when the buckles and optic fibers have been applied to the tendons—the measured forces cannot be used to isolate the forces or the movements of the contractile tissue from those of the tendon tissue. The methods can therefore be used to determinate the loading characteristics of the entire MTC only. It must be mentioned, however, that the fascicle F–V curves in isolated forms of maximal eccentric and concentric action resemble the classic F–V relationships quite well, and that the instantaneous F–V curve in SSC resembles that of the total MTC, but with a more irregular form.

TENDON TISSUE LOADING DURING DYNAMIC MOVEMENTS AS MEASURED BY ULTRASONOGRAPHY

Ultrasonography has been mostly applied to describe the behavior of the contractile tissue (fascicles) during human movement. As is evident from Fig. 8.6, changes in TT can be calculated simultaneously with the fascicle record. This isolation is important, because the fascicle displacement, pennation angle of muscle fibers, and tendon strain can substantially affect the entire MTC length, and has different implications for muscle–tendon function (Fukunaga *et al.* 2001; Ishikawa *et al.* 2003, 2005a,c). Figure 8.19 shows the fascicle–TT behavior during the different rebound intensity drop jumps. The extracted window of Fig. 8.19 shows the dramatic TT recoil at the end of the push-off phase with increasing rebound effort. This can then be transferred to the calculated F–V relationship of TT. Figure 8.20 represents how the tensile force is potentiated differently in the two DJ conditions (Ishikawa *et al.* 2005c). When the prestretch intensity was increased, the elastic potentiation increased with higher prestretch intensity (Fig. 8.20a). However, when the rebound intensity was increased, it primarily affected the elastic potentiation during the late push-off phase (Fig. 8.20b). It is indeed quite possible that in SSC, the performance potentiation results from the fascicle length changes, which operate effectively to make the tendon recoil possible during the push-off phase. Thus, the intensity of both prestretch and effort of push-off have considerable influence on the mechanical behavior of fascicle–TT interaction.

Clinical relevance and significance

Information available on loading characteristics on human tensile tissue *in vivo* conditions have revealed that in dynamic activities such as walking,

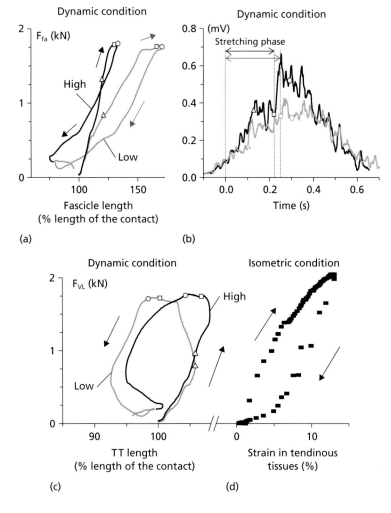

Fig. 8.19 The length changes of muscle–tendon complex (MTC), tendinous tissues and fascicle drawn together with ground reaction force and EMG recording during low and high rebound intensity jumps (Ishikawa 2005).

hopping, and running the tensile loading modes may be considerably different from those measured under isometric conditions. A wide range of tensile forces (1.4–9 kN) has been reported. The tendon force usually increases with movement intensity, but only to a certain submaximal level of effort, after which it may remain the same. However, the rate of tendon force development may be more relevant to characterize tendon loading, as this parameter increases linearly with activity (e.g. speed of running). Individual differences are large, and no representative values can be given for various age groups. This is partly because of the difficulties in using invasive tendon force measurements in large population studies. However, the data obtained are important for describing the tendon loading patterns within an individual, who can perform many different activities in one measurement session lasting 2–3 hours. These measurements have shown that each activity gives a specific loading pattern, which can be modified by intensity of effort within the specific joint as well as in the neighboring joints or muscles.

These individual responses make it more challenging to characterize the loading of the tensile tissue with respect to the injury mechanisms. It is of considerable clinical relevance that the rate of force increase during the braking phase of the loading is

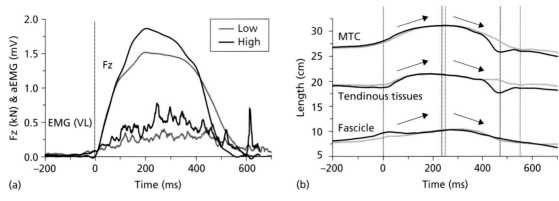

Fig. 8.20 Comparison of the instantaneous force–velocity (F–V) curves for tendinous tissues from vastus lateralis (VL) during contact of three different conditions on the sledge drop jump for one subject. (a) Reference jump (DJ_{ref}) vs. high drop jump (D_{High}); (b) DJ_{ref} vs. high rebound jump R_{High}). (Ishikawa *et al.* Contribution of the tendinous tissue to force enhancement during stretch–shortening cycle exercise depends on the prestretch and concentric phase intensities. *Journal of Electromyography and Kinesiology* [Epub ahead of print]. Copyright © 2005. Used with permission.)

probably much more related to tissue rupture and overuse than the simple loading amplitudes. This fact has to be taken into consideration also when artificial structures are being developed to replace the tendon or ligament.

Future directions

In general, tendon loading during normal locomotion is very dynamic. Consequently, tendon should be viewed as an "organ" which has considerable performance potential, but whose *in vivo* function is under the influence of other factors, such as the contractile tissue of the same MTC and related sensory and motor control. It must be emphasized that the tendon does not have much functional meaning, if it were not connected anatomically with the true "motor", the skeletal muscle. In this regard, the muscle (or its fascicles) makes it possible that TT can store considerable amount of elastic strain energy and that this energy can be utilized to potentiate the performance in the natural SSC action. However, it is not only the external force (e.g. gravity) that can regulate the TT loading. The fascicles have an important role in this task of elastic storage and utilization. As this interaction between fascicle and TT depends on several factors, such as intensity of effort (stretching and shortening velocity of the SSC

action) as well as task specificity, no general rules can be written to cover the loading characteristics of TT. This is another challenge, not only for clinical work, but also for modelling of musculoskeletal function in specific activities.

Thus, there is a continuous need for measurement of tensile (and muscular) forces during dynamic conditions. Despite the developed techniques and their applications, we still do not understand in detail the function of the aponeuroses and free tendon during natural locomotion. This is simply because the techniques are not yet precise enough to record their function separately while they are working together. Cadaver studies are not necessarily applicable for this problem. Perhaps a better solution could be to utilize sonomicrometers by placing them inside the free tendon for the recording of true tendon strain. This should be technically possible in humans, as it has been applied quite successfully in animal studies (Griffith 1991; Roberts *et al.* 1997).

The optic fiber technique has been proven successful in recording tendons that are easily accessible. The same is true for the recording of ligament forces. In addition, in the hands of a skillful surgeon, successful attempts have been made to apply the technique for deeper ligaments that are not easily accessible, such as the anterior talofibular (ATL) and calcaneofibular ligaments.

A preliminary report will soon become available on the ATL forces during normal walking and hopping (Lohrer *et al.*, in preparation). From the orthopaedic point of view, it is important to be able to characterize loading of many important ligaments that are crucial to sport activities and but also are injury prone. The anterior cruciate ligament is an example of a structure that needs to be replaced when completely ruptured by a sudden, unexpected stress. In this case, the loading characteristics of the anterior cruciate ligament should be known more precisely through *in vivo* dynamic activities so that the reconstructed tissue will have similar loading tolerance to the original.

Finally, the additional challenges to utilize the techniques presented in this chapter are the follow-up recording of both muscle architecture and tensile (and ligament) forces. Ultrasound has already proven its success in this regard both for training and aging studies (Narici *et al.* 2005); however, the optic fiber technique has not yet been applied for similar purposes. The technique itself is only slightly invasive and recovery from 1–2 hour measurements occurs quite quickly. The future should bring the optic fiber and the sonomicrometer together, especially with regard to more precise long-term recording of tendon adaptation during both training and aging.

References

Arndt, A.N., Komi, P.V., Brüggemann, G-P. & Lukkariniemi, J. (1998) Individual muscle contributions to the *in vivo* achilles tendon force. *Clinical Biomechanics* 13, 532–541.

Bocquet, J.-C. & Noel, J. (1987) Sensitive skin-pressure and strain sensor with optical fibres. In: *Proceeding of 2nd Congress on Structural Mechanics of Optical Systems*, 13–15 January 1987, Los Angeles, CA.

Bouisset, S. (1973) EMG and muscle force in normal motor activities. In: *New Developments in Electromyography and Clinical Neurophysiology* (Desmedt, J.E. ed.), Vol.1. Karger, Basel: 547–583.

Butler, D.L., Grood, E.S., Noyes, F.R., Zernicke, R.F. & Brackett, K. (1984) Effects of structure and strain measurement technique on the material properties of young human tendons and fascia. *Journal of Biomechanics* 17, 579–596.

Candau, R., Belli, A., Chatard, J.C., Carrez, J-P. & Lacour, J-R. (1993) Stretch shortening cycle in the skating technique of cross-country skiing. *Science et Motricité* 22, 252–256.

Fellows, S.J., & Rack, P.M. (1987) Changes in the length of the human biceps brachii muscle during elbow movements. *Journal of Physiology* 383, 405–412.

Finni, T. & Komi, P.V. (2002) Two methods for estimating tendinous tissue elongation during human movement. *Journal of Applied Biomechanics* 18, 180–188.

Finni, T., Hodgson, J.A., Lai, A.M., Edgerton, V.R. & Sinha, S. (2003b)

Nonuniform strain of human soleus aponeurosis–tendon complex during submaximal voluntary contractions *in vivo*. *Journal of Applied Physiology* 95, 829–837.

Finni, T., Ikegawa, S. & Komi, P.V. (2001c) Concentric force enhancement during human movement. *Acta Physiologica Scandinavica* 173, 369–377.

Finni, T., Ikegawa, S., Lepola, V. & Komi, P.V. (2001b) *In vivo* behavior of vastus lateralis muscle during dynamic performances. *European Journal of Sport Science* 1, 1.

Finni, T., Ikegawa, S., Lepola, V. & Komi, P.V. (2003a) Comparison of force–velocity relationships of vastus lateralis muscle in isokinetic and in stretch–shortening cycle exercises. *Acta Physiologica Scandinavica* 177, 483–491.

Finni, T., Komi, P.V. & Lepola, V. (2000) *In vivo* triceps surae and quadriceps femoris muscle function in a squat jump and counter movement jump. *European Journal of Applied Physiology* 83, 416–426.

Finni, T., Komi, P.V. & Lepola, V. (2001a) *In vivo* muscle mechanics during normal locomotion is dependent on movement amplitude and contraction intensity. *European Journal of Applied Physiology* 85, 170–176.

Finni, T., Komi, P.V. & Lukkariniemi, J. (1998) Achilles tendon loading during walking: application of a novel optic fiber technique. *European Journal of Applied Physiology* 77, 289–291.

Fornage, B.D. (1986a) Achilles tendon: US examination. *Radiology* b159, 759–764.

Fornage, B.D. & Deshayes, J.L. (1986b) Ultrasound of normal skin. *Journal of Clinical Ultrasound* 14, 619–622.

Fukashiro, S. & Komi, P.V. (1987) Joint moment and mechanical power flow of the lower limb during vertical jump. *International Journal of Sports Medicine* 8, 15–21.

Fukashiro, S., Itoh, M., Ichinose, Y., Kawakami, Y. & Fukunaga, T. (1995a) Ultrasonography gives directly but noninvasively elastic characteristic of human tendon *in vivo*. *European Journal of Applied Physiology and Occupational Physiology* 71, 555–557.

Fukashiro, S., Komi, P.V., Järvinen, M. & Miyashita, M. (1993) Comparison between the directly measured Achilles tendon force and the tendon force calculated from the ankle joint moment during vertical jumps. *Clinical Biomechanics* 8, 25–30.

Fukashiro, S., Komi, P.V., Järvinen, M. & Miyashita, M. (1995b) *In vivo* achilles tendon loading during jumping in humans. *European Journal of Applied Physiology* 71, 453–458.

Fukunaga, T., Ito, M., Ichinose, Y., Kuno, S., Kawakami, Y. & Fukashiro, S. (1996) Tendinous movement of a human muscle during voluntary contractions determined by real-time ultrasonography. *Journal of Applied Physiology* 813, 1430–1433.

Fukunaga, T., Kawakami, Y., Kubo, K. & Kanehisa, H. (2002a) Muscle and tendon interaction during human movements. *Exercise and Sport Sciences Reviews* 30, 106–110.

Fukunaga, T., Kawakarni, Y., Muraoka, T. & Kanehisa, H. (2002b) Muscle and tendon relations in humans: power enhancement in counter-movement exercise. *Advances in Experimental Medicine and Biology* **508**, 501–505.

Fukunaga, T., Kubo, K., Kawakami, Y., Fukashiro, S., Kanehisa, H. & Maganaris, C.N. (2001) *In vivo* behavior of human muscle tendon during walking. *Proceedings of the Royal Society London* **B268**, 229–233.

Fukunaga, T., Roy, R.R., Shellock, F.G., et al. (1992) Physiological cross-sectional area of human leg muscles based on magnetic resonance imaging. *Journal of Orthopaedic Research* **10**, 928–934.

Gollhofer, A., Schmidtbleicher, D. & Dietz, V. (1984) Regulation of muscle stiffness in human locomotion. *International Journal of Sports Medicine* **5**, 19–22.

Gregor, R.J., Komi, P.V., Browning, R.C. & Järvinen, M. (1991) A comparison of triceps surae and residual muscle moments at the ankle during cycling. *Journal of Biomechanics* **24**, 287–297.

Gregor, R.J., Komi, P.V. & Järvinen, M. (1984) Achilles tendon forces during cycling. *International Journal of Sports Medicine* **8** (Suppl.), 9–14.

Gregor, R.J., Roy, R.R., Whiting, W.C., Lovely, R.G., Hodgson, J.A. & Edgerton, V.R. (1988) Mechanical output of the cat soleus during treadmill locomotion *in vivo* vs. *in situ* characteristics. *Journal of Biomechanics* **21**, 721–732.

Grieve, D.W., Pheasant, S.Q. & Cavanagh, P.R. (1978) Prediction of gastrocnemius length from knee and ankle joint posture. In: *Biomechanics VI-A* (Asmissen, E. & Jörgensen, K., eds.) University Park Press, Baltimore: 405–412.

Griffiths, R.I. (1991) Shortening of muscle fibres during stretch of the active cat medial gastrocnemius muscle: the role of tendon compliance. *Journal of Physiology* **436**, 219–236.

Henriksson-Larsen, K., Wretling, M.L., Lorentzon, R. & Oberg, L. (1992) Do muscle fibre size and fibre angulation correlate in pennated human muscles? *European Journal of Applied Physiology and Occupational Physiology* **64**, 68–72.

Herbert, R.D. & Gandevia, S.C. (1995) Changes in pennation with joint angle and muscle torque: *in vivo* measurements in human brachialis muscle. *Journal of Physiology* **484**, 523–532.

Häkkinen, K. & Komi, P.V. (1983) Electromyographic changes during strength training and detraining. *Medicine & Science in Sports & Exercise* **15**, 455–460.

Hijikata, T., Wakisaka, H. & Niida, S. (1993) Functional combination of tapering profiles and overlapping arrangements in nonspanning skeletal muscle fibers terminating intrafascicularly. *Anatomical Record* **236**, 602–610.

Hill, A.V. (1938) The heat and shortening of the dynamic constant of muscle. *Proceedings of the Royal Society London* **B126**, 136–195.

Howry, D.H. (1965) A brief atlas of diagnostic ultrasonic radiologic results. *Radiologic Clinics of North America* **3**, 433–452.

Huijing, P.A. (1992) Elastic potential of muscle. In: *Strength and Power in Sport* (Komi, P.V., ed.) Blackwell Scientific Pulications, Oxford: 151–168.

Ikai, M. & Fukunaga, T. (1968) Calculation of muscle strength per unit cross-sectional area of human muscle by means of ultrasonic measurement. *Internationale Zeitschrift für angewandte Physiologie, einschliesslich Arbeitsphysiologie* **26**, 26–32.

Inoue, F. & Frank, G.B. (1962) Action of procaine on frog skeletal muscles. *Journal of Pharmacology and Experimental Therapeutics* **136**, 190–196.

Ishikawa, M. (2005). *In vivo muscle mechanics during human locomotion.* PhD thesis. University of Jyväskylä. Studies in Sport, Physical Education and Health, 107.

Ishikawa, M. & Komi, P.V. (2004) Effects of different dropping intensities on fascicle and tendinous tissue behavior during stretch–shortening cycle exercise. *Journal of Applied Physiology* **96**, 848–852.

Ishikawa, M., Finni. T., & Komi, P.V. (2003) Behaviour of vastus lateralis muscle–tendon during high intensity SSC exercises *in vivo.* *Acta Physiologica Scandinavica* **178**, 205–213.

Ishikawa, M., Komi, P.V., Grey, M.J., Lepola, V. & Bruggemann, G.P. (2005b) Muscle–tendon interaction and elastic energy usage in human walking. *Journal of Applied Physiology* **99**, 603–608.

Ishikawa, M., Komi, P.V., Finni, T. & Kuitunen, S. (2005c) Contribution of the tendinous tissue to force enhancement during stretch–shortening cycle exercise depends on the prestretch and concentric phase intensities. *Journal of Electromyography and Kinesiology* Nov 3: [Epub ahead of print].

Ishikawa, M., Niemela, E. & Komi, P.V. (2005a) The interaction between fascicle and tendinous tissues in short contact stretch–shortening cycle exercise with varying eccentric intensities. *Journal of Applied Physiology* **99**: 217–223.

Ito, M., Kawakami, Y., Ichinose, Y., Fukashiro, S. & Fukunaga, T. (1998) Nonisometric behavior of fascicles during isometric contractions of a human muscle. *Journal of Applied Physiology* **85**, 1230–1235.

Kawakami, Y., Abe, T. & Fukunaga, T. (1993) Muscle-fiber pennation angles are greater in hypertrophied than in normal muscles. *Journal of Applied Physiology* **74**, 2740–2744.

Kawakami, Y., Ichinose, M., Kubo, K., Ito, M., Imai, M. & Fukunaga, T. (2000) Architecture of contracting human muscles and its functional significance. *Journal of Applied Biomechanics* **16**, 88–98.

Kawakami, Y., Muraoka, T., Ito, S., Kanehisa, H. & Fukunaga, T. (2002) *In vivo* muscle fibre behaviour during counter-movement exercise in humans reveals a significant role for tendon elasticity. *Journal of Physiology* **540**, 635–646.

Kaya, M., Carvalho, W., Leonard, T. & Herzog, W. (2002) Estimation of cat medial gastrocnemius fascicle lengths during dynamic contractions. *Journal of Biomechanics* **35**, 893–902.

Komi, P.V. (1973) Measurement of the force–velocity relationship in human muscle under concentric and eccentric contraction. In: *Medicine and Sport, Biomechanics III* (Jokl, E., ed.) Karger, Basel: Vol. 8, 224–229.

Komi, P.V. (1983) Electromyographic mechanical and metabolic changes during static and dynamic fatigue. In: *Biochemistry of Exercise* (Knuttgen, H.G., Vogel, J.A. & Poortmans, J., eds.) Human Kinetics Publishers, Champaiign, IL: 197–215.

Komi, P.V. (1990) Relevance of *in vivo* force measurements to human biomechanics. *Journal of Biomechanics* **23** (Suppl. 1), 23–34.

Komi, P.V. (2000) Stretch–shortening cycle: a powerful model to study normal and fatigued muscle. *Journal of Biomechanics* **33**, 1197–1206.

Komi, P.V. & Bosco, C. (1978) Utilization of stored elastic energy in leg extensor muscles by men and women. *Medicine and Science in Sports and Exercise* **10**, 261–265.

Komi, P.V. & Buskirk, E.R. (1972) Effect of eccentric and concentricmuscle conditioning on tension and electrical activity of human muscle. *Ergonomics* **15**, 417–434.

Komi, P.V., Belli, A., Huttunen, V. & Partio, E. (1995) Optic fiber as a transducer for direct *in vivo* measurements of human tendomuscular forces. In: *Proceedings of the Xvth ISB, Jyväskylä, Finland* (Häkkinen, K., Keskinen, K.L., Komi, P.V. & Mero, A., eds.) 494–495.

Komi, P.V., Belli, A., Huttunen, V., Bonnejoy, R., Geyssant, A. & Lacour, J.R. (1996) Optic fiber as a transducer of tendomuscular forces. *European Journal of Applied Physiology* **72**, 278–280.

Komi, P.V., Fukashiro, S. & Järvinen, M. (1992) Biomechanical loading of Achilles tendon during normal locomotion. *Clinics in Sport Medicine* **11**, 521–531.

Komi, P.V., Salonen, M. & Järvinen, M. (1984) *In vivo* measurements of Achilles tendon forces in man. *Medicine and Science in Sports and Exercise* **16**, 165.

Komi, P.V., Salonen, M. & Järvinen, M. (1985) Measurement of *in vivo* Achilles tendon forces in man and their calibration. *Medicine and Science in Sports and Exercise* **17**, 263.

Komi, P.V., Salonen, M., Järvinen, M. & Kokko, O. (1987) *In vivo* registration of Achilles tendon forces in man. I. Methodological development. *International Journal of Sports Medicine* **8**, 3–8.

Kubo, K., Kanehisa, H., Takeshita, D., Kawakami, Y., Fukashiro, S. & Fukunaga, T. (2000) *In vivo* dynamics of human medial gastrocnemius muscle–tendon complex during stretch–shortening cycle exercise. *Acta Physiologica Scandinavica* **170**, 127–135.

Kubo, K., Kawakami, Y. & Fukunaga, T. (1999) Influence of elastic properties of tendon structures on jump performance in humans. *Journal of Applied Physiology* **87**, 2090–2096.

Kurokawa, S., Fukunaga, T. & Fukashiro, S. (2001). Behavior of fascicles and tendinous structures of human gastrocnemius during vertical jumping.

Journal of Applied Physiology **90**, 1349–1358.

Kurokawa, S., Fukunaga, T., Nagano, A. & Fukashiro, S. (2003) Interaction between fascicles and tendinous structures during counter movement jumping investigated *in vivo*. *Journal of Applied Physiology* **95**, 2306–2314.

Kyrolainen, H., Finni, T., Avela, J. & Komi, P.V. (2003) Neuromuscular behaviour of the triceps surae muscle–tendon complex during running and jumping. *International Journal of Sports Medicine* **24**, 153–155.

Maganaris, C.N. & Paul, J.P. (2000) Hysteresis measurements in intact human tendon. *Journal of Biomechanics* **33**, 1723–1727.

Moritani, T., Oddson, L. & Thorstensson, A. (1990) Electromyographic evidence of selective fatigue during the eccentric phase of stretch–shortening cycles in man. *European Journal of Applied Physiology and Occupational Physiology* **60**, 425–429.

Muraoka, T., Kawakami, Y., Tachi, M. & Fukunaga, T. (2001) Muscle fiber and tendon length changes in the human vastus lateralis during slow pedaling. *Journal of Applied Physiology* **91**, 2035–2040.

Narici, M.V., Binzoni, T., Hiltbrand, E., Fasel, J., Terrier, F. & Cerretelli, P. (1996) *In vivo* human gastrocnemius architecture with changing joint angle at rest and during graded isometric contraction. *Journal of Physiology* **496**, 287–297.

Narici, M.V., Magnaris, C. & Reeves, N. (2005) Myotendinous alterations and effects of resistive loading in old age. *Scandinavian Journal of Medicine and Science in Sport* **15**, 392–401.

Nicol, C. & Komi, P.V. (1998) Significance of passively induced stretch reflexes on Achilles tendon force enhancement. *Muscle and Nerve* **21**, 1546–1548.

Nicol, C., Komi, P.V., Belli, A., Huttunen, V. & Partio, E. (1995) Reflex contribution of achilles tendon forces: *in vivo* measurements with the optic fibre technique. In: *Proceedings of the Xvth ISB,*

Jyväskylä, Finland (Häkkinen, K., Keskinen, K.L., Komi, P.V. & Mero, A. eds.) 674–675.

Roberts, T.J., Marsh, R.L., Weyand, P.G. & Taylor, C.R. (1997) Muscular force in running turkeys: the economy of minimizing work. *Science* **275**, 1113–1115.

Rugg, S.G., Gregor, R.J., Mandelbaum, B.R. & Chiu, L. (1990) *In vivo* moment arm calculations at the ankle using magnetic resonance imaging (MRI). *Journal of Biomechanics* **23**, 495–501.

Rutherford, O.M. & Jones, D.A. (1992) Measurement of fibre pennation using ultrasound in the human quadriceps *in vivo*. *European Journal of Applied Physiology and Occupational Physiology* **65**, 433–437.

Sabbahi, M.A., De Luca, C.J. & Powers, W.R. (1979) Effect of ischemia, cooling and local anesthesia on the median frequency of the myoelectric signals. *Proceedings of 4th Congress International Society of Electrophysiology Kinesiology, Boston*, 94–95.

Salmons, S. (1969) The 8th International Conference on Medical and Biomechanical Engineering, meeting report. *Biomedical Materials and Engineering* **4**, 467–474.

Scott, S.H. & Winter, D.A. (1990) Internal forces of chronic running injury sites. *Medicine and Science in Sports and Exercise* **22**, 357–369.

Sherif, M.H., Gregor, R.J., Liu, M., Roy, R.R. & Hager, C.L. (1983) Correlation of myoelectric activity and muscle force during selected cat treadmill locomotion. *Journal of Biomechanics* **16**, 691–701.

Wilkie, D.R. (1950) The relation between force and velocity in human muscle. *Journal of Physiology* **110**, 249.

Yeh, H.C. & Wolf, B.S. (1978) A simple portable water bath for superficial ultrasonography. *American Journal of Roentgenology* **130**, 275–278.

Zajac, F.E. (1989) Muscle and tendon: properties, models, scaling, and application to biomechanics and motor control [Review]. *Critical Reviews in Biomedical Engineering* **17**, 359–411.

Chapter 9

Tendon Innervation: Understanding of Pathology and Potential Implications for Treatment

PAUL W. ACKERMANN, JOHAN DAHL, DANIEL K-I. BRING, AND PER A.F.H. RENSTRÖM

Both occupational and sports-related tendon pain and degeneration pose a huge problem, mainly because of the lack of specific treatment subsequent to limited knowledge of the pathomechanisms involved. Recent studies show that a variety of signal substances (e.g. neuropeptides) harbored by the peripheral nervous system have an important role in the regulation of pain, inflammation, vasoactivity, and tissue repair. This chapter presents novel findings considering tendon innervation, expression of neuropeptides, and neuronal response to injury as studied in the rat Achilles tendon.

Based on structural and quantitative analysis, the neuronal presence of autonomic, sensory, and opioid peptides in the tendon was disclosed. This is the first detection of a peripheral musculoskeletal anti-nociceptive system consisting of opioid ligands and receptors. Abundant nerve fibers were observed in the paratenon, whereas the proper tendon was practically devoid of nerves, suggesting that tendon pain and inflammation is regulated from the surrounding structures.

Nerve regeneration and neuropeptide expression at different time points (1–16 weeks) were analyzed in the healing of experimental Achilles tendon rupture. During weeks 1–2 (inflammatory phase), an extensive nerve fiber ingrowth into the rupture site (i.e. the tendon proper) was seen which peaked during weeks 2–6 (regenerative phase). Nerve ingrowth may represent a prerequisite for delivery of neuronal mediators required for tissue repair. During the regenerative phase, a peak expression of the sensory neuropeptides substance P (SP) and calcitonin gene-related peptide (CGRP) in the

proper tendon, seen as free sprouting nerve endings among fibroblasts and new vessels, may have a role in repair.

The present study demonstrates that tendons are supplied with a complex peptidergic network, which presumably takes part in maintaining tissue homeostasis, but also by its plasticity (i.e. nerve ingrowth and temporal alteration in neuropeptide expression) is capable of responding to injury. In a future perspective, neuronal mediators may prove to be useful in targeted pharmacotherapy and tissue engineering in painful and degenerative tendon disorders.

Introduction

Tendons exhibiting degeneration and eliciting pain represent a considerable part of the musculoskeletal disorders, which pose a tremendous burden on the health care system. According to the National Research Council, 1 million workers in the USA are affected each year, costing $54 billion in compensation expenditures, lost wages, and decreased productivity (Barnard 1997; Winnick 2001). During the past several years, the incidence of overuse injuries, mostly related to work and sports, has increased considerably (Mani & Gerr 2000; Jarvinen *et al.* 2001). Overuse injuries can be related to extrinsic and intrinsic factors (Renstrom & Johnson 1985). Among extrinsic factors, repetitive movement is considered a main cause. Repetitive microtraumas of the tissues are thought to exceed the repair capability of the cells (Renström & Kannus 1991; Leadbetter 1992; Archambault *et al.* 1995).

Intrinsic factors, some genetically determined, include obesity, extremity malalignment, joint laxity, muscle weakness, and disturbed blood supply. Mechanical risk factors solely cannot clarify the relationship to pain and inflammation, which thus still requires a biologic explanation (Neely 1998).

In inflammatory conditions of the locomotor apparatus, pain is almost a constant feature; however, in degenerative disorders it is highly variable. Whether inflammation is a prerequisite for pain in degenerative disease is unclear. Notably, spontaneous ruptures of tendons, presumed to be caused by degeneration, are often not preceded by pain. In a study by Kannus and Józsa (1991), at time of surgery, degenerative changes were found in 97% of all tendon ruptures, whereas signs of inflammation were rare. On the whole, the relationship between pain, inflammation, and degeneration of the locomotor system remains obscure, which can be attributed to the still poorly defined neuroanatomy and pathophysiology. In particular, this applies to tendons, which in their proper tissue show insignificant signs of inflammation and exhibit a high prevalence of degeneration and a considerable variation in the incidence and intensity of pain.

In chronic, painful conditions of tendons, histologic studies have shown that the proper tissues exhibit very few signs of inflammation. Therefore, the classic term tendinitis has been replaced by the term tendinopathy. Localized degenerative lesion is called tendinosis (Puddu et al. 1976) to denote collagen disorganization, increased ground substance, hypercellularity, and neovascularization (Józsa & Kannus 1997).

Although degeneration seems to be a prominent feature of chronic tendon conditions, this does not preclude an initial inflammatory phase. Moreover, it appears that histologic analyses of painful tendon tissues primarily have focused on the proper tendon, not always including the envelope (i.e. the paratenon and surrounding loose connective tissue). It may prove that degeneration of tendons is related to inflammatory changes in the surrounding structures. Notably, a recent study in rats showed that application of a prostaglandin, PGE_1, an inflammatory mediator, to the paratenon produced degenerative like changes in the proper tendon (Sullo et al. 2001).

Traditionally, tendon innervation has not yet been designated of major importance. Neuronal regulation has mostly been associated with afferent mediation of primarily mechanoceptive information, whereas efferent information has been related to autonomic muscular and vascular reflexes. It has been demonstrated that a wide variety of signal substances in the peripheral nervous system—also present in tendons—in balanced combinations regulate important biologic processes.

Tendon innervation

The nerves of tendons are composed of myelinated, fast transmitting Aα- and Aβ-fibers mediating mechanoception, and unmyelinated, slow transmitting Aγ-, Aδ-, B-, and C-fibers mediating deep tissue pain and hyperalgesia, which are characteristic features of tendon pain. The innervation of tendons originates from three neighboring sources: from nerve trunks in skin, muscle, and loose connective tissue. The paratenon is richly innervated and the nerve fibers send branches that penetrate the epitenon. Most nerve fibers do not enter the tendon proper.

It is now well established that the peripheral nervous system, in addition to classic functions such as nociception and vasoactivity, also participates in the regulation of a wide variety of efferent actions on cell proliferation, cytokine expression, inflammation, immune responses, and hormone release (Haegerstrand et al. 1990; Strand et al. 1991; Schwartz 1992; Brain 1997; Schaffer et al. 1998; Hökfelt et al. 2000; Onuoha & Alpar 2001). The paradoxical "efferent" role of afferent nociceptive fibers is now widely recognized (Bayliss 1901). So far, however, the innervation and neuronal regulation of periarticular tissues and especially tendons have received little attention. In particular, this applies to the specific neuronal mediators (i.e. the signal substances).

The mediators of the nervous system act principally through two ways:
1 With fast transmitters (i.e. classic neurotransmitters: monoamines, acetylcholine, amino acids), which directly effectuate muscle contractions or afferently relay information on painful stimuli.
2 With slow transmitters, neuropeptides, which

slowly regulate physiologic functions in the central as well as peripheral nervous system.

Neuropeptides

Neuropeptides act as chemical messengers in the central as well as peripheral nervous system. They differ from classic neurotransmitters in several respects. Peripheral neuropeptides are synthesized in the dorsal root ganglia and sympathetic chain and transported distally. In contrast, classic neuro-transmitters are synthesized in the axon terminals. The synthesis and turnover of neuropeptides is more prolonged than those of classic transmitters. Neuropeptides have been demonstrated in large, dense-core vesicles, while classic transmitters occur in small as well as in large vesicles, in the latter together with neuropeptides (Hökfelt *et al.* 1980). It has been shown that these vesicles are released differently, depending on the frequency of the action potentials. A low-impulse frequency selectively activates small vesicles releasing classic trans-mitters, whereas higher frequencies release neuro-peptides from large vesicles (Hökfelt *et al.* 1987). The large vesicles permit more than one func-tional neuropeptide to be processed and released, also together with classic transmitters (Hökfelt *et al.* 1980), which offers a variety of functional interactions.

A vast number of neuropeptides has been identi-fied in the central and peripheral nervous system. So far, however, research on the occurrence and functions of neuropeptides in tendons has been very limited. Given this, which neuropeptides could be of interest in the regulation of tendon pathology? Neuropeptides known to be of importance for noci-ception and tissue homeostasis can be classified in three groups: autonomic, sensory and opioid, according to their function and original nerve fiber type finding.

Autonomic neuropeptides

Autonomic fibers in the periphery contain several mediators. Neuropeptide Y (NPY) found in sym-pathetic fibers has been shown to be a potent vasoconstrictor. It often coexists with noradrenaline (NA) potentiating the vasoconstrictive action of NPY (Lundberg & Hökfelt 1986). Moreover, it has recently been reported that NPY at low levels has an angiogenetic effect (Grant & Zukowska 2000). In parasympathetic nerve fibers, vasoactive intestinal polypeptide (VIP) has been shown to be a potent vasodilator (Lundberg *et al.* 1980). In addition to the well-established vasoactive role of VIP, other important effects have been reported over recent years. Thus, VIP has been implicated in regulating immune cells and the expression of pro- and anti-inflammatory signal substances (cytokines) and growth factors. Recently, a study on experimental arthritis demonstrated an anti-inflammatory effect of VIP (Delgado *et al.* 2001).

Sensory neuropeptides

Sensory nerve endings contain SP (Hökfelt *et al.* 1975) claimed to transmit nociceptive signals (Hökfelt *et al.* 1975; Lembeck *et al.* 1981; Snijdelaar *et al.* 2000) and to exert pro-inflammatory effects such as vasodilation and protein extravasation (Brain *et al.* 1985; Nakamura-Craig & Smith 1989; Maggi 1995). CGRP coexists with and potentiates the effect of SP (Wiesenfeld-Hallin *et al.* 1984; Woolf & Wiesenfeld-Hallin 1986; Oku *et al.* 1987).

Sensory nerve fibers respond to noxious thermal, mechanical, and chemical stimuli in the periphery by SP release from C- and Aδ-fibers, both centrally and peripherally. Several studies have demon-strated that SP acts as a transmitter of pain in the spinal cord (Piercey *et al.* 1981; Snider *et al.* 1991; Snijdelaar *et al.* 2000). In the periphery, release of SP leads to sensitization of surrounding primary affer-ents by enhancing cellular release of prostaglandins, histamines, and cytokines (Schaible & Grubb 1993; Vasko *et al.* 1994). Recently, however, it was shown that SP also directly stimulates nociceptor endings (Ueda 1999). CGRP, often colocalized with SP in unmyelinated C fibers, facilitates the release of SP and delays SP degradation in the spinal cord, thereby potentiating the nociceptive effect (Le Greves *et al.* 1985; Woolf & Wiesenfeld-Hallin 1986; Schaible 1996). It is still unclear whether this poten-tiating mechanism also occurs in the periphery.

However, sensory nerve fibers also contain pep-tides with anti-nociceptive and anti-inflammatory effects counteracting the effects of SP and CGRP.

Thus, galanin (GAL), somatostatin (SOM) as well as opioids, all of which occur in primary afferents, have been shown to inhibit inflammation and nociception (Cridland & Henry 1988; Xu *et al.* 1991; Carlton & Coggeshall 1997; Szolcsanyi *et al.* 1998; Heppelmann *et al.* 2000). A number of studies suggest that these anti-nociceptive peptides exert their modulatory effect through inhibition of SP release (Brodin *et al.* 1983; Yaksh 1988; Xu *et al.* 1991; Green *et al.* 1992).

Opioid neuropeptides

The endogenous opioid peptides consist of three families (enkephalins, dynorphins, and endorphins), which contain several biologically active products (e.g. met-enkephalin-arg-phe [MEAP] and dynorphin B [DYN B]) that exert physiologic actions by interacting with opioid receptors. Enkephalins are thought to be the ligands for the δ-opioid receptor (DOR), whereas dynorphins are suggested to be ligands for the κ-receptor (KOR). Recent studies identified that in addition to endorphins and the enkephalins, endomorphins are endogenous ligands for μ-opioid receptors (MOR). Recent publications also show a fourth opioid receptor, which is genetically closely related to the others and responds to the endogenous agonist nociceptin (N/OFQ). Both opioids and opioid receptors are produced by the dorsal root ganglia and transported peripherally and to the central nervous system (CNS).

The endogenous opioids seem to provide a peripheral anti-nociceptive system. Thus, it was recently reported that locally administered intra-articular morphine had a significant analgesic effect in a dose–response manner. Notably, morphine has been reported to inhibit SP release from peripheral sensory nerve endings (Brodin *et al.* 1983; Yaksh 1988). The observations suggest that opioid receptors are not confined to the CNS, but also occur in the periphery and that pain can be inhibited at a peripheral level (Herz 1995). Opioid receptors have in fact been demonstrated on peripheral sensory nerve terminals of the skin (Stein *et al.* 1990; Coggeshall *et al.* 1997; Wenk & Honda 1999).

There are two principal sources of opioid peptides in the periphery. One is the immune cells, which have been shown to contain and release opioids and also to be implicated in mitigating inflammatory pain (Stein *et al.* 1993; Cabot 2001). The other source is most likely the peripheral nervous system. Notably, a recent study showed that approximately 17% of peripheral cutaneous axons contain enkephalins presumed to be of importance in regulating pain and inflammation (Carlton & Coggeshall 1997). As for tendons, the neuronal occurrence of endogenous opioids and receptors, has until recently not been explored.

Neuropeptides in tendons

As information on neuropeptide prevalence in connective tissue is still sparse, we decided to study the neuropeptide occurrence in tendons compared with ligaments and joint capsules. The results presented here are presented partly in a thesis called "Peptidergic innervation of periarticular tissue" (Ackermann 2001).

To explore the occurrence of neuropeptides in tendons both a quantitative and morphologic approach was applied. Radioimmunoassay (RIA) was employed for screening to detect and quantify three main classes of neuropeptides: autonomic, sensory, and opioid. Immunohistochemistry (IHC) was used to establish the neuronal occurrence and the distribution among different tissues of 14 peptides representing the three classes.

RIA analysis: occurrence and levels of neuropeptides

The RIA study focused on two autonomic (NPY, VIP), three sensory (SP, CGRP, GAL), and three opioid (MEAP, N/OFQ, DYN B) peptides in Achilles tendon, knee collateral ligaments, and joint capsule of the rat.

AUTONOMIC PEPTIDES

The analysis included one sympathetic (NPY) vasoconstrictive and one parasympathetic (VIP) vasodilatory neuropeptide. Measurable concentrations (0.11–5.63 pmol/g) of the two neuropeptides were obtained in all tissues analyzed (Ackermann *et al.* 2001b). The analysis showed that NPY consistently exhibited higher concentrations than VIP in the different tissues (Fig. 9.1a). The concentration of NPY compared to VIP was 15 times higher in ligaments and twice as high in tendons and in capsules. The observation seems to reflect that the sympathetic tonus is higher than the parasympathetic tonus in periarticular tissue. Such a difference between tissues may be assumed to be of importance for blood flow, and hypothetically for healing capacity, possibly also for susceptibility to degeneration and injury. Notably, ligaments are more prone to rupture than tendons (Woo *et al.* 2000).

Neuropeptides, in contrast to other transmitters, mediate more sustained changes in vascular resistance, possibly by prolonging the effect of other transmitters. Thus, NPY has been shown to potentiate the vasoconstrictive effect of the classic neurotransmitter NA. The latter was recently reported to reduce blood flow by more than 75% after topical administration (McDougall *et al.* 1997). The high ratio of NPY : VIP would seem to reflect that the vasoconstrictive capability is greater than the vasodilatory in periarticular tissue.

The tissue specific levels of vasoconstrictive and vasodilatory neuropeptides observed presumably represent a homeostatic state, which may be altered in response to external stress (Hökfelt *et al.* 2000). It has been suggested that impaired blood flow and hypoxic degeneration could be contributing factors in the genesis of atraumatic tendon ruptures (Józsa & Kannus 1997). Increased release of NPY and NA during stress and overtraining has been reported (Levenson & Moore 1998). Conceivably, a combination of poor vascularization, increased vasoconstriction, and repetitive mechanical load may lead to ischemia, necrosis, and rupture.

SENSORY PEPTIDES

The relative concentration of nociceptive and modulatory mediators, respectively, could suggest physiologic nociceptive thresholds. Among the sensory peptides screened for by radioimmunoassay, SP and CGRP have nociceptive and pro-inflammatory

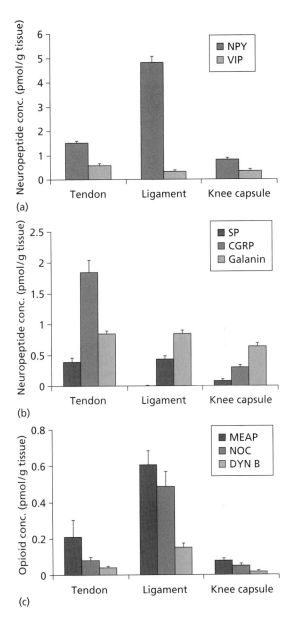

(a)

(b)

(c)

Fig. 9.1 Radioimmunoassay tissue concentrations (pmol/g) of sensory (SP, CGRP, and GAL) (a), autonomic (NPY and VIP) (b), opioid (MEAP, N/OFQ and DYN B) (c) neuropeptides in the Achilles tendon, collateral ligaments, and joint capsule of rat knee (mean ± standard error of the mean [SEM]). CGRP, calcitonin gene-related peptide; DYN B, dynorphin B; GAL, galanin; MEAP, met-enkephalin-arg-phe; N/OFQ, nociceptin; NPY, neuropeptide Y; SP, substance P; VIP, vasoactive intestinal polypeptide. (Reproduced with permission from Ackermann *et al.* 1999, 2001a,b.)

effects, whereas GAL is known to modulate these effects. The investigation disclosed that CGRP and GAL were present in all tissues analysed, whereas SP could not be demonstrated in ligaments (Fig. 9.1b). The highest concentrations of SP and CGRP were found in tendons, whereas GAL essentially exhibited the same levels in the different tissues (Ackermann *et al.* 1999). Thus, the highest rate of nociceptive versus modulatory neuropeptides was observed in the Achilles tendon. The relative concentrations observed may reflect a physiologic balance between sensory mediators and modulators. In painful and inflammatory conditions, it may prove that there is an altered balance between these neuropeptides, resulting in enhanced or perpetuated nociceptive and inflammatory responses. Several studies have demonstrated increased levels of sensory peptides in patients with rheumatoid arthritis (Menkes *et al.* 1993) and similar results were found in rats with experimentally induced arthritis (Ahmed *et al.* 1995). The higher concentrations of SP and CGRP in tendons compared to ligaments could reflect a greater susceptibility to pain and inflammation.

OPIOID PEPTIDES

The analysis comprised two opioid peptides (MEAP, DYN B) and one opioid-like peptide, nociceptin (N/OFQ). Among these opioid peptides, MEAP and DYN B belong to classic opioid peptide families, whereas N/OFQ has only lately been discovered and characterized (Meunier *et al.* 1995; Reinscheid *et al.* 1995; Darland *et al.* 1998). Both opioids and the opioid-like peptide have been shown to have anti-nociceptive effects (Millan 1986; Calo' *et al.* 2000).

The analysis disclosed that both MEAP and N/OFQ occurred in all tissues analyzed, but DYN B was below the detection limit of the assay (Fig. 9.1c). A significant proportion of samples with measurable concentrations of MEAP and N/OFQ was obtained from all tissues. The most conspicuous finding pertained to the higher concentrations of both MEAP and N/OFQ in ligaments compared to tendons and capsules (Ackermann *et al.* 2001a).

This is the first observation on the occurrence of opioids including nociceptin in periarticular tissues. Despite a somewhat high standard deviation, the results clearly demonstrate the existence of opioid peptides (enkephalin and nociceptin) in the periarticular tissues.

The physiologic role of enkephalins like MEAP can be assumed to be anti-nociceptive (Carlton & Coggeshall 1997; Machelska & Stein 2000), anti-inflammatory (Lembeck *et al.* 1982; Hong & Abbott 1995), vasodilatory (Florez & Mediavilla 1977; Moore & Dowling 1982), immunosuppressive (Brown & Van Epps 1985), and trophic (Willson *et al.* 1976; Zagon & McLaughlin 1991). Notably, it has been shown that the release of SP from nerve fibers in the cat knee joint is inhibited by intra-articular enkephalin–analog injections (Yaksh 1988).

As for nociceptin, the occurrence in peripheral tissues has not previously been demonstrated, to our knowledge. The physiologic role of nociceptin is largely unknown. In the spinal cord, low levels have been suggested to be anti-nociceptive and high levels nociceptive (Calo' *et al.* 2000). Recently, nociceptin was reported to reduce mechanosensitivity in the rat knee joint through inhibition of SP release (McDougall *et al.* 2000, 2001) possibly via receptor activation in the periphery.

Altogether, the present investigation shows that opioids are present in tendons. The lower concentrations of MEAP and N/OFQ in tendons and capsules compared to ligaments could reflect a greater susceptibility to pain and inflammation, in particular when considering also the high levels of SP found in tendons and capsules. Notably, pain syndromes in tendons are much more common than in ligaments. The combined quantitative data obtained suggest that there is a balance between nociceptive and anti-nociceptive peptides under normal conditions, which may prove to be altered under pathologic conditions.

Immunohistologic analysis: distribution of neuropeptides

Further exploration of the Achilles tendon was performed by immunohistochemistry to assess the neuronal occurrence of the neuropeptides detected by RIA and also to extend the investigation to other neuropeptides representing the three main sub-groups. Thus, the investigation included three autonomic (NA, NPY, VIP), five sensory (SP, CGRP, neurokinin A [NKA], GAL, SOM) and six opioid (MEAP, leucine-enkephalin [LE], met-enkephalin [ME], met-enkephalin-arg-gly-lys [MEAGL], DYN B, N/OFQ) mediators. Moreover, the occurrence of three different opioid receptors (DOR, KOR, MOR), was investigated.

AUTONOMIC FIBERS

Both sympathetic (NPY, NA) and para-sympathetic (VIP) fibers were identified in the tendon (Ackermann et al. 2001b). The autonomic fibers were mostly observed in the loose connective tissue around the proper tendon (Fig. 9.2). In the Achilles tendon, the fiber density was higher in the proximal musculotendinous junction than in the distal bone insertion. Overall, the autonomic fibers were predominantly seen as networks around blood vessels (Figs 9.2b & 9.3a). Among the three neuronal mediators, NPY was the most abundant and VIP the least.

As for the sympathetic fibers, NPY and NA immunoreactivities were almost exclusively observed as networks of varicose nerve terminals in the blood vessel walls (Fig. 9.3a). The vascular NPY-positive fibers were abundant in the paratenon as well as in the loose connective tissue. NA-positive fibers were confined to the surrounding loose connective tissues, mostly in large blood vessel walls, as also demonstrated in a study of human forearm muscle insertions (Ljung et al. 1999a). Overall, the observations seem to reflect that the regulation of blood flow to tendons predominantly occurs in the surrounding tissues (i.e. the paratenon and loose connective tissue).

The parasympathetic VIP-immunoreactive fibers, albeit scarce, were mostly observed as long, thin, varicose nerve terminals forming a "fence" in the paratenon (Fig. 9.3b). The fibers appeared to be evenly distributed between vascular and non-vascular structures. As opposed to NA/NPY mostly occurring in larger vessels, VIP was predominantly found around smaller vessels, which is in line with other reports (von During et al. 1995; Ljung et al. 1999a). This observation may reflect that NA

and NPY (vasoconstrictive) predominantly regulate the main blood flow to the tissues, whereas VIP (vasodilatory) is responsible for the fine-tuning of blood flow at a microlevel. The vascular and non-vascular distribution of VIP would seem to comply with an anti-ischemic and an anti-inflammatory effect in the periphery as reported earlier (Gherardini et al. 1998; Delgado et al. 2001). Notably, previous studies have suggested a strong anti-inflammatory role of VIP (Said 1998; Dickinson et al. 1999) through inhibition of T-cell proliferation and migration (Ottaway & Greenberg 1984).

Double-staining experiments disclosed coexistence of NPY and NA, mostly in vascular fibers, whereas coexistence of NPY and VIP was seen in both vascular and non-vascular fibers. Occasionally, some VIP-immunoreactivity could be seen colocalized with NA in nerve fibers of small blood vessels. This observed coexistence presumably reflects synergistic and/or inhibitory vasoactive effects in the tissues analyzed. NPY has been shown to potentiate the vasoconstrictive actions of NA (Lundberg & Hökfelt 1986), which is supported by NA and NPY being colocalized almost exclusively in fibers around blood vessels. Conversely, the coexistence of VIP with NA or NPY would seem to represent a modulatory mechanism (Li et al. 1999).

SENSORY FIBERS

Nerve fibers immunoreactive to SP, CGRP, NKA, GAL, and SOM were consistently identified in the Achilles tendon (Ackermann et al. 1999). The highest fiber density was observed in the surrounding tissues (i.e. the paratenon and loose connective tissue) (Fig. 9.2). The ratio of vascular to non-vascular fibers was higher in the surrounding loose connective tissue than in the paratenon, which exhibited a large number of non-vascular free nerve endings (Fig. 9.2c). Overall, there was no significant difference in the tissue distribution between the specific neuropeptides. However, the occurrence of CGRP-positive fibers was clearly higher than that of the other sensory neuropeptides.

The most conspicuous findings pertained to the abundance of sensory fibers in the surrounding tissues of the structures analyzed, whereas the

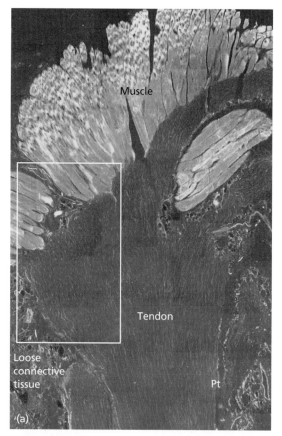

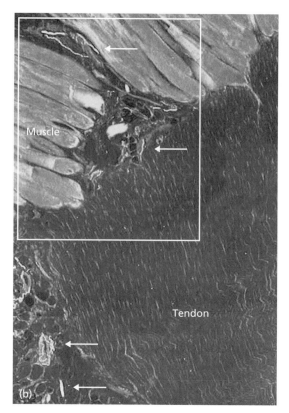

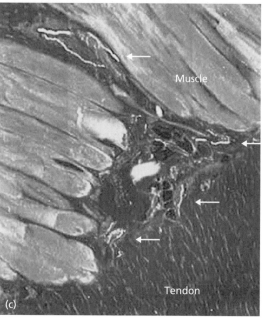

Fig. 9.2 Overview micrographs of longitudinal sections through the Achilles tendon built up by putting together computerized images of smaller micrographs. Incubation with antisera to general nerve marker PGP. Micrographs depict the proximal half of the Achilles tendon at increasing magnification in figures. Arrows denote varicosities and nerve terminals. The typical vascular localization of neuropeptide Y (NPY) is depicted in (b), whereas the free nerve endings are typical localization of substance P (SP) (c). The immunoreactivity is seen in the paratenon and surrounding loose connective tissue, whereas the proper tensinous tissue, notably, is almost devoid of nerve fibers. Pt, paratenon. (Reproduced with permission from Ackermann *et al.* 2002.)

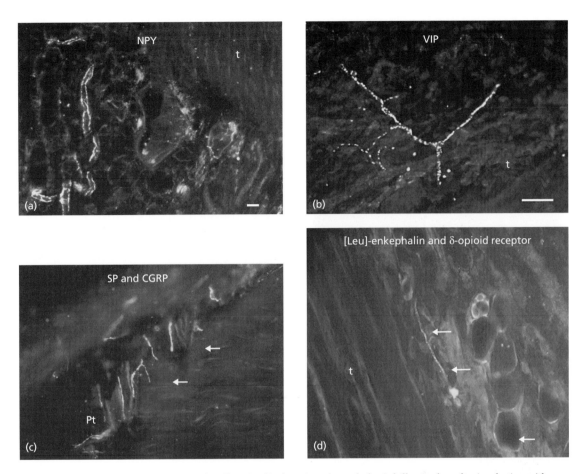

Fig. 9.3 Immunofluorescence micrographs of longitudinal sections through the Achilles tendon after incubation with antisera to neuropeptide Y (NPY) (a), vasoactive intestinal polypeptide (VIP) (b), and double staining (colocalization) of substance P (SP) and calcitonin gene-related peptide (CGRP) (c), leucine-enkephalin (LE) and δ-opioid receptor (DOR) (d). The NPY-positive fibers are arranged as nerve terminals in the vessel walls. VIP-positive nerves are arranged as a "fence", surrounding the proper tendon, of small varicosities in the paratenon. A coexistence of SP and CGRP is seen in the paratenon, indicating possible proinflammatory actions. The immunoreactivity displaying coexistence of LE and DOR is seen as free nerve endings in the paratenon, which indicates a potential peripheral anti-nociceptive system. t, tendon tissue; Pt, paratenon. Bar = 50 μm. (Reproduced with permission from Ackermann *et al.* 1999, 2001a.)

proper tendon, notably, was almost devoid of nerve fibers (Fig. 9.2). This would seem to reflect that the neuronal regulation of tendons highly depends on the innervation of the surrounding tissues. Thus, the abundance of immunopositive vascular fibers in the surrounding loose connective tissues may be assumed to reflect an important role in the regulation of blood flow to the proper structures. Both SP and CGRP, in particular the latter, have been reported to be potent vasodilators (Brain *et al.* 1985). In addition, they have also been

demonstrated to have pro-inflammatory effects (e.g. by enhancing protein extravasation and leukocyte chemotaxis). The occurrence of sensory free nerve endings unrelated to vessels predominantly seen in the paratenon suggests a nociceptive role.

The present investigation confirmed the well-known coexistence of SP and CGRP (Fig. 9.3c). However, each of these was also found to be colocalized with GAL and SOM. This has previously been demonstrated in dorsal root ganglia (Hökfelt *et al.* 1987) and in colon (Ekblad *et al.* 1988), but not in peripheral tissues of the locomotor apparatus. The observations of multiple coexistences strengthen the notion of functional interactions between sensory neuropeptides in the periphery (Hökfelt *et al.* 1987). Thus, CGRP has been reported to enhance the nociceptive effect of SP, whereas GAL and SOM are claimed to modulate nociception and pro-inflammation (Cridland & Henry 1988; Xu *et al.* 1991; Carlton & Coggeshall 1997; Szolcsanyi *et al.* 1998; Heppelmann *et al.* 2000).

OPIOID PEPTIDES AND RECEPTORS

The analyses established that all enkephalins tested (LE, ME, MEAP, and MEAGL) were present in peripheral nerve fibers of the Achilles tendon (Fig. 9.3d), whereas neither N/OFQ nor DYN B could be identified (Ackermann *et al.* 2001a). The failure of detecting N/OFQ in immune cells and nerve fibers by IHC, but the fact that measurable concentrations were obtained by RIA should be attributed to the latter being a more sensitive assay. As for DYN B, however, not identified by IHC or RIA, its non-existence or presence in low amounts in tendon tissue under normal physiologic conditions remains to be established. Notably, it has been shown that peripheral sensory nerves immunostain for dynorphin in inflammation, but not under normal conditions (Hassan *et al.* 1992).

Although the enkephalins differed in amount, their tissue distribution displayed a similar pattern. Thus, all four enkephalins predominantly occurred in the loose connective tissue, the paratenon and musculotendinous junction, whereas no enkephalins were found in the proper tendon tissue. Hypothetically, this difference in anatomic distribution might suggest that regulation of painful disorders of the Achilles tendon mainly occurs in the surrounding tissues, which during normal condition also harbor the sensory and autonomic neuropeptides.

In the loose connective tissue surrounding the tendon, the enkephalin-positive fibers appeared as small varicosities around the walls of both large and small blood vessels, which may reflect involvement in both vasodilatory actions (Moore & Dowling 1982) and anti-inflammatory responses (Lembeck *et al.* 1982; Hong & Abbott 1995). In the paratenon and the musculotendinous junction, the enkephalins

mostly occurred as varicosities in free nerve terminals without any relationship to blood vessels, suggesting a paracrine or an autocrine function in the regulation of nociception (Carlton & Coggeshall 1997; Machelska & Stein 2000). Such a regulation is probably executed in interaction with the sensory nervous system. Thus, it has been shown that the release of the sensory neuropeptide SP from afferents in the knee joint is inhibited by intra-articular enkephalin-analog injections (Yaksh 1988). It may prove that there is an inherent balance between opioid and sensory neuropeptides.

The existence of an opioid system in connective tissues as demonstrated by neuronal immunoreactivity to enkephalins is supported by our opioid receptor analyses based on binding assays and immunohistochemistry (Ackermann *et al.* 2001a). Of the three opioid receptors (DOR, KOR, MOR) studied, only DOR could be detected by immunohistochemistry (Fig. 9.3d). Double staining disclosed coexistence of each of the enkephalins with DOR in the nerve fibers (Fig. 9.3d), which complies with other studies suggesting that enkephalins are the main ligands for DOR (Dhawan *et al.* 1996). Thus, colocalization of enkephalins and DOR in paratenon, loose connective tissue and the musculotendinous junction was seen in small peripheral nerve terminals, suggesting C-fiber origin, which is in agreement with other reports demonstrating that both enkephalin (Carlton & Coggeshall 1997) and DOR (Coggeshall *et al.* 1997; Wenk & Honda 1999) are localized in unmyelinated afferent sensory axons in the skin. The major part of the enkephalins and DOR identified in the nerve fibers were found to be colocalized. The presence of peripheral opioid receptors was corroborated by the receptor binding analysis showing that tendon tissue could bind naloxone (a drug that binds to opiod receptors) in a specific and saturable way. DOR activity has been shown to have a potent inhibitory effect on SP release (Hirota *et al.* 1985; Yaksh 1988). There are several reports demonstrating that treatment with delta opioid agonists in the periphery elicit both anti-inflammatory and anti-nociceptive effects in models of inflammation (Taiwo & Levine 1991; Nozaki-Taguchi & Yamamoto 1998; Zhou *et al.* 1998). The anti-nociceptive actions have been shown to be mediated through DOR localized on unmyelinated afferent sensory axons (Zhou *et al.* 1998). Presumably, the coexistence of enkephalins and DOR in vascular nerve fibers reflects inhibition of neurogenic pro-inflammatory actions, whereas the coexistence in free nerve endings reflects inhibition of nociception.

Endogenous opioids, implicated in mitigating inflammatory pain, have been reported to be released by immune cells. However, data on the neuronal occurrence in the periphery are sparse so far. The present findings suggesting a neuronal source of opioids in the periphery would seem to reflect an anti-nociceptive system in connective tissues, which may be exploited in the therapeutic setting by drugs acting selectively in the periphery.

Altogether, there seems to exist a complex neuropeptidergic network in periarticular tissues, where each structure exhibits a specific expression of neuropeptides, as well as a specific ratio of potentiating and inhibitory mediators. The observations may be assumed to reflect unique tissue requirements of innervation under normal conditions, which includes tissue-specific susceptibilies to stress. The data obtained on normal tendons, ligaments, and joint capsules may be used as a neuroanatomic basis for studies of pathologic conditions of the locomotor apparatus.

Neuronal response to tendon injury

Besides cytokines and growth factors, neuropeptides in the periphery have been suggested to participate in tissue repair (Haegerstrand *et al.* 1990; Brain 1997; Schaffer *et al.* 1998; Onuoha & Alpar 2001). Having established the normal occurrence of nerve fibers and neuropeptides mainly localized in the surrounding structures of the tendon (i.e. the paratenon), further analyses were aimed at studying the occurrence of nerve fibers and their expression of neuropeptides after injury and during healing of tendinous tissue.

Neuropeptides and repair

One of the main functions of neuropeptides is to elicit and convey responses to stress and injury (Hökfelt *et al.* 2000). Neuropeptides have been shown to respond very specifically both in the central and peripheral nervous systems to inflammation and nerve injury, for example. A number of studies show that the expression of different neuropeptides in response to external stress follows a specific temporal pattern in accordance with the healing process. This would seem to reflect that neuropeptides have a regulatory role in nerve repair, possibly also in repair of other tissues including tendons.

So far there are very limited data on the peripheral expression of neuropeptides after injury of musculoskeletal tissues. Increased expression of SP and CGRP 2 weeks post-injury has been observed in fracture and skin healing (Kishimoto 1984; Hukkanen *et al.* 1993; Li *et al.* 2001). As for ligament healing, Grönblad *et al.* studied SP and CGRP expression 4 and 14 weeks after ligament rupture and found an increase at week 4 and a decrease at week 14. Altogether, the temporal expression of neuropeptides indicates that they are not only involved in the acute response to injury, but also in tissue regeneration.

It is well known that neuropathy in diabetes is associated not only with increased susceptibility to skin wounds but also with delayed tissue healing in general. A few investigators have reported a neuronal role in tissue healing over recent years (Haegerstrand *et al.* 1990; Brain 1997; Schaffer *et al.* 1998; Onuoha & Alpar 2001). Administration of SP and CGRP to the rat was shown to accelerate wound healing, while the combination of both neuropeptides accelerated healing even more. In fact, healing of wounds treated with SP and CGRP was completed 10 days earlier than controls (Khalil & Helme 1996). Conversely, capsaicin-induced sensory neuropeptide depletion causes delayed healing of corneal and skin ulcers (Gallar *et al.* 1990; Ko *et al.* 1998). Denervation of tendons or skin leads to decreased mechanical strength and collagen content (Aspenberg & Forslund 2000; Stelnicki *et al.* 2000). Notably, both SP and CGRP have been shown to participate in the regulation of proliferation of tendon proper cells (fibroblasts), tendon sheath cells (synoviocytes), and blood wall cells (endothelial cells) (Brain *et al.* 1985; Nilsson *et al.* 1985; Haegerstrand *et al.* 1990; Yule & White 1999), as well as in the synthesis or release of cytokines and growth factors (Broome & Miyan 2000; Monneret *et al.* 2000).

Neuronal plasticity during healing

Nerve regeneration during healing of experimental Achilles tendon rupture was studied by immunohistochemistry including a semi-quantitative assessment focusing on the rupture site of the proper tendinous tissue. Neuronal markers for regenerating and mature nerve fibers (i.e. growth associated protein 43 [GAP] and protein gene product 9.5 [PGP], respectively) were analyzed at different time points 1–16 weeks post-rupture. The morphologic distribution and expression of the neuronal markers over time were analyzed in relation to the three different phases of tissue healing: the inflammatory, the regenerative/proliferative, and the remodeling phase.

NEW NERVE FIBER INGROWTH—WEEK 1–2

In the first week post-rupture, which corresponds to the transition from the inflammatory to the regenerative phase, there was increased neuronal immunoreactivity to PGP and GAP, both in original nerve fibers of the surrounding loose connective tissue and, notably, in new nerve fibers in the proper tendon tissue of the rupture site (Ackermann *et al.* 2002) (Figs 9.4 & 9.5). In general, PGP positive fibers were predominantly observed in the surrounding loose connective tissue, predominantly seen around vessels. The vascular distribution of PGP in the loose connective tissue may be assumed to reflect the vasoregulatory role of the peripheral nervous system, but possibly also a proinflammatory role. In the proper tendinous tissue, normally GAP negative, there was a clear GAP immunoreactivity indicating new nerve fiber ingrowth, which is consistent with reports on GAP levels in dorsal root ganglia after peripheral nerve injury (Van der Zee *et al.* 1989; Chong *et al.* 1994, Bolden *et al.* 1997). GAP has been suggested to be involved in nerve regeneration by regulating growth cone motility and axon guidance signals (Frey *et al.* 2000; Gagliardini *et al.* 2000). Our observations of early nerve ingrowth are in line with observations on fracture and skin healing (Kishimoto 1984; Hukkanen *et al.* 1993; Li *et al.* 2001) indicating that this process is a fundamental feature of tissue healing.

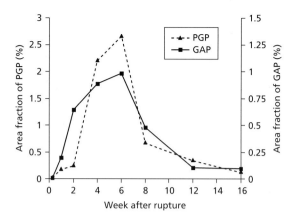

Fig. 9.4 Area occupied by nerve fibers (%) immunoreactive to growth associated protein 43 (GAP) and protein gene product 9.5 (PGP) in relation to total area, in the mid-third of the tendon, over 16 weeks post-rupture (mean ± SEM). (Reproduced with permission from Ackermann *et al.* 2002.)

NERVE FIBER PEAK EXPRESSION—WEEKS 2–6

During weeks 1–6 post-rupture of Achilles tendon, there was a striking shift in neuronal immunoreactivity from the surrounding loose connective tissue into the proper tendinous tissue (Figs 9.2 & 9.5). This would seem to reflect the transition of a predominantly inflammatory phase into a regenerative phase. The peak expression of GAP immunoreactivity in the rupture site occurred between weeks 2 and 6, while that of PGP occurred somewhat later (i.e. between weeks 4 and 6) (Fig. 9.4). The earlier peak of GAP should be explained by its trophic role in regulating growth cone formation. Analogously, the extensive ingrowth of GAP and PGP fibers into the rupture site may represent a neuronal involvement in tendon repair. The observed free nerve endings among fibroblasts in the tendinous tissue may reflect a stimulatory role in cell proliferation (McCarthy & Partlow 1976; Nilsson *et al.* 1985). The occurrence of free nerve endings around newly formed blood vessels in the rupture site suggests a role in vasoregulation, possibly also in angiogenesis (Haegerstrand *et al.* 1990).

NERVE FIBER WITHDRAWAL—WEEKS 6–16

During weeks 6–16 post-rupture (remodeling phase) the expression of the neuronal markers

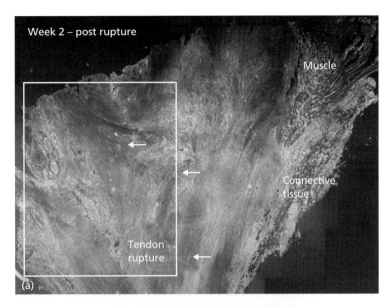

Week 2 – post rupture

Muscle

Connective tissue

Tendon rupture

(a)

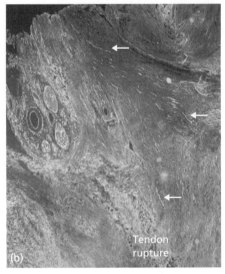

Tendon rupture

(b)

Fig. 9.5 Overview micrographs of longitudinal sections through the Achilles tendon 2 weeks post-rupture built up by putting together computerized images of smaller micrographs. Incubation with antisera to a nerve growth marker, GAP-43. Micrographs depict the proximal half of the Achilles tendon at increasing magnification in figures. Arrows denote varicosities and nerve terminals. The GAP positive fibers, indicating new nerve fiber ingrowth, are abundantly observed in the healing proper tendon tissue. Some GAP fibers are also located in the loose connective tissue; however, most are localized as free nerve endings within the healing proper tendon tissue. (Reproduced with permission from Ackermann *et al.* 2002.)

showed a significant decrease in the rupture site (Fig. 9.4). The nerve fibers appeared to withdraw from the healing area. While GAP immunoreactivity almost completely disappeared during this phase, that of PGP successively returned to normal in the paratenon and surrounding loose connective tissue. The process seemed to end simultaneously with the completion of paratenon repair.

The observations during tendon healing clearly demonstrate the capability of the peripheral nervous

system to respond and adapt to injury. This plasticity is characterized by nerve fiber ingrowth into the rupture site, a peak nerve fiber expression during the regenerative phase followed by nerve fiber withdrawal.

The experimental model employed appears to be highly appropriate and relevant for studies of the role of the peripheral nervous system in tissue repair. To our knowledge, no similar studies of repair are based on tissues normally devoid of a neuronal supply. The ingrowth and later with-drawal of nerve fibers in the proper Achilles tendon after rupture convincingly reflect that the neuronal supply is fundamental in the repair process. Although it may be argued that new nerve fiber ingrowth after injury merely represents a secondary phenomenon to neovascularization, this is contra-dicted by the abundant occurrence of free sprouting nerve endings unrelated to vessels in the healing area. Presumably, new nerve ingrowth provides a delivery system for neuronal mediators that are required for tissue repair.

Neuropeptidergic expression in tendon healing

The extensive nerve regeneration and ingrowth observed in tendon rupture prompted an immuno-histologic analysis of the specific neuropeptides involved. Thus, the temporal expression of different neuropeptides presumed to exert trophic actions was examined. The study included sensory (SP, CGRP), sensory modulating (GAL), and autonomic (NPY, VIP) mediators.

The analysis including semi-quantification de-monstrated an early (week 1) expression of SP and CGRP positive fibers, both in the loose connective tissue and the rupture site of the proper tendon (Figs 9.6 & 9.7). The expression peaked during the

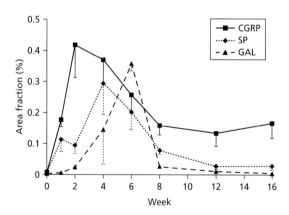

Fig. 9.6 Area occupied by nerve fibers (%) immunoreactive to substance P (SP), calcitonin gene-related peptide (CGRP), and galanin (GAL) in relation to total area, in the mid-third of the tendon, over 16 weeks post-rupture (mean ± SEM). (Reproduced with permission from Ackermann *et al.* 2003.)

regenerative phase. In contrast, GAL, NPY, and VIP positive fibers first emerged at the end of the regen-erative phase at weeks 4–6 (Fig. 9.6), most evidently in the border zone between loose connective tissue and proper tendon (Ackermann 2003).

INFLAMMATORY PHASE

One week post-rupture, corresponding to the end of the inflammatory phase, SP and CGRP fibers were predominantly located in blood vessel walls surrounded by inflammatory cells in the loose con-nective tissue (Fig. 9.7a). Only a weak and scanty expression of GAL, NPY, and VIP was observed. The findings comply with the nociceptive role of sensory neuropeptides, but also with a proinflam-matory role. Thus, SP release has been shown to enhance vasopermeability (Saria *et al.* 1983) and to stimulate recruitment of leukocytes (Carolan & Casale 1993; Bowden *et al.* 1994; Quinlan *et al.* 1998).

REGENERATIVE PHASE

During weeks 1–6, the expression of SP and CGRP peaked (Fig. 9.6). Notably, this peak occurred in the rupture site of the proper tendon, while the neuronal immunoreactivity in the surrounding loose con-nective tissue declined. The latter would seem to comply with decreased pain 3–4 weeks after injury. The most conspicuous finding, however, was the occurrence of SP and CGRP in free sprouting nerve endings among fibroblasts in the healing tendinous tissue (Fig 9.7b). The observation might reflect a stimulatory role of sensory neuropeptides on pro-liferation as has been demonstrated in cultered fibroblasts (Nilsson *et al.* 1985; Yule & White 1999). SP and CGRP are also known to stimulate proliferation of endothelial cells (Nilsson *et al.* 1985; Haegerstrand *et al.* 1990; Ziche *et al.* 1990). The observation of free sprouting SP and CGRP positive fibers around newly formed blood vessels in the rupture site would seem to comply with a role in angiogenesis (Fig. 9.7b).

During the regenerative phase, the occurrence of NPY, VIP, and GAL positive fibers was sparse until week 4. Subsequently, the expression increased to reach a peak at the end of the regenerative phase (i.e.

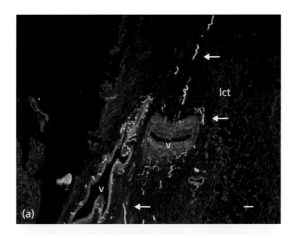

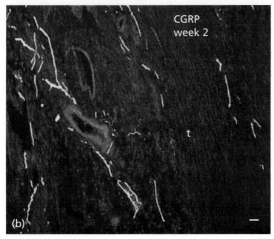

Fig. 9.7 Immunofluorescence micrograph of longitudinal sections through healing Achilles tendon (a) 1 and (b) 2 weeks post-rupture after incubation with antisera to calcitonin gene-related peptide (CGRP). Nerve fibers immunoreactive to CGRP are seen as vascular and free nerve endings in the loose connective tissue (a). CGRP immunoreactivity occurs mainly in the healing tendinous tissue as sprouting free nerve fibers. lct, loose connective tissue; t, proper tendon tissue; v, blood vessel. Bar = 50 μm. (Reproduced with permission from Ackermann *et al.* 2003.)

around week 6) followed by a successive decrease (Fig. 9.6). This pattern in temporal expression was assessed morphologically and semi-quantitatively for GAL (Fig. 9.6), whereas the assessment of NPY and VIP was confined to subjective morphology. Overall, the occurrence of NPY, VIP, and GAL was clearly lower than that of the sensory neuropeptides

during the first weeks, in particular at the rupture site of the proper tendon.

As for NPY, the observations would seem to reflect that vasoconstriction is downregulated during the regenerative phase. Notably, low levels of NPY have also been suggested to promote angiogenesis (Zukowska-Grojec *et al.* 1998). The initial low expression of VIP appears surprising considering the need for vasodilation during tissue repair given the predominant occurrence of VIP around small-sized vessels under normal conditions, where, hypothetically, it regulates the fine-tuning of vasoactivity. However, the demand for this function is probably low in the early phase of tissue repair. Another explanation for the low occurrence of VIP pertains to its inhibitory action on the proinflammatory effects of SP and CGRP as demonstrated by Delgado *et al.* (2001). Thus, the observation may represent less inhibition of SP and CGRP, which are presumed to be important regulators of early tissue repair (Gallar *et al.* 1990; Khalil & Helme 1996; Ko *et al.* 1998).

REMODELING PHASE

Between weeks 4 and 6, corresponding to the transition of the regenerative into the remodeling phase, there was a dramatic increase in the expression of GAL, VIP, and NPY, followed by decreased expression of SP and CGRP (Fig. 9.6). The increase in the immunoreactivity of GAL, VIP, and NPY was observed both around vessels and in free nerve endings in a "border zone" enveloping the healing tendon. The emergence of GAL, known to modulate the effect of sensory neuropeptides, would seem to comply with inhibition of the early inflammatory and nociceptive response to injury. Thus, GAL has been demonstrated to mitigate the proinflammatory and nociceptive effects of SP (Cridland & Henry 1988; Xu *et al.* 1991; Jancso *et al.* 2000; Heppelmann *et al.* 2000). Similarly, the increased occurrence of VIP may be explained by its inhibitory effect on immune cells expressing proinflammatoy cytokines (Delgado *et al.* 2001). The increased occurrence of NPY during this phase mostly seen around vessels should probably be attributed to its well-known vasoconstrictive actions. Notably, increased vasoconstriction leads to a relative hypoxia, which is known to enhance the tensile strength of the tendon by switching production of collagen from type III to type I (Steinbrech *et al.* 1999).

The early remodeling phase after tendon injury is characterized by an increased expression of GAL, VIP, and NPY, all of which are known to modulate the effects of SP and CGRP. It may prove that this modulation is required to end the nociceptive, inflammatory, and regenerative processes, thereby permitting entry to and maintenance of the remodeling phase.

On the whole, it seems that the temporal expression of the different neuropeptides studied complies with specific actions in injury, pain, and regeneration. Whether neuropeptides mainly act directly on the target tissues or indirectly by regulating the release of cytokines, growth factors, and chemokines from immune cells is unclear. Given the latter mechanisms it still remains to be clarified whether the effects on these cells pertain to chemotaxis, differentiation, or function.

Neuroanatomy in tendinopathy

Several studies have now established that the neuroanatomy of normal human tendons is comparable with the innervation of experimental animals (Ljung *et al.* 1999a,b, 2004; Ackermann & Renström 2001; Uchio *et al.* 2002; Schubert *et al.* 2005, 2006; Bjur *et al.* 2005; Lian *et al.* 2006). For example, under normal conditions, nerve fibers in the rat Achilles tendon are localized in the tendon envelope (i.e. the paratenon). This correlates well to the human Achilles tendon where under normal conditions nerve fibers also are localized in the tendon envelopes (i.e. the endotenon and paratenon). The proper tendon tissue, however, both in human and animals, is practically devoid of nerve fibers.

Recently, a number of studies demonstrated that in tendinopathy there exists a nerve ingrowth into the painful tendon proper that may reflect increased pain signaling as a response to repetitive mechanical stimuli. Thus, in patients with patellar tendinopathy (Lian *et al.* 2006), Dupuytren's contracture (Schubert *et al.* 2006) as well as Achilles tendinopathy (Schubert *et al.* 2005), sensory nerve ingrowth has been demonstrated. We speculate

that repeated microtrauma might be an initiator of the neuronal reactions because nerve ingrowth is known to occur as a response to tendon injury (Ackermann *et al.* 2002).

The ingrown nerves also express SP, which may be assumed to be involved in a number of actions. Vascular-related SP positive nerve fibers may reflect effects on vasodilation, plasma extravasation, and release of cytokines, but also a role in neovascularization has been shown for SP. The free sprouting SP positive nerve endings within the tendon proper may, in addition to their role in nociception (Ueda 1999), reflect a trophic role. SP has been reported to stimulate the production of transforming growth factor β in fibroblasts (Lai *et al.* 2003) and to directly enhance proliferation of fibroblasts (Nilsson *et al.* 1985) and endothelial cells (Haegerstrand *et al.* 1990). We therefore suggest that SP contributes to the morphologic changes observed in patients with tendinopathy (i.e. tenocyte transformation, hypercellularity, and presumably also neovascularization).

In addition to an upregulation of SP, we recently demonstrated a reduction in vasoregulatory NA in patients with tendinopathy. This suggests a decreased anti-nociceptive function because NA release leads to secretion of opioids from leukocytes (Rittner *et al.* 2005). Notably, patients with painful rheumatoid arthritis also exhibit a similar pattern with reduced NA and increased free SP nerve fibers (Straub *et al.* 2002). Altogether, the peripheral nervous system remains a promising target for further research.

Clinical relevance and significance

Tendon pathology, pain, degeneration, and rupture are major causes of sports-related morbidity, as well as sick leave. However, the actual pathomechanisms are still largely unknown, which makes rehabilitation an inexact and often prolonged process with slow returns to normal levels of activity.

The findings described in this chapter, concerning the involvement of the peripheral nervous system in tendon pathology, may open new doors to understanding the development of tendon disorders and provide new treatment regimes. Over the last decade, knowledge about specific neuronal signal substances involved in the regulation of pain, inflammation, and tissue repair has evolved. This chapter describes how these neuronal mediators, neuropeptides including opioids, for the first time were discovered in tendons. An endogenous peripheral system of pain inhibition was thus revealed. New data establish the involvement of the peripheral nervous system and neuropeptides in the development of painful tendinopathy. Moreover, recent findings on neuronal response to injury suggests new pathways for tendon repair.

The novel data presented in this chapter considering tendon innervation and neuronal response to injury, may suggest new targets for pain treatment and specific pharmacotherapy in tendon disorders to shorten recovery time until return to sports.

Future directions

Therapeutic potentials

The relevance of the present study pertains to the possibility of intervening in different efferent mechanisms of the peripheral nervous system, which presumably are implicated in a wide variety of functions such as nociception, inflammatory responses, vasoactivity, and regeneration. Specific neuronal intervention, however, presupposes that the innervation of the musculoskeletal system according to specific mediators is clarified. From the present study, it seems obvious that periarticular tissues are supplied with a complex peptidergic network, which presumably takes part in maintaining tissue homeostasis, but also by its plasticity (i.e. nerve ingrowth and temporal alteration in neuropeptide expression), is capable of responding to external injury. These findings raise the question whether manipulation of the nervous system and the neuropeptide expression could be used in the treatment of tendon disorders, both in pain management and to promote tissue healing and shorten rehabilitation.

ENHANCING NEUROPEPTIDE DELIVERY

Two possible strategies of optimizing the repair response comprise stimulation of the endogenous release of neuropeptides, and delivery of exogenous neuropeptides to the local healing area. Mimick-

ing as well as augmenting the endogenous release of neuropeptides could be carried out by means of an increased generation of delivery channels (i.e. stimulation of nerve ingrowth).

SUPPLEMENT OF NEUROPEPTIDES

Several experimental studies have been set up during the last decades to investigate the neuropeptide effect on tissue regeneration, with remarkable results on such tissue as skin and cornea. Administration of sensory neuropeptides, SP, or CGRP to rat skin accelerated wound healing, and the combination of both neuropeptides potentiated the effect. In fact, healing of wounds treated with SP and CGRP was completed 10 days earlier than controls (Khalil & Helme 1996). Conversely, capsaicin-induced sensory neuropeptide depletion leads to delayed healing, and blockade of the sympathetic nervous system actually causes degradation of the rat medial collateral ligament (MCL) (Dwyer et al. 2004).

Only recently, however, have neuropeptides been tested in the setting of connective tissue healing. It has been demonstrated that both sensory and autonomic neuropeptides administered to healing MCL accelerate tissue regeneration and reverse the effect of denervation. Subsequent to SP supplement the ligaments manifested an even greater tensile strength than the intact control (Dwyer et al. 2005). Recently, supplement of SP in physiologic concentrations to healing Achilles tendons proved to enhance fibroblast aggregation and to increase tensile strength more than 100% compared with controls (Burssens et al. 2005; Steyaert et al. 2006). These findings would denote SP as the most potent tissue growth stimulator known in tendon healing.

Interestingly enough, the cross-linking between collagen fibers did not increase by exogenous SP supplement during the early inflammatory phase. The cross-linking is accomplished during a later phase of tendon healing compared to longitudinal growth. SP is produced chiefly during the initial stages of tendon healing, followed by a withdrawal during the subsequent tendon remodeling phase. It may prove that a later supplement of additional neuronal growth factors (e.g. autonomic neuropeptides) would complement the effects of SP.

STIMULATION BY NERVE GROWTH FACTORS

One important factor for sensory nerve ingrowth, survival, and phenotype is the neuronal growth factor (NGF). It is normally secreted from different immune competent cells, fibroblasts, and smooth muscle cells, all present during tendon repair. The NGF concentration seems to be already elevated during the early inflammatory phase of healing. This implies that NGF in the early inflammatory phase of tendon healing could stimulate nerve ingrowth. Therefore, it should be possible to enhance neuronal ingrowth in the healing area through local NGF injections. In fact, repeated injections of NGF in mice muscle have been shown to increase the ingrowth of sensory but not of sympathetic nerves (Hopkins 1984). Additional nerve growth factors that might promote tendon healing are neurotrophins and laminins, which should be investigated.

PHYSICAL ACTIVITY TO PROMOTE NERVE INGROWTH

Physical activity and early mobilization are well known to be beneficial in the healing process following injury. This may, in part, be an effect of the increased neuronal ingrowth seen in tendon tissue stimulated by physical activity. One possible explanation for the increased neuronal ingrowth could be that cyclic stress stimulates the expression of NGF from smooth muscle cells (Clemow 2000), which might increase nerve ingrowth in the healing area. Both local application of NGF and early mobilization may lead to increased nerve ingrowth, thereby enhancing the endogenous delivery of neuropeptides to the repair site.

In order to investigate whether it would be possible to stimulate nerve ingrowth through graded physical activity, we designed an experiment where groups of rats were allowed to mobilize to different extents during healing. Preliminary results from these studies show an accelerated neuronal regeneration paralleled with an increased healing rate in rats with early mobilization compared with immobilized rats. This indicates an important role for early mobilization, possibly combined with NGF in the neuronal regulation of repair.

INTERMITTENT PNEUMATIC PRESSURE TREATMENT TO PROMOTE HEALING

Intermittent pneumatic compression (IPC), a treatment based on external cyclic pressure, has traditionally been used to promote circulation and prevent thrombosis. It has been stipulated that IPC may be useful in treating tissue damages and has proven effective in the treatment of skin wounds, venous ulcers, and recently even fractures, inducing increased bone strength and callus formation (Kumar & Walker 2002; Park & Silva 2003; Hewitt *et al.* 2005). In a recent study we have demonstrated that daily IPC treatment enhances the fibroblast aggregation and neurovascular ingrowth in healing Achilles tendons, based on an enhanced production of sensory neuropeptides. IPC acts as a passive exercise, with the greatest effect upon the venous circulation, but also by compressing the muscles effects the same cyclic stress as physical activity.

While the potential benefits of manipulations of the peripheral nervous system in the management of connective tissue injury are conceivable, several questions need to be addressed. Which technique will be the most efficient for delivery of neuropeptides to the repair site? Which neuropeptides are the most effective related to the different phases of healing? The appropriate dosage is a critical factor in optimizing repair. Moreover, the localization of neuropeptide delivery should most probably be applied according to the temporally and spatially determined phases of repair.

References

Ackermann, P. (2001) *Peptidergic innervation of periarticular tissue*. Thesis. Stockholm, Sweden.

Ackermann, P., Spetea, M., Nylander, I., Ploj, K., Ahmed, M. & Kreicbergs, A. (2001a) An opioid system in connective tissue: a study of achilles tendon in the rat. *Journal of Histochemistry and Cytochemistry* **49**, 1387–1396.

Ackermann, P.W. (2003) Neuronal plasticity in relation to nociception and healing of rat Achilles tendon. *Journal of Orthopaedic Research* **21**, 432–441.

Ackermann, P.W., Ahmed, M. & Kreicbergs, A. (2002) Early nerve regeneration after Achilles tendon rupture: a prerequisite for healing? A study in the rat. *Journal of Orthopaedic Research* **20**, 849–856.

Ackermann, P.W., Finn, A. & Ahmed, M. (1999) Sensory neuropeptidergic pattern in tendon, ligament and joint capsule. A study in the rat. *Neuroreport* **13**, 2055–2060.

Ackermann, P.W., Jian, L., Finn, A., Ahmed, M. & Kreicbergs, A. (2001b) Autonomic innervation of tendons, ligaments and joint capsules. A morphologic and quantitative study in the rat. *Journal of Orthopaedic Research* **19**, 372–378.

Ackermann, W.P. & Renström, A.F.H. (2001) Sensory neuropeptides in achilles tendinosis. *Arthroscopy: The Journal of Arthroscopic and Related Surgery*, 2001–07 (Vol. 17, Issue 6, Suppl. 2).

Ahmed, M., Bjurholm, A., Schultzberg, M., Theodorsson, E. & Kreicbergs, A. (1995) Increased levels of substance P and calcitonin gene-related peptide in rat adjuvant arthritis. A combined immunohistochemical and radioimmunoassay analysis. *Arthritis and Rheumatism* **38**, 699–709.

Archambault, J.M., Wiley, J.P. & Bray, R.C. (1995) Exercise loading of tendons and the development of overuse injuries. A review of current literature. *Sports Medicine* **20**, 77–89.

Aspenberg, P. & Forslund, C. (2000) Bone morphogenetic proteins and tendon repair. *Scandinavian Journal of Medicine and Science in Sports* **10**, 372–375.

Barnard, P. (1997) Musculoskeletal disords and workplace factors: a critical review of epidemiologic evidence for work-related musculoskeletal disorders of the neck, upper extremity, and low back. US Department of Health and Human Services (National Institute of Occuopational Safety and Health) A99, 97–628.

Bayliss, W.M. (1901) On the origin from the spinal cord of the vasodilator fibres of the hind limb and on the nature of these fibres. *Journal of Physiology* **26**, 173–209.

Bjur, D., Alfredson, H. & Forsgren, S. (2005) The innervation pattern of the human Achilles tendon: studies of the normal and tendinosis tendon with markers for general and sensory innervation. *Cell and Tissue Research* **320**, 201–206.

Bolden, D.A., Sternini, C. & Kruger, L. (1997) GAP-43 mRNA and calcitonin gene-related peptide mRNA expression in sensory neurons are increased following sympathectomy. *Brain Research Bulletin* **42**, 39–50.

Bowden, J.J., Garland, A.M., Baluk, P., *et al.* (1994) Direct observation of substance P-induced internalization of neurokinin 1 (NK1) receptors at sites of inflammation. *Proceedings of the National Academy of Sciences of the United States of America* **91**, 8964–8968.

Brain, S.D. (1997) Sensory neuropeptides: their role in inflammation and wound healing. *Immunopharmacology* **37**, 133–152.

Brain, S.D., Williams, T.J., Tippins, J.R., Morris, H.R. & MacIntyre, I. (1985) Calcitonin gene-related peptide is a potent vasodilator. *Nature* **313**, 54–56.

Brodin, E., Gazelius, B., Panopoulos, P. & Olgart, L. (1983) Morphine inhibits substance P release from peripheral sensory nerve endings. *Acta Physiologica Scandinavica* **117**, 567–570.

Broome, C.S. & Miyan, J.A. (2000) Neuropeptide control of bone marrow neutrophil production. A key axis for neuroimmunomodulation. *Annals of the New York Academy of Sciences* **917**, 424–434.

Brown, S.L. & Van Epps, D.E. (1985) Suppression of T lymphocyte chemotactic factor production by the opioid peptides beta-endorphin and met-enkephalin. *Journal of Immunology* **134**, 3384–3390.

Burssens, P., Steyaert, A., Forsyth, R., van Ovost, E.J., De Paepe, Y. & Verdonk, R. (2005) Exogenously administered substance P and neutral endopeptidase inhibitors stimulate fibroblast proliferation, angiogenesis and collagen organization during Achilles tendon healing. *Foot and Ankle International* **26**, 832–839.

Cabot, P.J. (2001) Immune-derived opioids and peripheral antinociception. *Clinical and Experimental Pharmacology and Physiology* **28**, 230–232.

Calo', G., Guerrini, R., Rizzi, A., Salvadori, S. & Regoli, D. (2000) Pharmacology of nociceptin and its receptor: a novel therapeutic target. *British Journal of Pharmacology* **129**, 1261–1283.

Carlton, S.M. & Coggeshall, R.E. (1997) Immunohistochemical localization of enkephalin in peripheral sensory axons in the rat. *Neuroscience Letters* **221**, 121–124.

Carolan, E.J. & Casale, T.B. (1993) Effects of neuropeptides on neutrophil migration through noncellular and endothelial barriers. *Journal of Allergy and Clinical Immunology* **92**, 589–598.

Chong, M.S., Reynolds, M.L., Irwin, N., *et al.* (1994) GAP-43 expression in primary sensory neurons following

central axotomy. *Journal of Neuroscience* **14**, 4375–4384.

Clemow, D.B. (2000) Stretch-activated signaling of nerve growth factor secretion in bladder and vascular smooth muscle cells from hypertensive and hyperactive rats. *Journal of Cellular Physiology* **183**, 289–300.

Coggeshall, R.E., Zhou, S. & Carlton, S.M. (1997) Opioid receptors on peripheral sensory axons. *Brain Research* **764**, 126–132.

Cridland, R.A. & Henry, J.L. (1988) Effects of intrathecal administration of neuropeptides on a spinal nociceptive reflex in the rat: VIP, galanin, CGRP, TRH, somatostatin and angiotensin II. *Neuropeptides* **11**, 23–32.

Darland, T., Heinricher, M.M. & Grandy, D.K. (1998) Orphanin FQ/nociceptin: a role in pain and analgesia, but so much more. *Trends in Neurosciences* **21**, 215–221.

Delgado, M., Abad, C., Martinez, C., Leceta, J. & Gomariz, R.P. (2001) Vasoactive intestinal peptide prevents experimental arthritis by downregulating both autoimmune and inflammatory components of the disease. *Natural Medicines* **7**, 563–568.

Dhawan, B.N., Cesselin, F., Raghubir, R., *et al.* (1996) International Union of Pharmacology. XII. Classification of opioid receptors. *Pharmacological Reviews* **48**, 567–592.

Dickinson, T., Mitchell, R., Robberecht, P. & Fleetwood-Walker, S.M. (1999) The role of VIP/PACAP receptor subtypes in spinal somatosensory processing in rats with an experimental peripheral mononeuropathy. *Neuropharmacology* **38**, 167–180.

Dwyer, K.W., Jensen, K.T. & Vanderby, R. (2005) Local delivery of neuropeptides reverses functional deficit in neuroapthic MCL healing. Proceedings of the 51th Annual meeting of the Orthopaedic Research Society. *Transactions* Vol. 30, Washington DC.

Dwyer, K.W., Provenzano, P.P., Muir, P., Valhmu, W.B. & Vanderby, R. (2004) Blockade of the sympathetic nervous system degrades ligament in a rat MCL model. *Journal of Applied Physiology* **96**, 711–718.

Ekblad, E., Ekman, R., Hakanson, R. & Sundler, F. (1988) Projections of peptide-containing neurons in rat colon. *Neuroscience* **27**, 655–674.

Florez, J. & Mediavilla, A. (1977) Respiratory and cardiovascular effects of met-enkephalin applied to the ventral surface of the brain stem. *Brain Research* **138**, 585–900.

Frey, D., Laux, T., Xu, L., Schneider, C. & Caroni, P. (2000) Shared and unique roles of CAP23 and GAP43 in actin regulation, neurite outgrowth, and anatomical plasticity. *Journal of Cell Biology* **149**, 1443–1454.

Gagliardini, V., Dusart, I. & Fankhauser, C. (2000) Absence of GAP-43 can protect neurons from death. *Molecular and Cellular Neurosciences* **16**, 27–33.

Gallar, J., Pozo, M.A., Rebollo, I. & Belmonte, C. (1990) Effects of capsaicin on corneal wound healing. *Investigative Ophthalmology and Visual Science* **31**, 1968–1974.

Gherardini, G., Gurlek, A., Evans, G.R., et al. (1998) Venous ulcers: improved healing by iontophoretic administration of calcitonin gene-related peptide and vasoactive intestinal polypeptide. *Plastic and Reconstructive Surgery* **101**, 90–93.

Grant, D.S. & Zukowska, Z. (2000) Revascularization of ischemic tissues with SIKVAV and neuropeptide Y (NPY) [In Process Citation]. *Advances in Experimental Medicine and Biology* **476**, 139–154.

Green, P.G., Basbaum, A.I. & Levine, J.D. (1992) Sensory neuropeptide interactions in the production of plasma extravasation in the rat. *Neuroscience* **50**, 745–749.

Haegerstrand, A., Dalsgaard, C.J., Jonzon, B., Larsson, O. & Nilsson, J. (1990) Calcitonin gene-related peptide stimulates proliferation of human endothelial cells. *Proceedings of the National Academy of Sciences United States of America* **87**, 3299–3303.

Hassan, A.H., Pzewlocki, R., Herz, A. & Stein, C. (1992) Dynorphin, a preferential ligand for kappa-opioid receptors, is present in nerve fibers and immune cells within inflamed tissue of the rat. *Neuroscience Letters* **140**, 85–88.

Heppelmann, B., Just, S. & Pawlak, M. (2000) Galanin influences the mechanosensitivity of sensory endings in the rat knee joint. *European Journal of Neuroscience* **12**, 1567–1572.

Herz, A. (1995) Role of immune processes in peripheral opioid analgesia. *Advances in Experimental Medicine and Biology* **373**, 193–199.

Hewitt, J.D., Harrelson, J.M., Dailiana, Z., Guilak, F. & Fink, C. (2005) The effect of intermittent pneumatic compression on fracture healing. *Journal of Orthopaedic Trauma* **19**, 371–376.

Hirota, N., Kuraishi, Y., Hino, Y., Sato, Y., Satoh, M. & Takagi, H. (1985) Met-enkephalin and morphine but not dynorphin inhibit noxious stimuli-induced release of substance P from rabbit dorsal horn *in situ*. *Neuropharmacology* **24**, 567–570.

Hökfelt, T., Broberger, C., Xu, Z.Q., Sergeyev, V., Ubink, R. & Diez, M. (2000) Neuropeptides: an overview. *Neuropharmacology* **39**, 1337–1356.

Hökfelt, T., Johansson, O., Ljungdahl, A., Lundberg, J.M. & Schultzberg, M. (1980) Peptidergic neurones. *Nature* **284**, 515–521.

Hökfelt, T., Kellerth, J.O., Nilsson, G. & Pernow, B. (1975) Substance p: localization in the central nervous system and in some primary sensory neurons. *Science* **190**, 889–890.

Hökfelt, T., Millhorn, D., Seroogy, K., et al. (1987) Coexistence of peptides with classical neurotransmitters. *Experientia* **43**, 768–780.

Hong, Y. & Abbott, F.V. (1995) Peripheral opioid modulation of pain and inflammation in the formalin test. *Eurpean Journal of Pharmacology* **277**, 21–28.

Hopkins, W.G. (1984) Effect of nerve growth factor on intramuscular axons of neonatal mice. *Neuroscience* **13**, 951–956.

Hukkanen, M., Konttinen, Y.T., Santavirta, S., et al. (1993) Rapid proliferation of calcitonin gene-related peptide-immunoreactive nerves during healing of rat tibial fracture suggests neural involvement in bone growth and remodelling. *Neuroscience* **54**, 969–979.

Jancso, G., Santha, P., Horvath, V. & Pierau, F. (2000) Inhibitory neurogenic modulation of histamine-induced cutaneous plasma extravasation in the pigeon. *Regulatory Peptides* **95**, 75–80.

Jarvinen, T.A., Kannus, P., Paavola, M., Jarvinen, T.L., Józsa, L. & Jarvinen, M. (2001) Work-related upper extremity musculoskeletal disorders. *Current Opinion in Rheumatology* **13**, 150–155.

Józsa, L. & Kannus, P. (1997) Pathophysiology of tendon overuse injuries. In: *Human Tendons*. Anonymous. Human Kinetics, Champaign, IL: 178–184.

Kannus, P. & Józsa, L. (1991) Histopathological changes preceding spontaneous rupture of a tendon. A controlled study of 891 patients. *Journal of Bone and Joint Surgery. American volume* **73**, 1507–1525.

Khalil, Z. & Helme, R. (1996) Sensory peptides as neuromodulators of wound healing in aged rats. *Journal of Gerontology* **51**, B354–3561.

Kishimoto, S. (1984) The regeneration of substance P-containing nerve fibers in the process of burn wound healing in the guinea pig skin. *Journal of Investigative Dermatology* **83**, 219–223.

Ko, F., Diaz, M., Smith, P., et al. (1998) Toxic effects of capsaicin on keratinocytes and fibroblasts. *Journal of Burn Care and Rehabilitation* **19**, 409–413.

Kumar, S. & Walker, M.A. (2002) The effects of intermittent pneumatic compression on the arterial and venous system of the lower limb: a review. *Journal of Tissue Viability* **12**, 58–60, 62–66.

Lai, X.N., Wang, Z.G., Zhu, J.M. & Wang, L.L. (2003) Effect of substance P on gene expression of transforming growth factor beta-1 and its receptors in rat's fibroblasts. *Chinese Journal of Traumatology* **6**, 350–354.

Le Greves, P., Nyberg, F., Terenius, L. & Hokfelt, T. (1985) Calcitonin gene-related peptide is a potent inhibitor of substance P degradation. *European Journal of Pharmacology* **115**, 309–311.

Leadbetter, W.B. (1992) Cell–matrix response in tendon injury. *Clinics in Sports Medicine* **11**, 533–578.

Lembeck, F., Donnerer, J. & Bartho, L. (1982) Inhibition of neurogenic vasodilation and plasma extravasation by substance P antagonists, somatostatin and [D-Met2, Pro5]enkephalinamide. *European Journal of Pharmacology* **85**, 171–176.

Lembeck, F., Folkers, K. & Donnerer, J. (1981) Analgesic effect of antagonists of substance P. *Biochemical and Biophysical Research Communications* **103**, 1318–1321.

Levenson, C.W. & Moore, J.B. (1998) Response of rat adrenal neuropeptide Y and tyrosine hydroxylase mRNA to acute stress is enhanced by long-term voluntary exercise. *Neuroscience Letters* **242**, 177–179.

Li, J., Ahmad, T., Spetea, M., Ahmed, M. & Kreicbergs, A. (2001) Bone reinnervation after fracture: a study in the rat. *Journal of Bone and Mineral Research* **16**, 1505–1510.

Li, Q., Johansson, H. & Grimelius, L. (1999) Innervation of human adrenal gland and adrenal cortical lesions. *Virchows Archiv* **435**, 580–589.

Lian, O., Dahl, J., Ackermann, P., Frihagen, F., Engebretsen, L. & Bahr, R. (2006) Pro- and anti-inflammatory neuromediators in patellar tendinopathy. *American Journal of Sports Medicine* Jun 30 [Epub ahead of print].

Ljung, B.O., Alfredson, H. & Forsgren, S. (2004) Neurokinin 1-receptors and sensory neuropeptides in tendon insertions at the medial and lateral epicondyles of the humerus. Studies on tennis elbow and medial epicondylalgia. *Journal of Orthopaedic Research* **22**, 321–327.

Ljung, B.O., Forsgren, S. & Friden, J. (1999a) Sympathetic and sensory innervations are heterogeneously distributed in relation to the blood vessels at the extensor carpi radialis brevis muscle origin of man. *Cells, Tissues, Organs* **165**, 45–54.

Ljung, B.O., Forsgren, S. & Friden, J. (1999b) Substance P and calcitonin gene-related peptide expression at the extensor carpi radialis brevis muscle origin: implications for the etiology of tennis elbow. *Journal of Orthopaedic Research* **17**, 554–559.

Lundberg, J.M., Anggard, A., Fahrenkrug, J., Hokfelt, T. & Mutt, V. (1980) Vasoactive intestinal polypeptide in cholinergic neurons of exocrine glands: functional significance of coexisting transmitters for vasodilation and secretion. *Proceedings of the National Academy of Sciences of the United States of America* **77**, 1651–1655.

Lundberg, J.M. & Hokfelt, T. (1986) Multiple co-existence of peptides and classical transmitters in peripheral autonomic and sensory neurons: functional and pharmacological implications. *Progress in Brain Research* **68**, 241–262.

Machelska, H. & Stein, C. (2000) Pain control by immune-derived opioids [In Process Citation]. *Clinical and Experimenal Pharmacology and Physiology* **27**, 533–536.

Maggi, C.A. (1995) Tachykinins and calcitonin gene-related peptide (CGRP) as co-transmitters released from peripheral endings of sensory nerves. *Progress in Neurobiology* **45**, 1–98.

Mani, L. & Gerr, F. (2000) Work-related upper extremity musculoskeletal disorders. *Primary Care* **27**, 845–864.

McCarthy, K.D. & Partlow, L.M. (1976) Neuronal stimulation of (3H)thymidine incorporation by primary cultures of highly purified non-neuronal cells. *Brain Research* **114**, 415–426.

McDougall, J.J., Ferrell, W.R. & Bray, R.C. (1997) Spatial variation in sympathetic influences on the vasculature of the synovium and medial collateral ligament of the rabbit knee joint. *Journal of Physiology* **503**, 435–443.

McDougall, J.J., Hanesch, U., Pawlak, M. & Schmidt, R.F. (2001) Participation of NK1 receptors in nociceptin-induced modulation of rat knee joint mechanosensitivity. *Experimental Brain Research* **137**, 249–253.

McDougall, J.J., Pawlak, M., Hanesch, U. & Schmidt, R.F. (2000) Peripheral modulation of rat knee joint afferent mechanosensitivity by nociceptin/orphanin FQ. *Neuroscience Letters* **288**, 123–126.

Menkes, C.J., Renoux, M., Laoussadi, S., Mauborgne, A., Bruxelle, J. & Cesselin, F. (1993) Substance P levels in the synovium and synovial fluid from patients with rheumatoid arthritis and osteoarthritis. *Journal of Rheumatology* **20**, 714–717.

Meunier, J.C., Mollereau, C., Toll, L., *et al.* (1995) Isolation and structure of the endogenous agonist of opioid receptor-like ORL1 receptor [see comments]. *Nature* **377**, 532–535.

Millan, M.J. (1986) Multiple opioid systems and pain. *Pain* **27**, 303–347.

Monneret, G., Pachot, A., Laroche, B., Picollet, J. & Bienvenu, J. (2000) Procalcitonin and calcitonin gene-related peptide decrease LPS-induced TNF production by human circulating blood cells. *Cytokine* **12**, 762–764.

Moore, R.H. & Dowling, D.A. (1982) Effects of enkephalins on perfusion pressure in isolated hindlimb preparations. *Life Sciences* **31**, 1559–1566.

Nakamura-Craig, M. & Smith, T.W. (1989) Substance P and peripheral inflammatory hyperalgesia. *Pain* **38**, 91–98.

Neely, F.G. (1998) Biomechanical risk factors for exercise-related lower limb injuries. *Sports Medicine* **26**, 395–413.

Nilsson, J., von Euler, A.M. & Dalsgaard, C.J. (1985) Stimulation of connective tissue cell growth by substance P and substance K. *Nature* **315**, 61–63.

Nozaki-Taguchi, N. & Yamamoto, T. (1998) Involvement of nitric oxide in peripheral antinociception mediated by kappa- and delta-opioid receptors. *Anesthesia and Analgesia* **87**, 388–393.

Oku, R., Satoh, M., Fujii, N., Otaka, A., Yajima, H. & Takagi, H. (1987) Calcitonin gene-related peptide promotes mechanical nociception by potentiating release of substance P from the spinal dorsal horn in rats. *Brain Research* **403**, 350–354.

Onuoha, G.N. & Alpar, E.K. (2001) Levels of vasodilators (SP, CGRP) and vasoconstrictor (NPY) peptides in early human burns. *European Journal of Clinical Investigation* **31**, 253–257.

Ottaway, C.A. & Greenberg, G.R. (1984) Interaction of vasoactive intestinal peptide with mouse lymphocytes: specific binding and the modulation of mitogen responses. *Journal of Immunology* **132**, 417–423.

Park, S.H. & Silva, M. (2003) Effect of intermittent pneumatic soft-tissue compression on fracture-healing in an animal model. *Journal of Bone and Joint Surgery. American volume* **85**, 1446–1453.

Piercey, M.F., Dobry, P.J., Schroeder, L.A. & Einspahr, F.J. (1981) Behavioral evidence that substance P may be a spinal cord sensory neurotransmitter. *Brain Research* **210**, 407–412.

Puddu, G., Ippolito, E. & Postacchini, F. (1976) A classification of Achilles tendon disease. *American Journal of Sports Medicine* **4**, 145–150.

Quinlan, K.L., Song, I.S., Bunnett, N.W., *et al.* (1998) Neuropeptide regulation of human dermal microvascular endothelial cell ICAM-1 expression and function. *American Journal of Physiology* **275**, C1580–C1590.

Reinscheid, R.K., Nothacker, H.P., Bourson, A., *et al.* (1995) Orphanin FQ: a neuropeptide that activates an opioidlike G protein-coupled receptor. *Science* **270**, 792–794.

Renström, P. & Johnson, R.J. (1985) Overuse injuries in sports. A review. *Sports Medicine* **2**, 316–333.

Renström, P. & Kannus P. (1991) Prevention of sports injuries. In: *Sports Medicine* (Strauss, R.H., ed.) Saunders, Philadelphia: 307–329.

Rittner, H.L., Machelska, H. & Stein, C. (2005) Leukocytes in the regulation of pain and analgesia. *Journal of Leukocyte Biology* **78**, 1215–1222.

Said, S.I. Anti-inflammatory actions of VIP in the lungs and airways. In: *Pro-Inflammatory and Anti-Inflammatory Peptides* (Said, S.I., ed.) Marcel Dekker, 1998.

Saria, A., Lundberg, J.M., Skofitsch, G. & Lembeck, F. (1983) Vascular protein linkage in various tissue induced by substance P, capsaicin, bradykinin, serotonin, histamine and by antigen challenge. *Naunyn-Schmiedeberg's Archives of Pharmacology* **324**, 212–218.

Schaffer, M., Beiter, T., Becker, H.D. & Hunt, T.K. (1998) Neuropeptides: mediators of inflammation and tissue repair? *Archives of Surgery* **133**, 1107–1116.

Schaible, H.G. (1996) On the role of tachykinins and calcitonin gene-related peptide in the spinal mechanisms of nociception and in the induction and maintenance of inflammation-evoked hyperexcitability in spinal cord neurons (with special reference to nociception in joints). *Progress in Brain Research* **113**, 423–441.

Schaible, H.G. & Grubb, B.D. (1993)

Afferent and spinal mechanisms of joint pain. *Pain* **55**, 5–54.

Schubert, T.E., Weidler, C., Borisch, N., Schubert, C., Hofstädter, F. & Straub, R.H. (2006) Dupuytren's contracture is associated with sprouting of substance P positive nerve fibres and infiltration by mast cells. *Annals of Rheumatic Diseases* **65**, 414–415.

Schubert, T.E., Weidler, C., Lerch, K., Hofstädter, F. & Straub, R.H. (2005) Achilles tendinosis is associated with sprouting of substance P positive nerve fibres. *Annals of Rheumatic Diseases* **64**, 1083–1086.

Schwartz, J.P. (1992) Neurotransmitters as neurotrophic factors: a new set of functions. *International Review of Neurobiology* **34**, 1–23.

Snider, R.M., Constantine, J.W., Lowe, J.A. 3rd, *et al.* (1991) A potent nonpeptide antagonist of the substance P (NK1) receptor. *Science* **251**, 435–437.

Snijdelaar, D.G., Dirksen, R., Slappendel, R. & Crul, B.J. (2000) Substance P. *European Journal of Pain* **4**, 121–135.

Stein, C., Gramsch, C., Hassan, A.H., *et al.* (1990) Local opioid receptors mediating antinociception in inflammation: endogenous ligands. *Progress in Clinical and Biological Research* **328**, 425–427.

Stein, C., Hassan, A.H., Lehrberger, K., Giefing, J. & Yassouridis, A. (1993) Local analgesic effect of endogenous opioid peptides [see comments]. *Lancet* **342**, 321–324.

Steinbrech, D.S., Longaker, M.T., Mehrara, B.J., *et al.* (1999) Fibroblast response to hypoxia: the relationship between angiogenesis and matrix regulation. *Journal of Surgical Research* **84**, 127–133.

Stelnicki, E.J., Doolabh, V., Lee, S., *et al.* (2000) Nerve dependency in scarless fetal wound healing. *Plastic and Reconstructive Surgery* **105**, 140–147.

Steyaert, A.E., Burssens, P.J., Vercruysse, C.W., Vanderstraeten, G.G. & Verbeeck, R.M. (2006) The effects of substance P on the biomechanic properties of ruptured rat Achilles' tendon. *Archives of Physical Medicine and Rehabilitation* **87**, 254–258.

Strand, F.L., Rose, K.J., Zuccarelli, L.A., *et al.* (1991) Neuropeptide hormones as neurotrophic factors. *Physiological Reviews* **71**, 1017–1046.

Straub, R.H., Günzler, C., Miller, L.E., Cutolo, M., Schölmerich, J. & Schill, S. (2002) Anti-inflammatory cooperativity of corticosteroids and norepinephrine in rheumatoid arthritis synovial tissue *in vivo* and *in vitro*. *FASEB Journal* **16**, 993–1000.

Sullo, A., Maffulli, N., Capasso, G. & Testa, V. (2001) The effects of prolonged peritendinous administration of PGE1 to the rat Achilles tendon: a possible animal model of chronic Achilles tendinopathy. *Journal of Orthopaedic Science* **6**, 349–357.

Szolcsanyi, J., Helyes, Z., Oroszi, G., Nemeth, J. & Pinter, E. (1998) Release of somatostatin and its role in the mediation of the anti-inflammatory effect induced by antidromic stimulation of sensory fibres of rat sciatic nerve. *British Journal of Pharmacology* **123**, 936–942.

Taiwo, Y.O. & Levine, J.D. (1991) Kappa- and delta-opioids block sympathetically dependent hyperalgesia. *Journal of Neuroscience* **11**, 928–932.

Uchio, Y., Ochi, M., Ryoke, K., Sakai, Y., Ito, Y. & Kuwata, S. (2002) Expression of neuropeptides and cytokines at the extensor carpi radialis brevis muscle origin. *Journal of Shoulder and Elbow Surgery* **11**, 570–575.

Ueda, H. (1999) *In vivo* molecular signal transduction of peripheral mechanisms of pain. *Japanese Journal of Pharmacology* **79**, 263–268.

Van der Zee, C.E., Nielander, H.B., Vos, J.P., *et al.* (1989) Expression of growth-associated protein B-50 (GAP43) in dorsal root ganglia and sciatic nerve during regenerative sprouting. *Journal of Neuroscience* **9**, 3505–3512.

Vasko, M.R., Campbell, W.B. & Waite, K.J. (1994) Prostaglandin E_2 enhances bradykinin-stimulated release of neuropeptides from rat sensory neurons in culture. *Journal of Neuroscience* **14**, 4987–4997.

von During, M., Fricke, B. & Dahlmann, A. (1995) Topography and distribution of nerve fibers in the posterior longitudinal ligament of the rat: an immunocytochemical and electron-microscopical study. *Cell and Tissue Research* **281**, 325–338.

Wenk, H.N. & Honda, C.N. (1999) Immunohistochemical localization of delta opioid receptors in peripheral tissues. *Journal of Comparative Neurology* **408**, 567–579.

Wiesenfeld-Hallin, Z., Hokfelt, T., Lundberg, J.M., *et al.* (1984) Immunoreactive calcitonin gene-related peptide and substance P coexist in sensory neurons to the spinal cord and interact in spinal behavioral responses of the rat. *Neuroscience Letters* **52**, 199–204.

Willson, N.J., Schneider, J.F., Roizin, L., Fleiss, J.F., Rivers, W. & Demartini, J.E. (1976) Effects of methadone hydrochloride on the growth of organotypic cerebellar cultures prepared from methadone-tolerant and control rats. *Journal of Pharmacology and Experimental Therapeutics* **199**, 368–374.

Winnick, E. (2001) Musculoskeletal workplace injuries cost US nearly $54 billion annually. *Royal Society of Health Journal*.

Woo, S.L-Y., An, K-N., Frank, C., Livesay, G., Ma, C.B. & Zeminski, J. (2000) Anatomy, biology, and biomechanics of tendon and ligament. In: *Orthopaedic Basic Science: Biology and Biomechanics of the Musculoskeletal System* (Buckwalter, J., Einhorn, T. & Simon, S., eds) American Academy of Orthopaedic Surgeons, Rosemont: **24**, 581–616.

Woolf, C. & Wiesenfeld-Hallin, Z. (1986) Substance P and calcitonin gene-related peptide synergistically modulate the gain of the nociceptive flexor withdrawal reflex in the rat. *Neuroscience Letters* **66**, 226–230.

Xu, X.J., Hao, J.X., Wiesenfeld-Hallin, Z., Hskanson, R., Folkers, K. & Hökfelt, T. (1991) Spantide II, a novel tachykinin antagonist, and galanin inhibit plasma extravasation induced by antidromic C-fiber stimulation in rat hindpaw. *Neuroscience* **42**, 731–737.

Yaksh, T.L. (1988) Substance P release from knee joint afferent terminals: modulation by opioids. *Brain Research* **458**, 319–324.

Yule, K.A. & White, S.R. (1999) Migration of 3T3 and lung fibroblasts in response to calcitonin gene-related peptide and bombesin. *Experimental Lung Research* **25**, 261–273.

Zagon, I.S. & McLaughlin, P.J. (1991) Identification of opioid peptides regulating proliferation of neurons and glia in the developing nervous system. *Brain Research* **542**, 318–323.

Zhou, L., Zhang, Q., Stein, C. & Schafer, M. (1998) Contribution of opioid receptors on primary afferent versus sympathetic neurons to peripheral opioid analgesia. *Journal of Pharmacological and Experimental Therapeutics* **286**, 1000–1006.

Ziche, M., Morbidelli, L., Pacini, M., Geppetti, P., Alessandri, G. & Maggi, C.A. (1990) Substance P stimulates neovascularization *in vivo* and proliferation of cultured endothelial cells. *Microvascular Research* **40**, 264–278.

Zukowska-Grojec, Z., Karwatowska-Prokopczuk, E., Rose, W., *et al.* (1998) Neuropeptide Y: a novel angiogenic factor from the sympathetic nerves and endothelium. *Circulation Research* **83**, 187–95.

Chapter 10

A Neuropathic Model to the Etiology and Management of Achilles Tendinopathy

NICK WEBBORN

The evolution of understanding of Achilles tendon pathology to be a largely degenerative process rather than inflammatory has stimulated debate on the possible etiology. Current theoretical models of Achilles tendinosis do not adequately explain the etiology, pathology, and response to exercise as treatment. Tendon rupture occurs predominantly in pathogenic tendons and is more common in sedentary subjects compared to athletes, casting doubt on exercise overload as the main causative factor.

However, new animal models show the importance of neural function for tendon and ligament healing and blocking neural function leads to collagen degradation. Human microdialysis studies show higher concentrations of excitatory neurotransmitters in painful tendons. Tendon pathology also appears to be associated with patients who have had sciatica. Clinical reports of altered neural dynamics in patients with tendinosis, together with anecdotal reports of treating altered neuropathic signs facilitating recovery, raise the question of a possible neuropathic etiology. Altered neural function may cause tendon degeneration in the human, as displayed in the animal models, and may also explain the presence or absence of pain accompanying tendinosis in some patients where pain-producing fibers are not involved. However, all these require further investigation.

This chapter discusses the rationale behind the theoretical basis for a neuropathic etiology of degenerative tendinopathy and outlines an appropriate clinical assessment and management protocol. Further research questions are identified and this chapter attempts to stimulate the academic debate on our shortcomings of current theoretical models.

Introduction

Achilles tendinopathy remains an enigma in modern medicine. Despite advances in basic medical sciences and imaging there is no clear evidence within the literature for the etiology of the condition or the rationale for management. The outcome of the condition remains unpredictable and provides significant morbidity within athletic and non-athletic populations. A major change in thinking has evolved from the understanding that the major lesion in chronic Achilles tendinopathy is a degenerative process characterized by an absence of inflammatory cells and a poor healing response (Åstrom & Rausing 1995). A reclassification of overuse conditions of tendinopathies was proposed by Bonar (Khan *et al*. 1999; Table 10.1).

It is suggested that the majority of overuse injuries of the Achilles are tendinosis, although it may coexist with inflammation of the paratenon (Khan *et al*. 1999). These changes are described in Chapter 6 of this textbook. However, the determination of degeneration being the primary pathology in the Achilles tendon puts into question many of our original beliefs and treatments. Most etiologic theories are based upon the following factors (Kvist 1994):

1 Mechanical
2 Degenerative—because of insufficient blood supply and oxygenation
3 Inflammatory

Table 10.1 Bonar's classification of overuse tendon conditions.

Pathologic diagnosis	Macroscopic pathology
Tendinosis	Intratendinous degeneration commonly resulting from aging, microtrauma, or vascular compromise
Partial rupture or tendinitis	Symptomatic degeneration of the tendon with vascular disruption, inflammatory repair response
Paratenonitis	Inflammation of the outer layer of the tendon (paratenon) alone whether or not the paratenon is lined by synovium
Paratenonitis with tendinosis	Paratenonitis associated with intratendinous degeneration

Previously, the clinician's management was aimed at reducing inflammation with anti-inflammatory electrotherapy modalities and medications (oral or injected). Therefore, it is not surprising that our treatment outcomes were poor. However, perhaps more importantly, it led us into a belief that the repetitive nature of an athlete's training was the causative factor producing a direct inflammatory effect on the Achilles tendon itself. Some have made the assumption that the exercise loading is now also directly responsible for the degeneration of the Achilles tendon but as yet no study proves this causation.

To explain this more fully in the context of Achilles tendinosis, we need to examine and rationalize:

1 The known effects of exercise and immobilization on the Achilles tendon;

2 The population affected by Achilles tendinosis and their activity levels;

3 Why Achilles tendinosis may be painful or pain-free; and

4 What is the contribution of imaging in Achilles tendinosis in understanding the presence or absence of pain.

In summary, there is no satisfactory theory that ties in etiology, histologic findings, clinical findings, radiologic findings, treatment, and prevention strategies. Over the course of this chapter the author highlights the weaknesses in the current theories of Achilles tendinosis and describes the potential for a neuropathic process that may provide a logical explanation for *one* of the processes leading to Achilles tendinosis and a model to apply to other tendinopathies.

Methods and results

Effects of exercise and immobilization on tendons

Tendons are composed of 70% water and 21% collagen, of which 95% is type I collagen. In the healthy state, tendons are able to sustain considerable loads and deformation. Collagen fibrils can have an 8–10% increase in length before failure point is reached and forces of approximately 4000 N can be absorbed by the Achilles tendon. Peak Achilles tendon forces have been recorded at 2233 N in the squat jump and 3786 N when hopping (Komi *et al.* 1992; Fukashiro *et al.* 1995a,b). Mechanical loading of tendons influences local collagen synthesis, and microdialysis studies indicate that exercise elevates type I collagen production in the human tendon (Heinemeier *et al.* 2003). Exercise also increases the cross-linkages between collagen fibrils. As aging occurs, the amount of type III collagen increases, producing an increase in stiffness and a decrease in the elasticity of tendon–aponeurosis structures. Low-load resistance training can increase the elasticity of tendon–aponeurosis structures in middle-aged and elderly women (Kubo *et al.* 2003).

Animal models showing the effects of mobilization or immobilization on tendon healing after surgical tenotomy and repair show consistently that tendon properties are enhanced by controlled mobilization and impaired by immobilization. A variety of studies have shown that immobilization causes tendon atrophy but the effects are slower than in muscle and make study more difficult. Both the density and the size of collagen fibers decrease and there is impaired tensile strength (Kvist 1994). In

Kvist's review, the only negative report of tendon adaptation to exercise reports that "strenuous training may be harmful because of delayed collagen maturation." However, this statement was from an animal study derived from research on 3-week-old White Leghorn roosters. The authors reported: "Runners were subjected to a progressive treadmill running program for 8 weeks, 5 days/week at 70–80% maximal O_2 consumption ($VO_{2\ max}$). The exercise program induced a significant increase in tendon collagen deposition (46%) without any changes in DNA, proteoglycan, and collagen concentrations or tendon dry weight. Also, tendon collagen from runners contained fewer (50%) pyridinoline cross-links. These results suggest that high-intensity exercise causes greater matrix–collagen turnover in growing chickens, resulting in reduced maturation of tendon collagen." This is an unconvincing argument for strenuous training being harmful to the Achilles tendon of a human adult athlete in training. Kvist highlights the paucity of research into the effects strength training on tendon tissue but it also appears to be the most successful of conservative therapies used in the management of Achilles tendinosis. Eccentric training drills have been shown to have a positive outcome in tendon strengthening by stimulating mechanoreceptors in tenocytes to produce collagen. Several researchers have highlighted the importance of eccentric training as an effective treatment of Achilles tendinosis (Stanish et al. 1986; Fyfe & Stanish 1992; Alfredson et al. 1998; Fahlstrom et al. 2003). More recent research also demonstrates the ability to normalize tendon structure and decrease tendon thickness in long-term follow-up of tendinosis treated with eccentric exercise (Öhberg et al. 2004).

In summary, the Achilles tendon is an inherently strong structure that is able to withstand considerable force. It becomes weaker with immobilization and is improved by exercise which forms the mainstay of conservative treatment. So how do we explain the link between tendon degeneration and exercise? Can it be that athletes are purely "overloading" the tissue and that this is the cause of tendinosis or do there need to be other factors that combined with overload result in tissue degeneration?

Population affected by Achilles tendinosis

Let us next examine the population that develops this condition as this may help to give some indication as to etiology. The sports medicine community tends to see active and sporting patients and their perception of those who have this condition may be skewed. Cook et al. (2002) state that: "Achilles tendon injury (tendinopathy) and pain occur in active individuals, when the tendon is subject to high or unusual load." However, the evidence available on the epidemiology of Achilles tendinopathy (or using tendinitis as a search term for older references) is limited but does not clearly support this view (Kvist 1994). Significantly greater information is available on rupture of the Achilles tendon. Ruptured and tendinopathic tendons are histologically significantly more degenerated than control tendons with the general pattern of degeneration common to the ruptured and tendinopathic tendons (Tallon et al. 2001). Kannus and Józsa (1991) found that at rupture, 97% of Achilles tendons in 891 cases showed degenerative changes. Thirty four percent of cadavers at postmortem also show these changes. From research over a 15-year period concerning Achilles tendon rupture it is clear that there are a bimodal peaks of incidence at around age 39 and age 80 years, with a steady rise after age 60 (Maffulli et al. 1999). In the older group, regular physical activity is a minor factor as is sporting activity at the time of injury. However, it is clear that the changes in tendinosis are different and a separate process from aging alone (Ippolito et al. 1975). With increasing age, the human tendon shows an increase of collagen and a diminution of mucopolysaccharides and glycoproteins whereas the tendinopathic tendon shows a marked diminution of collagen and an increase of acid mucopolysaccharides and structural glycoproteins. Furthermore, although sport is commonly the activity at time of rupture in the younger age group (75–80%), researchers suggest that rupture is usually a sequel to a sedentary lifestyle and participation in unaccustomed sports activities.

In summary, degenerative tendinopathy occurs in a wide age range but is commonly in older adults and in a sedentary population and is not restricted to those in regular sporting activity. Sudden forces in unaccustomed sporting activity in a largely sedentary population precipitates a rupture and so to postulate that physical activity is the main cause of the degenerative process leading to the tendinotic state is not well founded. Furthermore, two-thirds of these subjects will not have experienced any preceding symptoms in their Achilles tendon prior to their rupture and so although pain will cause the patient to seek medical attention, many people with tendinosis will have a "silent disease" which results in significant morbidity when rupture occurs.

Pain in Achilles tendinosis

For the athlete it is pain and loss of performance that brings them to seek medical attention but for the two-thirds of patients with tendinosis leading to rupture, preceding pain is not an issue. While 34% of cadavers show signs of tendinosis at postmortem, it is not recorded that this proportion of the population are complaining of Achilles pain prior to death! Histologically it is now generally accepted that inflammation is not a component of Achilles tendinosis and so we cannot blame inflammatory mediators as the cause of pain unless inflammation of the paratenon coexists with the tendinopathy. So how can we explain why pain occurs at all and why some patients have pain and some do not for the same histologic process? If inflammation is the initial process, why do these patients experience no pain in the majority of the cases that go on to rupture?

There have been several models proposed for the cause of pain in Achilles tendinosis. Khan and Cook (2000) discuss the potential origins of pain and state, "although collagen fiber injury is almost certainly involved in production of pain in tendinopathies, it may not explain the mechanism of pain completely." The "mechanical" model of collagen separation is too simplistic given the variability in symptoms or lack thereof in many patients. It may be acceptable at a macroscopic level with an acute injury but not for the degenerate and disordered fibers in the chronic state at the microscopic level. Also it does not explain the absence of pain in some subjects or the causation in sedentary sufferers. The "biochemical" model focuses on examining the

chemical and cellular appearances in tendons and proposes chemical irritations that "aggravate peritendinous nociceptors." It is suggested that chondroitin sulfate may be exposed by tendon damage and stimulate nociceptors (Khan et al. 2000). No explanation is offered as to why these biochemical factors do not uniformly produce pain in subjects with tendinosis.

For those patients who do experience pain, can we provide an explanation? First, pain is very subjective and is influenced by many factors. Pain does not always signal injury, as in the common headache, and injury does not always generate pain. For those patients with painful Achilles tendinosis, there is persistent or chronic pain that can last many months. The pain of Achilles tendinosis can be aggravated by activity but can also be present at rest, particularly in the morning on waking. Athletes who have been forced to cease training can continue to experience pain for several months even though they have stopped the activity that has produced the changes in the tendon. So we need to go back to some basic questions and ask, "What can cause ongoing pain?" Gunn (1995) says "persistent pain can occur in the presence of the following conditions:

1 Ongoing nociception or persistent inflammation (e.g. rheumatoid arthritis). Inflammation results in the local release of algogenic substances.
2 Psychologic factors such as somatization disorders, depression, or adverse operant learning processes.
3 Abnormal functioning in the nervous system—neuropathic pain."

Having excluded inflammation histologically, and assuming that the cause is not psychologic, it would be reasonable to consider the possibility of neuropathy as a possible source of ongoing pain in Achilles tendinosis.

Neuropathy is a disorder in peripheral nerve function that can be multifactorial and can vary from being asymptomatic to severe pain or muscular paralysis. Gunn (1980) states the neurologic properties of receptor organs, neurons, and their interconnections determine whether or not pain occurs and also that these structures may develop a "supersensitivity" following denervation. It is suggested that the most common cause of neuropathy is radiculopathy with degeneration of the intervertebral disc leading to pressure or stretch on the nerve root. This may be asymptomatic because "small-diameter pain fibers may not initially be involved despite the attenuation of the other component fibers of the nerve." He uses a term "prespondylosis" to describe the "unrecognized phase of insidious attrition to the other functions of the nerve, especially the trophic aspect." Thus, Gunn describes a situation where pain may or may not be present but there may be trophic effects on the end organs of affected nerves. Affected nerves are still able to conduct nerve impulses and evoke both muscle action potentials and muscle contraction. Disturbance of the trophic function of the nerve leading to dystrophy or atrophy of the end organ occurs as a result of destruction of microtubules within the axons disrupting axoplasmic flow. Irritation of the peripheral nerve can affect fibers other than those of pain, "producing insidious neuropathy, the effects of which are projected onto the dermatomal, myotomal, and sclerotomal target structures supplied by the segmental nerve." Gunn states that pain fibers are smaller and less liable to mechanically caused ischemia and as such pain may not be present.

If a neuropathic model can explain the presence or absence of pain, can it also show evidence in the histochemistry, histology, clinical features, and treatment factors? The function of the peripheral nervous system (PNS) is said to be threefold (Dwyer *et al.* 2003):

1 To relay sensorimotor information to and from the central nervous system (CNS);
2 To control local blood flow; and
3 To influence inflammatory, proliferative, and reparative processes in injured tissue.

Perhaps the functions of the PNS in points 2 and 3 above are less well known. Neuropeptides and neurotransmitters are chemical agents that are thought to mediate these functions and may modulate immune cell and cytokine responses and also local blood flow (Schaffer *et al.* 1998). The effects on cell proliferation and angiogenesis, for example, may last from hours to days after release from nerve endings (Felten *et al.* 1987). Vascular endothelial growth factor (VEGF) is a key signal in the induction of new vessel growth and its role in the unexplained neovascularization of Achilles tendinosis has not been

studied (Öhberg *et al.* 2001; Alfredson *et al.* 2003). Although injections of sclerosant therapy have been used to treat these new vessels (Öhberg & Alfredson 2002, 2003) in an attempt to manage painful tendinosis, little consideration was given to why the new vessel formation might be occurring. Experimental sciatic nerve crush injury has produced a significant increase in the expression of VEGF and its receptor Flt-1 on the injured side of the lumbar spinal cord (Islamov *et al.* 2004). The effect of nerve injury distal to the lesion on VEGF expression has not been investigated but if a similar increase in VEGF expression is seen, then it may account for the neovascularization seen in Achilles tendinosis. It has also been suggested that VEGF is a neuroprotectant (Storkebaum *et al.* 2004) and as such the increased levels may cause neovascularization as a byproduct of attempting to maintain neural health in tissues affected by disorders of the PNS.

Evidence is accumulating in animal model studies for the importance of a functioning PNS for maintenance of ligament, joint, and tendon wellbeing and for healing after injury (Ivie *et al.* 2002; Salo *et al.* 2002). Ackerman *et al.* (2001) describe the neuronal occurrence of autonomic transmitters; noradrenaline (NA), neuropeptide Y (NPY) and vasoactive intestinal polypeptide (VIP), in the Achilles tendon in the rat. The researchers postulated "dysregulation of autonomic transmitters in hypovascularized tissues subjected to repetitive mechanical load may contribute to tissue hypoxia leading to degeneration and rupture of tendons and ligaments." Subsequent work on nerve regeneration during healing of Achilles tendon rupture in the rat showed the appearance of nerve fibers expressing neuropeptides early in the repair process. The authors suggest that neuronal regeneration and neuropeptide expression may be a prerequisite for healing (Ackermann *et al.* 2002). Other researchers used femoral nerve transection as a model to determine the role of sensory and autonomic innervation in the initial outcome of repair of the injured medial collateral ligament (MCL) (Ivie *et al.* 2002). The force required for ultimate failure at 6 weeks post-injury was found to be 50% higher in normally innervated MCLs compared to denervated MCLs. They concluded that intact innervation makes a critical contribution to the early healing responses of the MCL of adult rabbits.

More recently, Dwyer *et al.* (2003) examined the effect of blocking the sympathetic nervous system on collagen degradation in the medial collateral ligament in the rat. Type I collagen forms 95% of collagen in normal tendons. The process of remodeling and degradation of this collagen is regulated by proteases from fibroblasts, and, in particular, cysteine proteases and matrix metalloproteinases have been associated with collagen type I degradation. After 10 days, rats treated with guanethidine increased the expression of proteases MMP-13 and cathepsin K in the MCL. Although macroscopically there was no apparent difference between treated and control ligaments, ultimate stress values and strain at failure were reduced in treated ligaments. There was also increased ligament vascularity and disappearance of VIP in treated ligaments and greatly reduced levels of NPY, while substance P levels were increased (Fig. 10.1). The authors suggest that "sympathetic peripheral nerves influence ligament homeostasis by altering vascularity and levels of neuropeptides, while mediating levels of degradative enzymes."

Other researchers, using a microdialysis technique for *in vivo* studies of human tendons, have found that significantly higher concentrations of the excitatory neurotransmitter glutamate exists in painful tendons opposed to normal, non-painful tendons (Alfredson *et al.* 2001). Biopsies of the Achilles tendons were also made for immunohistochemical analysis. This showed that the glutamate *N*-methyl-D-aspartate receptors (NMDAR) were present in nerve structures within the tendon. Alfredson *et al.* suggested that this indicates "glutamate might be involved in chronic tendon pain and that this might have implications for treatment." However, rather than just viewing this as a potential pain management issue, it may also be that the findings in the nerve structures within the damaged tendons indicate the neural structures are involved in the degenerative process. To test this hypothesis further one could repeat Alfredson *et al.*'s study but in this instance choose subjects with painless tendinosis (diagnosed on ultrasound or MRI). If the same findings of glutamate and glutamate NMDAR1 immunoreaction were present then this would show whether glutamate was involved in chronic tendon pain or whether neural transmitters were reflecting neuropathy in the process of tendinosis.

Further work would be helpful to support the neuropathic model of tendinosis but it is clear that we have undervalued the importance of neural well-

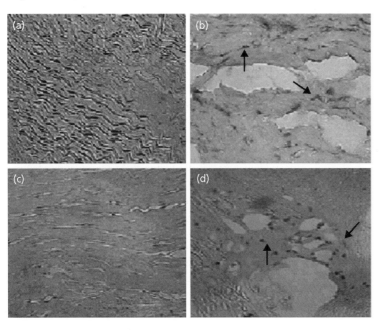

Fig. 10.1 After 10 days of treatment, histologic sections of rat medial collateral ligaments (MCLs), were labeled for collagenolytic enzymes. Guanethidine-treated animals had an increase in proteolytic enzymes (indicated by arrows) compared with controls. Tartrate-resistant acid phosphatase (TRAP; b) and cathepsin K (d) were observed in guanethidine-treated MCLs but not in control MCLs (a and c, respectively). Both TRAP and cathepsin K have potent collagenolytic activity and may contribute to tissue degradation in guanethidine-treated ligaments.

being in collagen regulation, neuropeptide expression, tissue vascularity, and mechanical properties.

Imaging and Achilles tendinosis

It is also important to consider if the presence of pain is an important factor when considering imaging appearances of Achilles tendons? Haims *et al.* (2000) described a significant overlap of magnetic resonance imaging (MRI) findings in symptomatic and asymptomatic Achilles tendons. The significance of finding abnormalities of tendinopathy on ultrasound or MRI in asymptomatic patients is raised by several authors (Husson *et al.* 1994; Åstrom *et al.* 1996; Archambault *et al.* 1998; Blankstein *et al.* 2001; Khan *et al.* 2003). Khan *et al.* describe ultrasonic and MRI changes in 57 symptomatic patients diagnosed with tendinopathy but suggest there is only moderate correlation with clinical assessment of chronic Achilles tendinopathy at 12 months. However, this assumes that pain or dysfunction is the only important factor in assessment and that the presence of abnormal findings on imaging without symptoms are not significant. Having established that two-thirds of patients who go on to rupture their Achilles tendon have no preceding symptoms, it would seem prudent to look for precipitating factors and advise on an appropriate *pre*-habilitation regime in athletes with imaging findings of tendinosis. Indeed, Åstrom *et al.* (1996) suggest that ultrasonography and MRI "may have their greatest potential as prognostic instruments." If you are caring for an elite, possibly multimillion dollar, athlete with radiologic evidence of tendinopathy, then it would seem prudent for any clinician to try to reduce the chance of a potentially career-threatening injury (i.e. tendon rupture).

Clinical relevance and significance

The histologic appearance of the completely neuropathic tendon shows appearances similar to the degenerative Achilles seen in athletes (Kannus & Józsa 1997). Some might ascribe the changes purely to disuse but other research points towards the clinical association between established neuropathy

and the risk of developing Achilles tendinosis leading to rupture (Maffulli *et al.* 1998). Thirty-five out of 102 patients had experienced sciatic pain before Achilles tendon rupture, compared with only 15 out of 128 individuals in the control group. This supports the possibility that a known neuropathic insult may be linked to the development of the degenerative changes seen in Achilles tendinosis. However, in most patients with Achilles tendinopathy we do not have such a clear-cut history of sciatica but perhaps we should be looking for subtler signs of neural involvement that may produce "silent" tendinosis.

Considering a possible neuropathic origin has led some clinicians to take a wider view in the patient with Achilles tendinosis. Gunn's pre-spondylosis theory points toward the potential spinal origin of the problem. Maffuli noticed the correlation between Achilles tendon rupture and sciatica. Terms such as "dural tension" (Cyriax 1978), "adverse mechanical tension" (Butler 1989), and "neurodynamics" (Shacklock 1995) have developed over the last 25 years, introducing the concept of considering dysfunction of the nervous system as a mechanical and physiologic entity. This involves manually assessing neural structures and treating them as part of rehabilitation. An appreciation of the potential for pathophysiologic changes in peripheral nerves subjected to stretch, compression, or vibration is required (Rempel *et al.* 1999) rather than looking for evidence of large disc prolapses, electromyography (EMG) changes or loss of tendon reflexes. Routine nerve conduction studies, which measure only the few fastest conducting and largest fibers and take no account of the majority of smaller fibers. In focal neuropathy, nerve conduction velocities remain within the wide range of normal values, but F-wave latency may be prolonged. EMG is not specific either but may show increased insertional activity. As such there is no simple objective test to confirm the diagnosis other than history and clinical examination.

Disc degeneration is well reported in association with sporting activity. The incidence of low back pain (LBP) in runners is high and relates to the road surface causing impact forces of three times body weight being imposed upon the lumbar spine with each stride (Woolf *et al.* 2002). A study of 539 runners gave a previous history of LBP in 74% of respondents overall. Prevalence of LBP at the time of survey completion was 13.6%. In the older population, the incidence of lumbar spondylosis increases with age, leading to a progressive reduction in disc space and the potential for nerve root pressure, traction, or stretch. Potentially, the impact loading of running, jumping, weight lifting, and other athletic activities could be causing stretch, traction, or pressure on the nerve root leading to peripheral neuropathy.

Another location where sciatic nerve stretch or compression can occur is in the buttock where the piriformis muscle specifically (Durrani & Winnie 1991; Douglas 1997) or other deep gluteal muscles (McCrory & Bell 1999; Meknas *et al.* 2003) have been associated with production of sciatic pain. Some are reported to be in association with anatomic anomalies of the sciatic nerve or piriformis muscle (Sayson *et al.* 1994; Ozaki *et al.* 1999). Grant's *Atlas of Anatomy* reports that in 12.2% of the population the peroneal division of the sciatic nerve passes through the pirifomis, giving 1 in 8 of the population an anatomic variant. The sciatic nerve is closely associated with the obturator internus muscle in particular and the potential for other muscles to be the source of symptoms has led to the suggested term "deep gluteal syndrome" (McCrory & Bell 1999). McCrory describes that external hip rotators are weak and tight and there is an increased discomfort with passive internal rotation and hip flexion. A more effective test of deep gluteal tightness is described later under clinical examination (Webborn's test). Release of piriformis tightness with acupuncture to treat piriformis syndrome has been successfully documented (Shu 2003).

Thus, it is possible that the changes of tendinopathy result from this indirect cause rather than by a direct effect of exercise on the tendon as currently thought, or a combination of the two (i.e. increased loading on neurally compromised tissue). So far we have considered the potential of a direct neuropathic effect on tendon tissue but there are also influences on muscle. Gunn's explanation states that "muscle tone may be increased at the muscle spindle whose intrafusal fibers, innervated from higher centers by the gamma motoneurons, may be subjected to increased impulse traffic. Hypersensitivity of the primary and secondary endings, which are sensitive to stretch of the central portion of the spindle, may also over-stimulate the essential feedback mechanism by which skeletal muscle and resting muscle tonus are controlled. The afferent discharge of the spindle via the dorsal root on the motoneurons of the same muscle is excitatory" (Gunn 1980). This disordered response of the muscle spindle system, which sets the resting tone of the muscle, produces chronic shortening that is often clinically described as "poor flexibility" and is treated with stretching exercises. However, in addition to the change in length there is also an accompanying increased tenderness to palpation which is maximal at the "motor point" of the muscle. This is where nociceptors are most abundant around the principal blood vessels and nerves as they enter the deep surface of the muscle to reach the muscle's motor zone of innervation. With regard to the triceps surae in patients with Achilles tendinopathy, this is most easily felt within the medial head of the mid-portion of the gastrocnemius muscle but the whole of the muscle belly will have increased tone compared to the unaffected side. This is important to appreciate when considering the load-strain characteristics of the Achilles tendon and the muscle aponeurosis. Researchers using the human medial gastrocnemius *in vivo* found no significant difference in strain between the Achilles tendon and aponeurosis of the gastrocnemius (Muramatsu *et al.* 2001). A sustained increase in resting tension in the muscle will cause a constant but low level of load in the tension of the tendon and this may influence the degenerative or healing process. Constant low load could affect blood flow in tissue already poorly vascularized. Increased tightness of the of the gastrocnemius has been found to be a risk factor for Achilles tendonitis in military recruits (Kaufman *et al.* 1999).

The tightness in the gastrocnemius may have other effects. Two branches of the sural nerve arise above the knee and pierce the medial head of the gastrocnemius muscle before joining the peroneal communicating nerve. The association between posterior thigh pain, grade 1 hamstring injuries, and impaired neural mobility has been reported and effectively treated using neural mobilizing slump stretches (Kornberg & Lew 1989; Turl & George 1998). It is possible that a similar phenomenon occurs as the sural nerve passes through the tightened medial head of the gastrocnemius muscle further aggravating the situation. Interestingly, reports of piriformis syndrome mimicking sural nerve entrapment have been reported in the literature (Murphy 1997). Despite multiple variations of the nerve and its branches, the course of a typical nerve trunk shows the nerve lying in close proximity to the Achilles tendon at a level of 7 cm above the tip of the lateral malleolus (Lawrence & Botte 1994). Lying in such close proximity to the Achilles tendon, the nerve is easily compressed by the palpating physician and may produce pain that is attributed to the Achilles. Furthermore, the nerve can also be examined at this point using diagnostic ultrasound and is found adjacent to the Achilles tendon and the short saphenous vein. The concept of impaired nerve movement leading to pain and injury is well established in particular regard to carpal tunnel syndrome. Researchers are able to use diagnostic ultrasound or spectral Doppler ultrasound to measure longitudinal movement of nerve and muscle (Hough *et al.* 2000a,b; Dilley *et al.* 2001; Dilley *et al.* 2003; Erel *et al.* 2003). Restriction in sural nerve motion has been established in preliminary investigations of patients with Achilles tendinosis by the author but further work is required with examinations of motion with different lower limb movements (Fig. 10.2).

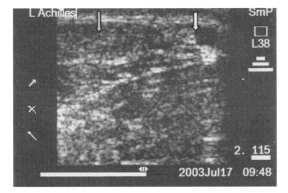

Fig. 10.2 Ultrasound of sural nerve.

It is unfortunate that the long-held belief that Achilles tendinopathy was inflammatory in origin generally appears to have lead clinicians to look at local factors around the Achilles as the potential source of the problem. That, combined with time constraints of many health services, meant that few clinicians looked farther in examination than palpation of the Achilles and basic biomechanical examination. Considering the potential for altered neural function leading to lower limb symptoms is important in the taking of the history of the tendinopathic patient. As a result of these observations, the author has found it relevant to ask directly about a previous history of low back pain, recurrent buttock, hamstring, or calf pain with activity (structures also innervated by the L5 or S1 nerve roots).

The physical examination of the patient should also extended to include a more thorough assessment of spinal mobility as well as any other test that may expose limitations in neural mobility into the lower limb. The clinical tests in Table 10.2 have been included in the examination in addition to standard examination of gait, foot mechanics, and the tendon itself. A test of hip flexion and adduction with lumbopelvic rotation (Webborn's test) is performed to assess deep gluteal muscle tightness (Fig. 10.3).

In summary, the neuropathic model proposes that evidence exists biochemically and histologically for the changes that are observed in tendinopathy and furthermore may explain the presence or absence of pain in the condition and the epidemiology of the condition. The history and clinical examination are directed towards potential causes of neuropathy by a thorough neurodynamic assessment. This may include a spinal, deep gluteal, or calf component as the most common causes in the author's experience, although tethering in the posterior thigh has also been seen. However, we need to examine how this fits in with successful treatment rationales to support the theory. Achilles tendinopathy is notoriously difficult and frustrating to treat. Previously held beliefs of its inflammatory nature lead to the use of anti-inflammatory modalities (e.g. therapeutic ultrasound, injection of corticosteroid) (Speed 2001) or non-steroidal anti-inflammatory drugs (NSAIDs) (Åstrom & Westlin 1992) with poor results (other than ultrasound after

Table 10.2 Clinical tests included in the examination in addition to standard examination of gait, foot mechanics, and the tendon.

Examination protocol
Lumbar motion—in particular flexion range (Schober's test) (Gill *et al.* 1988)
Posteroanterior (PA) compression of the lumbar spinal processes for stiffness of movement and subjective sensation of discomfort or pain on the PA compression
Palpation of the paraspinal musculature for increased tone—muscle hyperalgesia as described by Gunn
Dynamic tests of the sacroiliac joint in lumbar flexion and ipsilateral hip flexion abnormal movement may indicate tightness in the deep gluteal muscles causing neural restriction
Palpation of the piriformis muscle as the sciatic nerve passes across (or through) the muscle in the pelvis
Straight leg raise (SLR) ± added dorsiflexion and inversion to load the sural nerve. Hip adduction can also be added to further sensitise the test (Butler 2000)
The seated SLR or "slump" test. Performed looking for side-to-side differences in pain responses and restriction of movement
Palpation of the calf musculature for increased resting tone and areas of hyperalgesia (or trigger points). This is most easily performed with the patient lying supine and the knee flexed to 90° and a side-to-side comparison made

surgical repair (Ng *et al.* 2003)). Surgery loomed for those failing treatment, with long recovery rates and doubt over the ability to return to full performance. Without doubt the most successful treatment reported in clinical trials is that of eccentric calf exercise programs (Stanish *et al.* 1986; Alfredson *et al.* 1998; Fahlstrom *et al.* 2003; Öhberg *et al.* 2004). Öhberg *et al.*'s most recent study showed a localized decrease in tendon thickness and a normalized tendon structure in most patients treated with the exercise program at a mean of 3.8 years follow-up. Persistent tendon abnormalities in more than 20% of patients were associated with residual pain in the tendon (i.e. the condition had not resolved). We have established previously the beneficial effects of exercise on collagen and should not be totally be surprised by the potential for improvement with exercise. However, the key issue may be that eccentric exercises provide maximum stimulation for tendon healing while minimizing impact loading of the lumbar spine during the activity. In the neuropathic model it would be important to reduce pressure, angulation, or stretch on the neural structures while continuing to stimulate the tendon to repair. If neuronal regeneration and neuropeptide expression is a prerequisite for healing as previously discussed, then providing the optimum environment for tendon healing would include limitation of aggravating factors such as spinal loading or impact. However, can we further enhance the healing process if the neuropathic model is correct?

The aims of such a treatment would be to:

1 Identify and treat any "supersensitivity" in paraspinal or peripheral muscle groups.

2 Identify and treat any restriction in neural mobility (e.g. spinal segmental stiffness).

3 Perform eccentric exercise loading of the tendon while emphasizing spinal and/or core stability during the exercise.

4 Enhance core stabilizing muscles and integrate into sport-specific activity.

The Gunn approach to treatment uses a dry needling approach termed intramuscular stimulation (IMS). Palpable muscle bands that are tender to digital pressure are distributed in a segmental or myotomal fashion, in muscles of both anterior and posterior primary rami of that segment. Acupuncture needles are place in the paraspinal muscles and in the peripheral muscles of that segment which in the case of Achilles tendinosis involves the L5–S1 levels and the calf muscles. When the needle penetrates normal muscle, it meets with little resistance and produces no response; when it penetrates a muscle in the neuropathic state there may be an insertional twitch or firm resistance. The needle is grasped by the muscle causing a cramping sensation and the needle cannot be withdrawn. After a period of minutes, usually dependent upon severity and duration

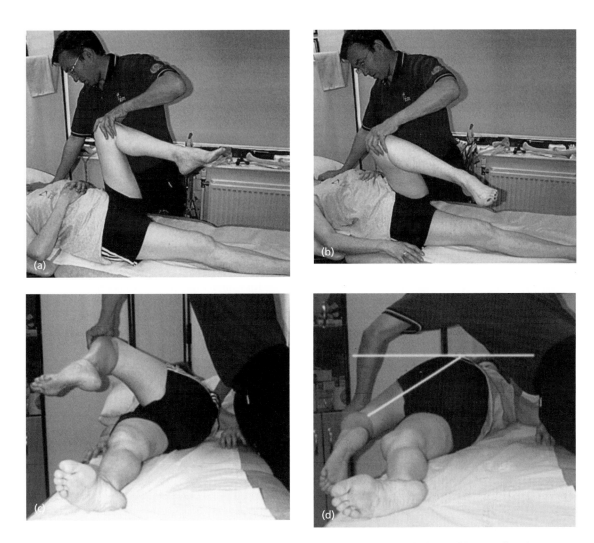

Fig. 10.3 Webborn's test of hip flexion and adduction with lumbopelvic rotation. (a) The hip and knee are flexed to 90°. (b) Start with hip adduction and flow into pelvic and lumbar rotation while maintaining shoulder position. (c) Maintaining shoulder continue motion to end point or pain "Where is it tight/stretching?" Measure angle of femur relative to horizontal. Record as degrees + or –. (d) Positive test—feel resistance to rotation with restricted range compared to other side. Normal usually = negative value. Any value above horizontal is abnormal. Clinician can treat spinal component or pelvic and record change in motion to determine the contribution of each to the limitation of range.

of symptoms, the muscle will relax and can be easily withdrawn without resistance. This may take up to 30 minutes in the chronic or more severe cases initially. Afterwards, the muscle feels loose and relaxed and there is often a dramatic increase in range of motion on repeat testing. When the needle pierces the muscle, it disrupts the cell membrane of individual muscle fibers, mechanically discharging

an outburst of injury potentials. Unlike external forms of stimulation such as stretching or massage, the stimulation from a needle lasts for several days until the cell membrane heals. Treatments are repeated at increasing intervals according to response as the tissues desensitize and the time taken for relaxation of the muscle diminishes. A reduction in pain follows needling and may occur within minutes. The reduction in pain facilitates the ability to perform the eccentric exercise program and as such may enhance adherence to the exercise.

The reduction in paraspinal tone now facilitates manual mobilization of the spinal segments and progression is made to the core stabilizing exercise program. Examination of the mobility of the thoracic spine is also performed and treated as required. If deep gluteal muscles are tight and tender to palpation and there is restriction in range on Webborn's test, then these may be similarly palpated and needled. The patient is taught neural mobilizing exercises (e.g. in slump stretch with knee extensions). As rehabilitation through the eccentric program progresses and the patient becomes pain free, then more dynamic exercises can be introduced with the focus on quality of movement and ensuring trunk stabilization. For example, a Pilates reformer with a jump board could be used to progress the level of activity without full body weight resistance. A biomechanical assessment of running is performed to assess trunk and pelvic stabilization and any tendency to overpronation corrected.

The author's personal experience of managing the Achilles patient in this fashion has accelerated return to sporting activity but long-term follow-up of greater numbers of patients is required. It is also believed that the core stabilizing muscles of the athlete tend to fatigue before the lower limb muscles or the cardiorespiratory system of the athlete (distance runners in particular) and this predisposes to loss of lumbopelvic control and development of LBP or the potential for "prespondylosis" and tendinopathy. For athletes with radiologic evidence of tendinosis without pain, a similar assessment and management strategy would be instigated to prevent the risk of Achilles tendon rupture.

Does the neuropathic model work for other tendinopathies?

Several studies have already established the link between lateral epicondyle pain and loss of radial nerve mobility (Albrecht *et al.* 1997; Drechsler *et al.* 1997). A similar model can be applied to patellar tendinopathy where it is the quadriceps (rectus femoris predominantly) that is tight and overactive with spinal segmental findings at the L3–L4 level. Findings of reduced neural mobility may be seen on prone knee bend or slump knee bend. Poor trunk stability on take off or landing from jumps can load higher lumbar segments than the simple impact loading of running on the L5–S1 disc and may help explain why this condition is more common in jumping sports. A similar protocol of management can be applied.

Future directions

The principle of parsimony states that one should not make more assumptions than the minimum needed to support a theory. This underlies all scientific modeling and is sometimes known as Occam's razor, a logical principle attributed to the medieval philosopher William of Occam. The traditional model of exercise-induced tendinopathy fails to explain histologic findings, histochemistry, pain patterns, epidemiology, imaging studies and the effect of treatment modalities. To accept exercise overload on the Achilles alone as causation requires too many assumptions to accept this theory logically. The neuropathic model offers an explanation that combines etiology, clinical assessment, management, and preventive strategies that have been the most successful in the author's 25 years of practice but further work is required to confirm or refute this theory. However, the opportunity to share these views through this chapter will allow clinicians and scientists to test the model more thoroughly.

What do we need to know?

There is a clear need for better epidemiologic data on Achilles tendinosis and not just on those subjects who rupture their Achilles. It is also clear that the process starts long before rupture occurs and for many people this is a painless and insidious process and they may not present early for treatment. If we are able to identify those predisposed to this condition, we may be able to introduce preventive strategies and prehabilitation to avoid the disastrous consequences of Achilles' rupture. A variety of animal studies have started to show the link between the neural health of tissues and well-being and recovery from injury but these need to be extended. Further histologic and histochemical studies could help to confirm the neuropathic link but we also need to be aware of research in other areas which may alert us to other pathologic mechanisms. For example, research into the mechanisms of the neovascularization that occurs in the diabetic eye may help us in our understanding of the process within the Achilles. Raising the awareness of a possible neuropathic etiology will alert other clinicians to expand their history taking and examination assessment in an attempt to duplicate the findings of adverse neural mobility seen in those with tendinosis by the author.

How do we get there?

Good epidemiologic evidence is time-consuming, laborious, and not markedly stimulating to researchers or financially appealing for grants but is invaluable for greater understanding of the population affected and possible etiological factors for the condition. A coordinated approach between institutions to data collection on the epidemiology of Achilles tendinosis would greatly assist in improving the quality of evidence available.

Further research in animal models of the effect of blocking the nerve supply to the Achilles tendon in the healthy and damaged tendon needs to be performed with examination of the effect on the mechanical properties, neurotransmitters and neuropeptides, and vascular endothelial growth factor. Comparative work with other conditions associated with peripheral neuropathy and neovascularization (e.g. diabetes) may increase our understanding of the degenerative process.

Further assessment of neural mobility in patients with Achilles tendinosis is required both clinically and ultrasonically. A greater attention to neural mobility assessment is required to see if wider clinical observation matches the author's. Assessment of sural nerve motion on ultrasound in patients with Achilles tendinosis can be made to see if there is any restriction compared with normal subjects. Lastly, a randomized clinical trial comparing treatment outcomes of eccentric exercise alone against combined intramuscular stimulation with eccentric exercise would assess the added effect of IMS on pain reduction and return to activity.

References

Ackermann, P.W., Ahmed, M. & Kreicsberg, A. (2002) Early nerve regeneration after Achilles tendon rupture: a prerequisite for healing? A study in the rat. *Journal of Orthopedic Research* **20**, 849–856.

Ackermann, P.W., Li, J., Finn, A., Ahmed, M. & Kreicsberg, A. (2001) Autonomic innervation of tendons, ligaments and joint capsules. A morphologic and quantitative study in the rat. *Journal of Orthopedic Research* **19**, 372–378.

Albrecht, S., Cordis, R., Kleihues, H. & Noack, W. (1997) Pathoanatomic findings in radiohumeral epicondylopathy. A combined anatomic and electromyographic study. *Archives of Orthopaedic and Trauma Surgery* **116**, 157–163.

Alfredson, H., Forsgren, S., Thorsen, K., Fahlstrom, M., Johansson, H. & Lorentzon, R. (2001) Glutamate NMDAR1 receptors localised to nerves in human Achilles tendons. Implications for treatment? *Knee Surgery, Sports Traumatology, Arthroscopy* **9**, 123–126.

Alfredson, H., Öhberg, L. & Forsgren, S. (2003) Is vasculo-neural ingrowth the cause of pain in chronic Achilles tendinosis? An investigation using ultrasonography and colour Doppler, immunohistochemistry, and diagnostic injections. *Knee Surgery, Sports Traumatology, Arthroscopy* **11**, 334–338.

Alfredson, H., Pietila, T., Jonsson, P. & Lorentzon, R. (1998) Heavy-load eccentric calf muscle training for the treatment of chronic Achilles tendinosis. *American Journal of Sports Medicine* **26**, 360–366.

Archambault, J.M., Wiley, J.P., Bray, R.C., Verhoef, M., Wiseman, D.A. & Elliot, P.D. (1998) Can sonography predict the outcome in patients with achillodynia? *Journal of Clinical Ultrasound* **26**, 335–339.

Åstrom, M. & Rausing, A. (1995) Chronic Achilles tendinopathy. A survey of surgical and histopathologic findings. *Clinical Orthopaedics* **316**, 151–164.

Åstrom, M. & Westlin, N. (1992) No effect of piroxicam on achilles tendinopathy. A randomized study of 70 patients. *Acta Orthopaedica Scandinavica* **63**, 631–634.

Åstrom, M., Gentz, C.F., Nilsson, P., Rausing, A., Sjoberg, S. & Westlin, N. (1996) Imaging in chronic achilles tendinopathy: a comparison of ultrasonography, magnetic resonance imaging and surgical findings in 27 histologically verified cases. *Skeletal Radiology* **25**, 615–620.

Blankstein, A., Cohen, I., Diamant, L., et al. (2001) Achilles tendon pain and related pathologies: diagnosis by ultrasonography. *Israel Medical Association Journal* **3**, 575–578.

Butler, D.S. (1989) Adverse mechanical tension in the nervous system: a model for assessment and treatment. *Australian Journal of Physiotherapy* **35**, 227–238.

Butler, D.S. (2000) *The Sensitive Nervous System*. Noigroup Publications, Adelaide.

Cook, J.L., Khan, K.M. & Purdam, C. (2002) Achilles tendinopathy. *Manual Therapy* **7** (3), 121–130.

Cyriax, J. (1978) Dural pain. *Lancet* **1**, 919–921.

Dilley, A., Greening, J., Lynn, B., Leary, R. & Morris, V. (2001) The use of cross-correlation analysis between high-frequency ultrasound images to measure longitudinal median nerve movement. *Ultrasound in Medicine and Biology* **27**, 1211–1218.

Dilley, A., Lynn, B., Greening, J. & DeLeon, N. (2003) Quantitative *in vivo* studies of median nerve sliding in response to wrist, elbow, shoulder and neck movements. *Clinical Biomechanics (Bristol, Avon)* **18**, 899–907.

Douglas, S. (1997) Sciatic pain and piriformis syndrome. *Nurse Practitioner* **22**, 166–8, 170, 172 passim.

Drechsler, W.I., Knarr, J.F. & Snyder-Mackler, L. (1997) A comparison of two treatment regimens for lateral epicondylitis. *Journal of Sport Rehabilitation* **6**, 226–234.

Durrani, Z. & Winnie, A.P. (1991) Piriformis muscle syndrome: an underdiagnosed cause of sciatica. *Journal of Pain and Symptom Management* **6**, 374–379.

Dwyer, K.W., Provenzano, P.P., Muir, P., Valhmo, W.B. & Vanderby, R. Jr. (2004) Blockade of the sympathetic nervous system degrades ligament in a rat MCL model. *Journal of Applied Physiology* **96**, 711–718.

Erel, E., Dilley, A., Greening, J., Morris, V., Cohen, B. & Lynn, B. (2003) Longitudinal sliding of the median nerve in patients with carpal tunnel syndrome. *Journal of Hand Surgery [Br]* **28**, 439–443.

Fahlstrom, M., Jonsson, P., Lorentzon, R. & Alfredson, H. (2003) Chronic Achilles tendon pain treated with eccentric calf-muscle training. *Knee Surgery, Sports Traumatology, Arthroscopy* **11**, 327–333.

Felten, D.L., Felten, S.Y., Bellinger, D.L., *et al.* (1987) Noradrenergic sympathetic neural interactions with the immune system: structure and function. *Immunological Reviews* **100**, 225–260.

Fukashiro, S., Itoh, M., Ichinose, Y., Kawakami, Y. & Fukunaga, T. (1995a) Ultrasonography gives directly but noninvasively elastic characteristic of human tendon *in vivo*. *European Journal of Applied Physiology and Occupational Physiology* **71**, 555–557.

Fukashiro, S., Komi, P.V., Jarvinen, M. & Miyashita, M. (1995b) *In vivo* Achilles tendon loading during jumping in humans. *European Journal of Applied Physiology and Occupational Physiology* **71**, 453–458.

Fyfe, I. & Stanish, W.D. (1992) The use of eccentric training and stretching in the treatment and prevention of tendon injuries. *Clinics in Sports Medicine* **11**, 601–624.

Gill, K., Krag, M.H., Johnson, G.B., Haugh, L.D. & Pope, M.H. (1988) Repeatability of four clinical methods for assessment of lumbar spinal motion. *Spine* **13**, 50–53.

Gunn, C.C. (1980) "Prespondylosis" and some pain syndromes following denervation supersensitivity. *Spine* **5**, 185–192.

Gunn, C. C. (1995) Musculoskeletal pain. *Journal of the Royal Society of Medicine* **88**, 302.

Haims, A.H., Schweitzer, M.E., Patel, R.S., Hecht, P. & Wapner, K.L. (2000) MR imaging of the Achilles tendon: overlap of findings in symptomatic and asymptomatic individuals. *Skeletal Radiology* **29**, 640–645.

Heinemeier, K., Langberg, H., Oleson, J.L. & Kjaer, M. (2003) Role of TGF-beta1 in relation to exercise-induced type I collagen synthesis in human tendinous tissue. *Journal of Applied Physiology* **95**, 2390–2397.

Hough, A.D., Moore, A.P. & Jones, M.P. (2000a) Measuring longitudinal nerve motion using ultrasonography. *Manual Therapy* **5**, 173–180.

Hough, A.D., Moore, A.P. & Jones, M.P. (2000b) Peripheral nerve motion measurement with spectral Doppler sonography: a reliability study. *Journal of Hand Surgery [Br]* **25**, 585–589.

Husson, J.L., De Korvin, B., Polard, J.L., Attali, J.Y. & Duvauferrier, R. (1994) [Study of the correlation between magnetic resonance imaging and surgery in the diagnosis of chronic Achilles tendinopathies]. *Acta Orthopaedica Belgica* **60**, 408–412.

Ippolito, E., Postacchini, F. & Ricciardi-Pollini, P.T. (1975) Biochemical variations in the matrix of human tendons in relation to age and pathological conditions. *Italian Journal of Orthopaedics and Traumatology* **1**, 133–139.

Islamov, R.R., Chintalgattu, V., Pak, E.S., Katwa, L.C. & Murashov, A.K. (2004) Induction of VEGF and its Flt-1 receptor after sciatic nerve crush injury. *Neuroreport* **15**, 2117–2121.

Ivie, T.J., Bray, R.C. & Salo, P.T. (2002) Denervation impairs healing of the rabbit medial collateral ligament. *Journal of Orthopedic Research* **20**, 990–995.

Kannus, P. & Józsa, L. (1991) Histopathological changes preceding spontaneous rupture of a tendon. A controlled study of 891 patients. *Journal of Bone and Joint Surgery. American volume* **73**, 1507–1525.

Kannus, P. & Józsa, L. (1997) *Human Tendons: Anatomy, Physiology & Pathology*. Human Kinetics, New York.

Kaufman, K.R., Brodine, S.K., Shaffer, R.A., Johnson, C.W. & Cullison, T.R. (1999) The effect of foot structure and range of motion on musculoskeletal overuse injuries. *American Journal of Sports Medicine* **27**, 585–593.

Khan, K.M. & Cook, J.L. (2000) Overuse tendon injuries: Where does the pain come from? In: *Sports Medicine and Arthroscopy Review* (Maffulli, N., ed.) Williams & Wilkins, Philadelphia: **8**: 17–31.

Khan, K.M., Cook, J.L., Bonar, F., Harcourt, P. & Åstrom, M. (1999) Histopathology of common tendinopathies. Update and implications for clinical management. *Sports Medicine* **27**, 393–408.

Khan, K.M., Cook, J.L., Maffulli, N. & Kannus, P. (2000) Where is the pain coming from in tendinopathy? It may be biochemical, not only structural, in origin. *British Journal of Sports Medicine* **34**, 81–83.

Khan, K.M., Forster, B.B., Robinson, J., *et al.* (2003) Are ultrasound and magnetic resonance imaging of value in assessment of Achilles tendon disorders? A two year prospective study. *British Journal of Sports Medicine* **37**, 149–153.

Komi, P.V., Fukashiro, S. & Jarvinen, M. (1992) Biomechanical loading of Achilles tendon during normal locomotion. *Clinics in Sports Medicine* **11**, 521–531.

Kornberg, C. & Lew, P. (1989) The effect of stretching neural structures on grade 1 hamstring injuries. *Journal of Orthopaedic and Sports Physical Therapy* (June), 481–487.

Kubo, K., Kanehisa, H., Miyatani, M., Tachi, M. & Fukunaga, T. (2003) Effect of low-load resistance training on the tendon properties in middle-aged and elderly women. *Acta Physiologica Scandinavica* **178**, 25–32.

Kvist, M. (1994) Achilles tendon injuries in athletes. *Sports Medicine* **18**, 173–201.

Lawrence, S.J. & Botte, M.J. (1994) The sural nerve in the foot and ankle: an anatomic study with clinical and surgical implications. *Foot and Ankle International* **15**, 490–494.

Maffulli, N., Irwin, A.S., Kenward, M.G., Smith, F. & Porter, R.W. (1998) Achilles tendon rupture and sciatica: a possible correlation. *British Journal of Sports Medicine* **32**, 174–177.

Maffulli, N., Waterston, S.W., Squair, J., Reaper, J. & Douglas, A.S. (1999) Changing incidence of Achilles tendon rupture in Scotland: a 15-year study. *Clinical Journal of Sport Medicine* **9**, 157–160.

McCrory, P. & Bell, S. (1999) Nerve entrapment syndromes as a cause of pain in the hip, groin and buttock. *Sports Medicine* **27**, 261–274.

Meknas, K., Christensen, A. & Johansen, O. (2003) The internal obturator muscle may cause sciatic pain. *Pain* **104**, 375–380.

Muramatsu, T., Muraoka, T., Takeshita, D., Kawakami, Y., Hirano, Y. & Fukunga, T. (2001) Mechanical properties of tendon and aponeurosis of human gastrocnemius muscle *in vivo*. *Journal of Applied Physiology* **90**, 1671–1678.

Murphy, B.P. (1997) Piriformis syndrome mimics sural nerve entrapment. *Journal of the American Podiatric Medical Association* **87**, 183–184.

Ng, C.O., Ng, G.Y., See, E.K. & Leung, M.C. (2003) Therapeutic ultrasound improves strength of achilles tendon repair in rats. *Ultrasound in Medicine and Biology* **29**, 1501–1506.

Öhberg, L. & Alfredson, H. (2002) Ultrasound guided sclerosis of neovessels in painful chronic Achilles tendinosis: pilot study of a new treatment. *British Journal of Sports Medicine* **36**, 173–175; discussion 176–177.

Öhberg, L. & Alfredson, H. (2003) Sclerosing therapy in chronic Achilles tendon insertional pain-results of a pilot study. *Knee Surgery, Sports Traumatology, Arthroscopy* **11**, 339–343.

Öhberg, L., Lorentzon, R. & Alfredson, H. (2001) Neovascularisation in Achilles tendons with painful tendinosis but not in normal tendons: an ultrasonographic investigation. *Knee Surgery, Sports Traumatology, Arthroscopy* **9**, 233–238.

Öhberg, L., Lorentzon, R. & Alfredson, H. (2004) Eccentric training in patients with chronic Achilles tendinosis: normalised tendon structure and decreased thickness at follow up [Commentary]. *British Journal of Sports Medicine* **38**, 8–11.

Ozaki, S., Hamabe, T. & Muro, T. (1999) Piriformis syndrome resulting from an anomalous relationship between the sciatic nerve and piriformis muscle. *Orthopedics* **22**, 771–772.

Rempel, D., Dahlin, L. & Lundborg, G. (1999) Pathophysiology of nerve compression syndromes: response of peripheral nerves to loading. *Journal of Bone and Joint Surgery. American volume* **81**, 1600–1610.

Salo, P.T., Hogervorst, T., Seerattan, R.A., Rucker, D. & Bray, R.C. (2002) Selective joint denervation promotes knee osteoarthritis in the aging rat. *Journal of Orthopaedic Research* **20**, 1256–1264.

Sayson, S.C., Ducey, J.P., Maybrey, J.B., Wesley, R.L. & Vermillion, D. (1994) Sciatic entrapment neuropathy associated with an anomalous piriformis muscle. *Pain* **59**, 149–152.

Schaffer, M., Beiter, T., Becker, H.D. & Hunt, T.K. (1998) Neuropeptides: mediators of inflammation and tissue repair? *Archives of Surgery* **133**, 1107–1116.

Shacklock, M. (1995) Neurodynamics. *Physiotherapy* **81**, 9–16.

Shu, H. (2003) Clinical observation on acupuncture treatment of piriformis syndrome. *Journal of Traditional Chinese Medicine* **23**, 38–39.

Speed, C.A. (2001) Fortnightly review: Corticosteroid injections in tendon lesions. *British Medical Journal* **323**, 382–386.

Stanish, W.D., Rubinovich, R.M. *et al.* (1986) Eccentric exercise in chronic tendinitis. *Clinical Orthopaedics and Related Research* **208**, 65–68.

Storkebaum, E., Lambrechts, D. & Carmeliet, P. (2004) VEGF: once regarded as a specific angiogenic factor, now implicated in neuroprotection. *Bioessays* **26**, 943–954.

Tallon, C., Maffulli, N. & Ewen, S.W. (2001) Ruptured Achilles tendons are significantly more degenerated than tendinopathic tendons. *Medicine and Science in Sports and Exercise* **33**, 1983–1990.

Turl, S.E. & George, K.P. (1998) Adverse neural tension: a factor in repetitive hamstring strain? *Journal of Orthopaedic and Sports Physical Therapy* **27**, 16–21.

Woolf, S.K., Barfield, W.R., Nietert, P.J., Mainous, A.G. 3rd & Glaser, J.A. (2002) The Cooper River Bridge Run Study of low back pain in runners and walkers. *Journal of the Southern Orthopaedic Association* **11**, 136–143.

Chapter 11

An Integrative Therapeutic Approach to Tendinopathy: Biomechanic and Biological Considerations

LOUIS C. ALMEKINDERS AND ALBERT J. BANES

Studies on chronic tendon problems, addressing the histopathology, epidemiology, and efficacy of traditional treatment, have yielded results that question the traditional view of "tendonitis." Tendinopathy cannot be easily explained as a simple overuse injury as a result of repeated tensile loads on the involved tendon.

Histopathologic studies on tendinopathy have shown mostly non-inflammatory, degenerative features in the tendon. Growth factors have been shown to positively influence tendon fibroblast metabolism. As such, they hold great promise in the treatment of tendinopathy. Initial studies with the injection of platelet concentrate, which contains a high concentration of platelet-derived growth factors, have yielded promising results in the treatment of tendinopathy.

Insertional tendinopathy is one of the most common forms of tendinopathy. Biomechanical studies on tendon insertion sites suggest that tensile stress-shielding or even compressive force may be more important than tensile forces in the development of insertional tendinopathy. Physical therapy treatment and preventative biomechanical measures for tendinopathy may need to be changed, based on these biomechanical studies, in order for them to be more effective.

Introduction

Musculoskeletal pathology can affect bones, muscles, tendons, ligaments, and cartilage in a variety of ways. Often, musculoskeletal pathology is categorized by etiologic factors such as acute trauma, chronic overuse, and intrinsic disorders. Acute traumatic events are obvious, single events that dramatically overwhelm the mechanical strength of the affected structure. These include events such as falls, collisions, and other obvious mishaps. Such acute events can cause injuries to these structures resulting in fractures, strains, sprains, or cartilage tears. Chronic overuse is thought to cause only minor mechanical damage to the affected structures. With continued overuse, the body may not be able to heal the repeated micro-injuries and eventually through accumulation of these micro-injuries, a macro-injury develops. These overuse injuries are frequently described as subacute and chronic conditions such as stress fractures, ligament laxity, and "tendonitis." Finally, there are intrinsic musculoskeletal disorders. These disorders are thought to develop within the affected structure regardless of its use. Rheumatoid arthritis, bone and soft tissue tumors are classic examples of intrinsic disorders.

The categorization of musculoskeletal disorders in this manner is helpful in order to initiate the diagnostic process if a patient presents with a musculoskeletal complaint. For instance, when the history clearly indicates a single traumatic event, the differential diagnostic possibilities are mostly limited to acute traumatic disorders. Chronic tendon problems have classically been designated as "tendonitis" and categorized as a chronic overuse injury (James et al. 1978; Clement et al. 1984; Karlsson et al. 1991). Tendonitis in this etiologic approach is thought to result from repeated micro-trauma from overuse. Once the accumulated micro-trauma has resulted in a clinically significant macro-injury, the body is thought to respond to this with an inflammatory response, hence the suffix-itis (Curl 1990).

Treatment of tendonitis has traditionally been non-surgical. Based on the above-mentioned concept of tendonitis, the treatment aims have been twofold: decreasing the mechanical stress and decreasing the anti-inflammatory response.

Decreasing the mechanical stress can be accomplished in a number of ways. Quite simply, prescribing rest, or at least relative rest, should accomplish this goal. Relative rest has been a popular concept in tendonitis in an attempt to avoid the ill effects of absolute rest (Clement *et al.* 1984). Absolute rest, such as bed rest or cast immobilization, is associated with several side-effects such as muscle atrophy, joint stiffness, and loss of conditioning. Relative rest refers to the concept of allowing continued activities but avoiding those that mechanically overload the affected tendon. For instance, runners with lower extremity tendonitis are switched to a training program that decreases their runner mileage and speed and increases exercises such as pool running and cycling. In some patients with tendonitis there are intrinsic mechanical factors that are thought to contribute to the mechanical overload on the tendon. Joint malalignment such as flat feet, muscle weakness, and imbalance and inflexibility are frequently implicated in the generation of a tendonitis problem. If present, these factors can be addressed through braces, shoe inserts, and, at times, physical therapy. Finally, the mechanical overload on the tendon can be associated with faulty training techniques, coaching errors, or improper equipment. Evaluation and correction of these factors can also lead to a decrease of the mechanical load on the tendon affected by tendonitis.

Decreasing the inflammation is a second major aim of traditional treatment of tendonitis. Several methods are utilized to accomplish this goal. Physical modalities such as cryotherapy, elevation, and compression are traditionally used for this purpose. Pharmacologic approaches also have enjoyed great popularity among treating physicians. Oral non-steroidal anti-inflammatory drugs (NSAIDs), such as aspirin, ibuprofen, and naproxen have been used extensively for this purpose (James *et al.* 1995;

Meyerson & Biddinger 1995). For more resistant cases of tendonitis, anti-inflammatory corticosteroids are frequently used by injecting them directly around the affected tendon. Because of a concern that corticosteroids contribute to weakening and potentially rupturing of the tendon, they are generally only used in the non-weight-bearing tendons of the upper extremity.

In the past decade, the etiology as well as the efficacy of treatment of tendonitis has been questioned. Because of these questions, the concepts of tendonitis are undergoing a fairly dramatic evolution. As a result, most experts in the field now designate these problems as tendinopathy rather than tendonitis. This chapter addresses some of the basic and clinical science aspects that cast doubt on the traditional view of tendonitis. In addition, it suggests possible newer avenues to improve treatment based on more recent research in this area.

Materials and methods

More recent, basic research studies have focused on evaluating the traditional concept of tendonitis both with regards to its biomechanical etiology and the traditional treatment approach. The following chapters review the research in this field as well as our own studies.

Biomechanical studies

Several research studies have supported the possibility that chronic mechanical overuse is not the sole etiologic factor in tendinopathy problems. Imaging as well as biopsy studies have indicated that tendinopathic changes can be seen in human tendons without necessarily causing symptoms (Shalaby & Almekinders 1999; Cook *et al.* 2001). Such changes can be seen in the patellar, Achilles, and supraspinatus tendons of asymptomatic subjects who are not specifically involved in strenuous, repetitive activities involving these tendons. These changes appear to correlate more specifically with age. Pronounced age-related tendon degeneration is particularly common in the Achilles tendon and supraspinatus tendon. Catastrophic mechanical failure of these tendons through the area of degeneration is not uncommon. These complete tendon tears do not clearly correlate with overuse and are actually frequently seen in relatively sedentary patients (Józsa *et al.* 1989).

Basic biomechanical studies have also questioned the role of repetitive mechanical overload in the development of tendinopathy. In the traditional view of tendonitis, repetitive tensile loads were thought to cause micro-injuries to the collagenous matrix. Extensive studies have been carried out in ligaments and tendons to determine the loads needed to cause such plastic deformation in soft tissue. Biomechanical studies have attempted to characterize the *in vivo* mechanical events in tendon, particularly in areas where tendinopathic changes are frequently seen (Almekinders *et al.* 2002). Careful examination of imaging studies of insertional tendinopathy appeared to reveal a consistent pattern. Tendinopathy of the tendon insertion is one of the most common forms of tendinopathy. Lateral epicondylitis, supraspinatus tendinopathy, patellar tendinopathy (jumper's knee), and Achilles tendinopathy at the calcaneal insertion are all examples of this type of tendinopathy. Magnetic resonance imaging (MRI), ultrasound, and histologic images show similar features in all these types of insertional tendinopathy. Pathologic tendon changes are generally found on the joint-side of the tendon insertion (Fig. 11.1). The tendon on the opposite side, away from the joint space, generally appears healthy and well maintained. If mechanical factors have a role in the etiology of insertional tendinopathy, then biomechanical studies should give an indication what mechanical loads are associated with this pathology. Several types of studies have been performed to study this issue. An MRI-based study of the supraspinatus tendon indicated that the joint-side of the tendon is subjected to lower strains than the remainder of the tendon (Bey *et al.* 2002). Cadaveric studies of the patellar tendon insertion on the patella and the Achilles tendon insertion on the calcaneus have been carried out (Almekinders *et al.* 2002; Lyman *et al.* 2004). Both indicated lower tensile strains on the joint-side of the tendons. These studies show that the area most frequently affected by tendinopathic changes is subjected to lower tensile strains compared with the rest of the tendon.

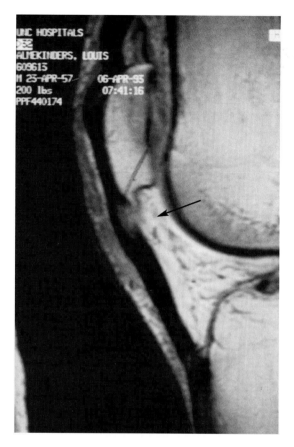

Fig. 11.1 Magnetic resonance imaging (MRI) of a knee with a typical lesion of insertional patellar tendinopathy at the joint side of the patellar insertion (arrow).

This suggests that tensile strains are not a major etiologic factor in insertional tendinopathy. However, this cannot be stated with certainty as the material properties of these different sites have not been determined at this point. Nevertheless, this concept is supported by histologic studies that frequently have noted cartilaginous changes within these tendon areas (Benjamin & Ralph 1998). It is well known that cartilaginous metaplasia within tendon occurs in response to compressive loads.

Mechanical load *in vitro* study is also stimulatory in itself (Almekinders *et al.* 1995). It should be noted that this stimulation is tensile loading of the fibroblasts with resulting elongation of the cell. Interestingly, tensile loading with surface strains as much as 25% was stimulatory and well tolerated by tendon fibroblasts. *In vivo*, such levels of strain would clearly result in mechanical failure of tendon tissue. The *in vitro* findings suggest that tensile loading of tendon *in vivo* is unlikely to cause any damage to the tendon fibroblasts as large strains are well tolerated by these cells. In fact, the cells appear to be positively stimulated by large tensile strains. A more extensive discussion of the cellular and molecular effects of mechanical stimulation can be found in Chapter 3.

From a biomechanical point of view, these results suggest that certain tensile forces are not necessarily injurious to the tendon, while compressive forces may be. Physical therapy approaches that emphasize the tensile forces but avoid compressive forces would logically be preferred for a tendinopathic tendon. No specific clinical studies have been completed that investigate this concept. It is possible that success of newer therapy approaches that emphasize eccentric exercise (Alfredson *et al.* 1998) is related to this concept, as it is know that eccentric exercise creates high tensile loads in the muscle–tendon unit.

Biologic studies

Recent biologic research has also cast significant doubt on the relatively simplistic view of chronic tendon problems as a result of repetitive mechanical overload with a subsequent injury and inflammatory response (Almekinders & Temple 1998). As early as the 1980s, it became known that surgical biopsies of tendons affected by "tendonitis" rarely if ever showed features of a classic inflammatory response (Fukuda *et al.* 1990; Józsa *et al.* 1990; Kannus & Józsa 1991; Åstrom & Westlin 1992). Instead, the histology was more consistent with a degenerative picture. Mucoid degeneration, lack of inflammatory cells, disorganized collagen matrix, and metaplasia of tendon fibroblasts were reported in conditions such as lateral epicondylitis, rotator cuff, Achilles, and patellar tendonitis. Some have argued that these surgical specimens were mostly degenerative in nature as the result of the fact that these particular patients had a failed healing response and therefore required surgery. This group possibly represents only one extreme end

of the spectrum of tendonitis. On the other hand, this raised the possibility that tendonitis is not just a chronic overuse injury, but possibly a primary, intrinsic, degenerative disorder. With the etiology and exact pathology in dispute, many have advocated designating these chronic tendon problems as tendinopathy and not tendonitis.

Although the exact role of all possible etiologic factors in the development of tendinopathy are not known, it appears that the simple, repetitive, tensile overload model does not explain the more recent findings in histologic, imaging, and biomechanical studies. The possibility that tendinopathy has a multifactorial etiology, which includes both extrinsic mechanical factors as well as intrinsic degenerative features, may also explain why our traditional treatment of tendinopathy is frequently not efficacious. In the traditional view of tendonitis, it was obvious that restriction of activities should be the mainstay of treatment (Clement *et al.* 1984). In addition, pharmaceutical intervention is frequently used. Oral NSAIDs have been generally recommended to treat the presumed inflammatory component of tendonitis (James *et al.* 1978; Meyerson & Biddinger 1995). Consistent with lack of inflammatory changes in biopsy studies, NSAID treatment of tendinopathy has not been shown to be superior when compared with simple analgesics or even placebo treatment in controlled studies (Petri *et al.* 1987; Åstrom & Westlin 1992). Prompted by the results of clinical studies, some basic studies were carried out investigating the potential role of NSAIDs in tendon cells and tissue. An *in vivo* study indicated that repetitive tensile loading of tendon fibroblasts resulted in an increase in prostaglandin levels (Almekinders *et al.* 1995). In a subsequent study, it appeared that these eicosanoids had a role in both cell division and matrix synthesis as NSAIDs had a mild stimulatory effect on protein synthesis *in vitro*, whereas the mitogenic response to mechanical load was inhibited (Almekinders *et al.* 1995). This was consistent with other animal studies where increased collagen synthesis was seen as a result of NSAID administration (Vogel 1997). These studies make clear that NSAIDs do not require the presence of an inflammatory response in order to have effects on the tendon tissue. Direct effects on the tendon fibroblasts were shown in these *in vitro* studies. Whether these effects in the clinical situation are beneficial or not remains unclear. The explant tendon studies clearly showed an age-dependent mitogenic and protein synthesis response (Almekinders 1999). Older specimens clearly had inferior responses in this regard.

Injections of corticosteroids into areas of symptomatic tendinopathy have also been frequently used, particularly for upper extremity tendinopathy such as lateral epicondylitis and supraspinatus tendinopathy. Corticosteroids are potent anti-inflammatory drugs and therefore were thought to be appropriate for the presumed inflammatory component of tendonitis. However, similar to NSAIDs, corticosteroids have not been shown to improve the natural history of tendinopathy (DaCruz *et al.* 1988; Price *et al.* 1991; Vecchia *et al.* 1993). The lack of efficacy of NSAIDs and corticosteroids adds questions to the validity of the traditional overuse tendonitis model with a subsequent inflammatory response. Similar to NSAIDs, relatively little is known about the direct effects of corticosteroids on tendon cells and tissue. In tendon tissue explants, dexamethasone had a small negative effect on the mitogenic response of tendon fibroblasts (Almekinders 1999). There was also a trend towards decreased protein synthesis with dexamethasone. These results indicate that direct effects of corticosteroids on tendon fibroblasts are not suggestive of positive clinical effects.

Physical therapists and athletic trainers frequently use physical modalities for chronic tendon problems. Cryotherapy, heat, ultrasound, and electrical stimulation have all been advocated for tendinopathy. Again, few scientific studies have documented their effects on tendon tissue or tendon fibroblasts. An *in vitro* study on the effects of ultrasound revealed no changes in tendon fibroblast mitogenesis and protein synthesis following ultrasound application (Almekinders 1999). There are no additional studies that document any beneficial effects of ultrasound treatment on tendon cells or tissue.

New treatment approaches

With the new findings with regards to the etiology of tendinopathy and the lack of clear efficacy or scientific rationale of commonly used treatment approaches, a new treatment paradigm for tendinopathy seems appropriate. The previously discussed studies suggest that drug treatment of tendinopathy should be aimed at generating a healing response within the tendon rather than treating a presumed inflammatory response. It could be argued that an inflammatory response within a tendinopathic area is actually needed, because an inflammatory response appears to be predictably followed by a proliferative healing response in collagenous tissues. Although a full-blown inflammatory response may not be desired, it seems attractive to identify those factors within the inflammatory response that are vital to progression to a proliferative healing response. Studies in our laboratory have attempted to focus on the role of growth factors in this process. If we are able to identify the exact role of growth factors in this process, they may present us with a biologic option for the treatment of tendinopathy.

Although not yet clinically used, the effects of growth factors in tendon have been studied in a number of basic science studies. The effects of epidermal growth factor, insulin, and transferrin have been tested *in vitro* on avian tendon cells (Gauger *et al.* 1985). The factors promoted cell replication as well as matrix synthesis. In addition, fibroblast growth factor has been investigated (Chan *et al.* 1997). In our laboratory, platelet-derived growth factor (PDGF) and insulin-like growth factor (IGF) were tested *in vitro* and *in vivo* with avian tendon fibroblasts (Banes *et al.* 1995; Bynum *et al.* 1997)). We know from other studies that tendon cells have growth factor receptors (Tsuzaki *et al.* 2000). Tendon fibroblasts consist of different populations: epitenon surface cells (TSC) and tendon internal fibroblasts (TIF) (Banes *et al.* 1988). They most likely have different roles in both maintenance and repair of tendons. They also have different growth rates when grown *in vitro*. The growth factor studies also showed different responses to growth factors. PDGF-BB was able to promote TSC cell division. There was a synergistic effect with mechanical load and IGF-1. The stimulation by PDGF-BB of TIF was lower but still measurable. In further experiments, it was found that PDGF-BB was able to induce novel genes when used in conjunction with mechanical load (Banes *et al.* 1999). Other investigators also have found stimulatory effects of PDGF in tendon tissue (Spindler *et al.* 1996). Based on these studies, it appears that selected growth factors show promising effects in these *in vitro* studies. However, mode of administration, timing, and dosing of these proteins are going to be crucial if they are to be used in human tendinopathy.

Ideally, animal studies would be carried out first to investigate the potential effects as well as determine dosing regimens. Unfortunately, it has been difficult to develop an animal model that closely resembles human tendinopathy (Backman *et al.* 1990; Archambault *et al.* 1995). Attempts with prolonged, repetitive motion do not clearly yield a tendinopathy picture. Enzyme-induced tendon changes with collagenase have been reported but not fully tested. Lately, it has been shown that antibiotics belonging to the group of flouroquinolones can give a tendinopathic picture in both rodents as well as humans (Kashida & Kato 1997; Khaliq & Zhanel 2003). Animal models with fluoroquinolones are being tested but it is too early to know whether they can be used to test new treatment methods.

In the absence of reliable animal models, there have been some initial attempts to utilize the effects of growth factors in human tendinopathy. Although growth factors are available in purified or recombinant form, it will be difficult to use them as such in humans with animal data. In order to avoid some potential risks with the use of purified or recombinant factors, our research group initiated a clinical project to use autologous platelets as a potential source of PDGF and other growth factors. Platelet-rich plasma (PRP) has been use extensively in as a source of growth factors in grafting procedures for maxillofacial surgery and spine surgery. Others have shown that besides PDGF, PRP contains significant amounts of other growth factors such as transforming growth factor β1 (TGF-β1) and IGF (Marx *et al.* 1998; Weibrich *et al.* 2002). This has a resulted in stimulation of bone grafts as well as human mesenchymal stem cells. Its direct effect on tendon cells and tissues is not entirely clear. PRP used in an animal model of Achilles tendon repair resulted in improved strength and repair tissue (Aspenberg & Virchenko 2004). Lately, small tabletop units have become commercially available, which can produce PRP in a one-step centrifugation process (Fig. 11.2). Based on the degenerative histologic picture of tendinopathy, injection of affected tendon areas with PRP seems a logical next step. Initial clinical studies have been started with this approach. Patients with lateral epicondylitis, patellar tendinopathy, and insertional Achilles tendinopathy who fail to respond to conservative treatment after 4–6 months are considered candidates for this approach. The affected area of the tendon is identified through a soft tissue imaging study. MRI will generally show the affected area in great detail; however, it cannot be used for real-time imaging. Therefore, diagnostic ultrasound is often used to not only identify the affected area but also control placement of the needle during PRP injection. In order to obtain the PRP, 20 mL venous blood is drawn from the patient through venipuncture in a citrate-containing syringe. The anticoagulated blood is placed in a multichambered centrifuge

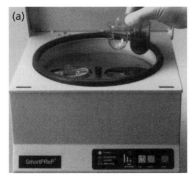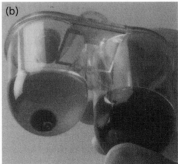

Fig. 11.2 Automated centrifuge system (a) for preparation of platelet-rich plasma (b). (Harvest Technologies, Plymouth, MA, USA.)

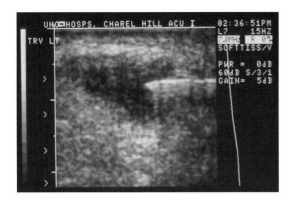

Fig. 11.3 Ultrasound guided injection while the needle is advanced into a tendinopathic tendon.

insert (Fig. 11.2). Using a pre-programmed centrifuge, the plasma and platelets are separated from the red blood cells in about 14 minutes. After the centrifugation, the plasma is discarded and approximately 3 mL PRP is available for injection. Usually, no more than 1–2 mL is injected in the tendon. Placement of the needle can be confirmed by sterile ultrasound probe (Fig. 11.3). The tip of the needle is purposely placed *in* the tendon, unlike the recommendation for corticosteroid injections. It is unlikely that the large growth factor proteins are transported well beyond the injection site. Therefore, it may be important to place the injection as close as possible to the affected tendon tissue. Injections directly into the tendon can be painful, most likely as a result of expansion of the tissues. We have not mixed the PRP with a local anesthetic because of the fear of losing growth factor activity. Generally, the pain dissipates rapidly following the injection. In general, we do not expect any significant improvement in the tendon pain until at least 4–6 weeks following the injection. If a partial improvement has occurred at that time, we have considered a second injection. Two out of four patients with patellar tendinopathy resolved completely with one PRP injection. One soccer player, whose patellar tendinopathy failed to improve after two surgical procedures, was treated with PRP and eventually resolved after three PRP injections. In the initial part of a double-blinded study on PRP injection for chronic epicondylitis,

three out of four patients injected with PRP improved at the 6-week follow-up point. Three patients injected with corticosteroids also had initial improvement but two out of three had already recurred at the 6-week time point. Although not all patients injected with PRP have responded, one should remember that these initial patients represent a worst case scenario. Several patients had failed corticosteroid injections or even surgery. PRP injection earlier in the course of treatment as well as multiple injections need to be considered to potentially improve the response rate. No PRP-injected patient indicated worsening of their pain at follow-up. This may be important because corticosteroid has been associated with increased problems after the initial effects are worn off. Follow-up imaging studies have been obtained in some patients. Resolution of the pain was associated with complete normalization of the imaging study. More recently, Mishra & Pavelko (2005) reported the result of this treatment approach in a study of patients with failed traditional treatment for lateral epicondylitis. One group received a single percutaneous injection of PRP, whereas the control group received a bupivicaine injection. At 8 weeks following the injection, the PRP-injected patients noted a 60% improvement of their pain on a visual analog scale. In the control group, only a 16% improvement was noted. This difference was highly statistically significant. At that point, most control patients withdrew from the study. The PRP-injected patients continued to improve with an 81% improvement of their pain at 6 months. Although it is too early to propose a treatment algorithm that includes PRP, it appears that it may be useful after initial conservative treatment has failed and prior to considering corticosteroid injection or surgery.

The *in vitro* mechanical studies suggest that tendon fibroblast respond favorably to tensile strain. Even large strains that would normally damage the structurally integrity of tendon tissue as a whole are well tolerated by individual fibroblasts. Therefore, flexibility exercises that exert controlled tensile strains on tendons and fibroblasts may remain important for both prevention and treatment. However, cadaveric studies suggest that the traditional exercises may need to be altered in order to place these strains on the most commonly affected area of the tendon in cases of insertional tendinopathy (Almekinders *et al.* 2002; Lyman *et al.* 2004). For instance, the posterior aspect of the patellar tendon at the inferior pole of the patella is most commonly affected by patellar tendinopathy or jumper's knee. This area of the tendon exhibits relatively little strain as the knee goes into more flexion. Traditionally, patellar tendon flexibility exercises are performed with the knee in maximum flexion. The biomechanical study indicates this position results in stress shielding of the affected area. If the exercises could be performed with the knee closer to full extension the involved area may be more likely to be mechanically stimulated. Similarly, the anterior portion of the Achilles tendon is most likely involved in insertional Achilles tendinopathy. This area of the tendon exhibits the lowest strains with the ankle in dorsiflexion. Again, this is the most common position of the ankle when athletes are performing Achilles stretching exercises. A plantar flexed position is more likely to place mechanical tensile stress on the affected area based on the biomechanical studies. As stated before, this hypothesis has not been tested in clinical studies. Other physical therapy approaches such as eccentric exercise (Alfredson *et al.* 1998) should be considered in conjunction with these findings. Additional details of this approach are described in Chapter 12.

Clinical relevance and significance

My research is focused on both the biomechanical and biologic events of the tendon insertion. Tendon insertion sites are one of the most common sites of tendon problems in athletes. Rotator cuff problems, tennis elbow, jumper's knee, and some Achilles tendon problems are all examples of insertional tendinopathy. Current treatment methods for these problems are largely based on theory and tradition. Very few scientific data are available that directly support these traditional treatments. Follow-up studies indicated that traditional treatment is often not effective. If we can gain a better understanding of the mechanical and biologic events that take place in the tendon insertion site, then we can formulate more logical approaches for these problems. These approaches could include both treatment and preventative strategies.

The treatment of tendinopathy with an injection of a platelet concentrate is an example of such a scientific approach. Histopathologic studies of tendinopathy suggested a degenerative picture. Growth factors were able to generate positive metabolic response in tendon cells when tested in the laboratory. Such metabolic responses evoked by growth factors could improve degenerative changes in the tendon. The currently used anti-inflammatory medication appears to be totally ineffective in that regard. As platelets contain these growth factors, injection of platelet concentrate could be a logical next step. Although the initial results are encouraging, more work needs to be carried out before this treatment can be recommended.

Future directions

It is too early to determine whether modification of the biomechanical and biologic approach to tendinopathy will result in improved prevention and treatment of this problem. At this point, it is premature to present a defined treatment algorithm that encompasses these newer approaches. However, both have supporting basic science studies, which have clearly been missing for some of the traditional treatment approaches. Continued investigation should focus on these new possibilities with larger groups of patients in a controlled manner.

In summary, tendinopathy may not be a simple mechanical failure of the tendon followed by an inflammatory response. Unfortunately, current treatment methods appear to have poor efficacy. Therefore, in order to improve the treatment of tendinopathy, we need to know the exact pathophysiology of tendinopathy with an emphasis on the early stages rather than the final end-stage. In addition, we need to further investigate treatment approaches such as growth factor application. The first step in this process will be to develop a reliable animal model. Next, new treatment approaches need to be tested in an animal model. Finally, comprehensive multicenter studies will need to be conducted on tendiopathy patients in all stages.

References

Alfredson, H., Pietila, T., Jonsson, P. *et al.* (1998) Heavy-load eccentric calf muscle training for treatment of chronic Achilles tendinosis. *American Journal of Sports Medicine* **26**, 360–366.

Almekinders, L.C. & Temple, J.D. (1998) Etiology, diagnosis and treatment of tendonitis: an analysis of the literature. *Medicine and Science in Sports and Exercise* **30**, 1183–1190.

Almekinders, L.C., Banes, A.J. & Bracey, L.W. (1995) An *in vitro* investigation into the effects of repetitive motion and nonsteroidal anti-inflammatory medication on human tendon fibroblasts. *American Journal of Sports Medicine* **23**, 119–123.

Almekinders, L.C. & Dere, G. (1999) The effects of aging, anit-inflammatory drugs and ultrasound on the *in vitro* response of tendon tissue. *American Journal of Sports Medicine* **27**, 417–421.

Almekinders, L.C., Vellema, J.H. & Weinhold, P.S. (2002) Strain patterns in the patellar tendon and the implications for patellar tendinopathy. *Knee Surgery, Traumatology, Arthroscopy* **10**, 2–5.

Archambault, J.M., Wiley, J.P. & Bray, R.C. (1995) Exercise loading of tendons and the development of overuse injuries. A review of current literature. *Sports Medicine* **20**, 77–89.

Aspenberg, P. & Virchenko, O. (2004) Platelet concentrate injection improves Achilles tendon repair in rats. *Acta Orthopaedica Scandinavica* **75**, 93–99.

Åstrom, M. & Westlin, N. (1992) No effect of piroxicam on Achilles tendinopathy: a randomized study of 70 patients. *Acta Orthopaedica Scandinavica* **63**, 631–634.

Backman, C., Boquist, L., Friden, J., Lorentzon, R. & Toolanen, G. (1990) Chronic Achilles paratenonitis with tendinosis: an experimental model in rabbit. *Journal of Orthopaedic Research* **8**, 541–547.

Banes, A., Link, G.W., Bevin, A.G., *et al.* (1988). Tendon synovial cells secrete fibronectin *in vivo* and *in vitro. Journal of Orthopaedic Research* **6**, 73–82.

Banes, A.J., Horesovsky, G., Larson, C., *et al.* (1999) Mechanical load stimulates expression of novel genes *in vivo* and *in vitro* in avian flexor tendon cells. *Osteoarthritis and Cartilage* **7**, 141–153.

Banes, A.J., Tsuzaki, M., Hu, P., *et al.* (1995) PDGF-BB, IGF-I and mechanical load stimulate DNA synthesis in avian tendon fibroblasts *in vitro. Journal of Biomechanics* **28**, 1505–1513.

Benjamin, M. & Ralph, J.R. (1998) Fibrocartilage in tendon and ligaments: an adaptation to compressive load. *Journal of Anatomy* **193**, 481–494.

Bey J.B., Kwon Song. H., Wehrli, F. & Soslowsky, L.J. (2002) Intratendinous strain fields of the intact supraspinatus tendon: the effect of glenohumeral joint position and tendon region. *Journal of Orthopaedic Research* **20**, 869–874.

Bynum, D., Almekinders, L., Benjamin, M., *et al.* (1997). Wounding *in vivo* and PDGF-BB *in vitro* stimulate tendon surface migration and loss of connesin-43 expression. *Transactions of the Orthopaedic Research Society* **22**, 26.

Chan, B.P., Chan, K.M., Maffulli, N., Webb, S. & Lee, K.H.K. (1997) Effect of basic fibroblast growth factor. An *in vitro* study of tendon healing. *Clinical Orthopaedics and Related Research* **342**, 239–247.

Clement, D.B., Taunton, J.E. & Smart, G.W. (1994) Achilles tendinitis and peritendinitis: etiology and treatment. *American Journal of Sports Medicine* **12**, 179–184.

Cook, J.L., Khan, K.M., Kiss, Z.S., *et al.* (2001) Asymptomatic hyperechoic regions on the patellar tendon ultrasound: A 4-year clinical and ultrasound followup of 46 tendons. *Scandinavian Journal of Medicine and Science in Sports* **11**, 321–327.

Curl, W. (1990) Clinical relevance of sports-induced inflammation. In: *Sports Induced Inflammation* (Leadbetter, W.B., Buckwalter, J.A., Gordon, S.L., eds.) AAOS, Park Ridge, IL.

Dacruz, D.J., Geeson, M., Allen, M.J. & Phair, I. (1988) Achilles paratenonitis: evaluation of steroid injection. *British Journal of Sports Medicine* **22**, 64–65.

Fukuda, H., Hamada, K. & Yamanaka, K. (1990) Pathology and pathogenesis of bursal side rotator cuff tears viwed from en bloc histologic sections. *Clinical Orthopaedics and Related Research* **254**, 75–80.

Gauger, A., Robertson, C., Greenlee, T.K. & Riederer-Henderson, M.A. (1985) A low-serum medium for tendon cells: effects of growth factors on tendon cells and collagen production. *In Vitro Cellular and Developmental Biology* **21**, 291–296.

James, S.L., Bates, B.T. & Osterning, L.R. (1978) Injuries to runners. *American Journal of Sports Medicine* **6**, 40–49.

Józsa, L., Kvist, M., Balint, B.I., *et al.* (1989) The role of recreational sport activity in

Achilles tendon rupture: A clinical, pathoanatomical and sociological study of 292 cases. *American Journal of Sports Medicine* **17**, 338–343.

Józsa, L., Reffy, A. & Kannus, P. (1990) Pathological alterations in human tendons. *Archives of Orthopaedic and Trauma Surgery* **110**, 15–21.

Kannus, P. & Józsa, L. (1991) Histopathological changes preceding spontaneous rupture of a tendon. *Journal of Bone and Joint Surgery. American volume* **73**, 1507–1525.

Karlsson, J., Lundin, O., Lossing, I.W. & Peterson, L. (1991) Partial rupture of the patellar ligament. *American Journal of Sports Medicine* **19**, 403–408.

Kashida, Y. & Kato, M. (1997) Characterization of fluoroquinolone-induced Achilles tendon toxicity in rats: a comparison of toxicities of 10 fluorquinolones and effects of anti-inflammatory compounds. *Antimicrobial Agents and Chemotherapy* **41**, 2389–2393.

Khaliq, Y. & Zhanel, G.G. (2003) Fluoroquinolone-associated tendinopathy: a critical review of the literature. *Clinical Infectious Diseases* **36**, 1404–1410.

Lyman, J., Weinhold, P.S. & Almekinders, L.C. (2004). Strain behavior in the distal Achilles tendon: implications for Achilles tendinopathy. *American Journal of Sports Medicine* **32**, 457–461.

Marx, R.E., Carlson, E.R., Eichstaedt, R.M., Schimmele, S.R., Strauss, J.E. & Georgeff, K.R. (1998) Platelet-rich plasma. Growth factor enhancement for bone grafts. *Oral Surgery, Oral Medicine, Oral Pathology, Oral Radiology, and Endodontics* **85**, 638–646.

Meyerson, M.S. & Biddinger, K. (1995) Achilles tendon disorders: practical management strategies. *Journal of Physical Sports Medicine and Physical Fitness* **23**, 24–54.

Mishra, A.K. & Pavelko, T. (2005) Treatment of severe elbow tendinosis with platelet rich plasma. Proceedings of the 2005 Annual Meeting of the American Academy of Orthopaedic Surgeons. 565.

Petri, M., Dubow, R., Neiman, R., Whiting-O'Keefe, Q. & Seaman, W.E. (1987) Randomized, double-blind, placebo-controlled study of the treatment of the painful shoulder. *Arthritis and Rheumatism* **30**, 1040–1045.

Price, R., Sinclair, M., Heinrick, I. & Gibson, T. (1991) Local injection treatment of tennis elbow. Hydrocortisone, triamcinolone and lignocaine compared. *British Journal of Rheumatology* **30**, 39–44.

Shalaby, M. & Almekinders, L.C. (1999) Patellar tendonitis: the significance of magnetic resonance imaging findings. *American Journal of Sports Medicine* **27**, 345–349.

Spindler, K.P., Imro, A.K., Mayes, C.E. & Davidson, J.M. (1996) Patellar tendon and anterior cruciate ligament have different mitogenic responses to platelet-derived growth factor and

transforming growth factor beta. *Journal of Orthopaedic Research* **14**, 542–546.

Tsuzaki, M., Xiao, H., Brigman, B., *et al.* (2000). IGF-I is expressed by avian flexor tendon cells. *Journal of Orthopaedic Research* **8**, 546–556.

Vecchia, P.C., Hazleman, B.L. & King, R.M. (1993) A double-blind trial comparing subacromial methyl prednisolone and lignocaine in acute rotator cuff tendonitis. *British Journal of Rheumatology* **32**, 743–745.

Vogel, H.G. (1977) Mechanical and chemical properties of various connective tissue organs in rats as influenced by non-steroidal antirheumatic drugs. *Connective Tissue Research* **5**, 91–95.

Weibrich, G., Kleis, W.K., Hafner, G. & Hitzler, W.E. (2002) Growth factor levels in platelet-rich plasma and correlations with donor age, sex, and platelet count. *Journal of Craniomaxillofacial Surgery* **30**, 97–102.

Chapter 12

The Chronic Painful Achilles Tendon: Basic Biology and Treatment—Results of the New Methods of Eccentric Training and Sclerosing Therapy

HÅKAN ALFREDSON

The etiology and pathogenesis of chronic tendon pain is unknown. Although tendon biopsies have shown an absence of inflammatory cell infiltration, non-steroidal anti-inflammatory agents (NSAIDs, corticosteroidal injections) are commonly used. We have demonstrated that it is possible to use intratendinous microdialysis to investigate human tendons, and found normal prostaglandin E_2 (PGE_2) levels in chronic painful tendinosis (Achilles and patellar) tendons. Furthermore, gene technologic analyses of biopsies showed no upregulation of pro-inflammatory cytokines. These findings show that there is no PGE_2-mediated intratendinous inflammation in the chronic stage of these conditions. The neurotransmitter glutamate (a potent modulator of pain in the central nervous system) was, for the first time, found in human tendons. Microdialysis showed significantly higher glutamate levels in chronic painful tendinosis (Achilles and patellar) tendons, compared with pain-free normal control tendons. The importance of that finding is under evaluation. Treatment is considered to be difficult, and often surgery is needed. However, recent research on non-surgical methods has shown promising clinical results. Painful eccentric calf-muscle training has been demonstrated to give good clinical short- and mid-term results in patients with chronic painful mid-portion Achilles tendinosis. Good clinical results were associated with decreased tendon thickness and a structurally more normal tendon with no remaining neovessels. Using ultrasonography (US) and color Doppler (CD), and immunohistochemical analyses of biopsies, we have recently demonstrated a vasculoneural (substance P [SP] and calcitonin gene-related peptide [CGRP] nerves) ingrowth in the chronic painful tendinosis tendon, but not in the pain-free normal tendon. A specially designed treatment, using US and CD guided injections of the sclerosing agent polidocanol, targeting the neovessels outside the tendon, in pilot studies has been shown to cure tendon pain in the majority of patients. A recent, randomized, double-blind study verified the importance of injecting the sclerosing substance polidocanol.

Introduction

The Achilles tendon has a high capacity to withstand tensional forces, and is one of the strongest tendons in the human body. However, chronic painful conditions in the tendon are relatively common, not only among middle-aged recreational athletes (Kvist 1994), but also among top-level elite athletes. The etiology and pathogenesis are unknown. There is a wide range of suggested etiologic factors, but the scientific background to most of these is lacking, and they are to be considered as non-proven theories. An association with overuse from repetitive loading is most often stated as being the etiologic factor (Curwin & Stanish 1984; Archambault et al. 1995; Kannus & Józsa 1997); however, these conditions are also seen in physically non-active individuals (Movin 1998; Alfredson & Lorentzon 2000). This was further emphasized in a study on a large group of patients with chronic Achilles tendinopathy (342 tendons with tendinosis), where it was demonstrated that physical activity was not correlated to the histopathology, suggesting that physical activity could be more important in provoking the symptoms than being the cause of the actual lesion (Åström 1998). Among other suggested etiologic factors are: aging, with a decreased blood supply and decreased tensile strength; muscle weakness and imbalance; and insufficient flexibility (Welsh & Clodman 1980; Clement et al. 1984; Nichols 1989; Galloway et al. 1992).

The nomenclature around the painful Achilles tendon is somewhat confusing. Chronic painful conditions in the Achilles tendon have been given many names, and the definition, of the same condition, is often different in different studies. The nomenclature for the chronic painful condition often does not reflect the pathology of the tendon disorder (Movin 1998), making it difficult to evaluate scientific articles and compare the results of different treatment regimens. Quite often, the terms "tendinitis" and "tendonitis" are used (Schepsis & Leach 1987; Nelen et al. 1989; Leadbetter et al. 1992; Myerson & McGarvey 1999), despite the absence of scientific evidence demonstrating a prostaglandin-mediated chemical inflammation. The terminology "chronic tendinopathy" is often used for patients with a long duration of a painful condition located in the Achilles tendon region (Åström 1997; Movin 1998; Khan et al. 1999). However, that term only indicates a condition with pain, but says nothing about its character. Puddu et al. (1976) suggested the term "tendinosis" to be used for local "degenerative" changes in the Achilles tendon. However, the term "degenerative" did not have a standard description, but was associated with a variety of histologic entities. Movin et al. (1997) demonstrated the characteristic morphologic features of "tendinosis" to be changes in the collagen fiber structure and arrangement, an increased amount of interfibrillar glycosaminoglycans (GAGs), vascular ingrowth and abscence of inflammatory cell infiltrates. It has now been generally accepted that the definition of tendinosis is a chronic painful condition in the mid-portion of the tendon, where examination (ultrasound, magnetic resonance imaging [MRI], or possibly biopsy) shows tendon changes corresponding to the painful area in the tendon.

Methods and results

Basic biology

Most studies on the intratendinous biology in humans have been performed on tissue specimens taken through biopsies. Information from biopsies is important, but not optimal. It is of significant importance to be able to study events inside the tendon over a period of time but, for ethical reasons, repeated biopsies from the same tendon cannot be justified.

MICRODIALYSIS

In situ microdialysis has been shown to be a useful technique to study metabolism of substances in different types of human tissue (Darimont et al. 1994; Thorsen et al. 1996), but the method had never before been used in human tendon tissue. The microdialysis technique allows continuous measurements of concentrations in vivo of substances with molecular size below the cut-off limit (20 kD) of the dialysis membrane. Therefore, it was of interest to investigate whether the microdialysis technique could be used to study certain metabolic events in the Achilles tendon. In patients with chronic painful conditions in the Achilles tendon, it has, despite the absence of inflammatory cell infiltration in tendon biopsies, been a common opinion that there is involvement of an inflammatory reaction (Leadbetter et al. 1992; Kvist 1994; Schrier et al. 1996; Myerson & McGarvey 1999). However, during recent years, the role of an intratendinous inflammation in the chronic stage of this condition has been questioned. It is well known that prostaglandins have a central role in inflammatory reactions (Solomon et al. 1968), and treatment is often focused on medication with prostaglandin antagonists. Therefore, the concentrations of PGE_2, which are known to be involved in chemical inflammation, were studied in tendinosis and normal Achilles tendons. The excitatory neurotransmitter glutamate, known to be a potent and very important pain modulator in the central nervous system (Dickenson et al. 1997) but never identified in human tendons, was also investigated.

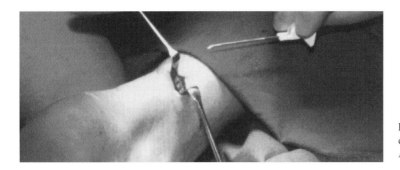

Fig. 12.1 Insertion of a microdialysis catheter into the mid-portion of an Achilles tendon.

Here we describe the first experiment using the microdialysis technique to detect and study the local concentrations of PGE$_2$ and glutamate in human tendons (patients with painful mid-portion chronic Achilles tendinosis and normal pain-free Achilles tendons) (Alfredson *et al.* 1999). A microdialysis catheter was introduced into the tendon through a small skin incision (Fig. 12.1), and placed longitudinally and parallel to the tendon fibers into the area of tendon changes (tendinosis), and in the controls into the central part of the tendon. The microdialysis pump has a fixed infusion rate of 0.3 μL·min, and samples were taken every 15 minutes during a 4-hour period. PGE$_2$ was analyzed using radioimmunoassay (RIA) technique and glutamate was analyzed with high-performance liquid chromatography (HPLC) technique. In four patients (mean age 40.7 years) with chronic symptoms from a painful area in the mid-portion of the Achilles tendon corresponding to tendon changes on ultrasonography, and in five controls (mean age 37.2 years) with normal Achilles tendons (verified by US), the local concentrations of glutamate and PGE$_2$ were recorded for 4 hours under resting conditions. The results showed that there were no significant differences in the mean concentrations of PGE$_2$ between tendons with tendinosis and normal tendons. Surprisingly, glutamate was found in the Achilles tendons, and there were significantly higher concentrations of glutamate in tendons with tendinosis compared with normal tendons (35 ± 6 vs. 9 ± 0.8 μmol/L [mean $\pm$ SD]; $P < 0.05$). There were no significant changes in glutamate concentration over the duration of investigation. The finding of the excitatory neurotransmitter glutamate in a human tendon had never before been reported. In recent years, the importance of glutamate as a mediator of pain in the human central nervous system has been emphasized (Dickenson *et al.* 1997), and from animal studies it is known that glutamate receptors, including the ionotrophic glutamate receptor *N*-metyl-D-aspartate (NMDA), are present in unmyelinated and myelinated sensory axons (Coggeshall & Carlton 1998). Furthermore, peripherally administered NMDA and non-NMDA glutamate receptor antagonists have been demonstrated to diminish the response to formalin-induced nociception in the rat (Davidson *et al.* 1997).

In conclusion, the microdialysis technique can be used for *in vivo* studies in the human Achilles tendon, and the results showed that there were no signs of inflammation (normal PGE$_2$ levels) but high levels of the excitatory neurotransmitter glutamate in tendons from patients with chronic, painful mid-portion Achilles tendinosis. These results further underline that there is no PGE$_2$ mediated inflammation involved in the chronic stage of this condition. However, there might well be a so-called neurogenic inflammation, involving neuropeptides such as SP and CGRP. Also, it is important to know that there is no knowledge about the situation in the early (acute or subacute) stages of the condition. A prostaglandin-mediated inflammation might possibly have a role in the early stage.

The possibility of using the microdialysis technique to study metabolic events in tendons is an interesting field for future research. Recently, the microdialysis technique was used to study the concentrations of lactate in Achilles tendons with painful mid-portion tendinosis, and in normal pain-free tendons. The results showed that tendons with tendinosis had significantly higher concentrations of lactate compared with normal tendons (Alfredson *et al.* 2002). The findings indicate that there might be anaerobic conditions, expressed as higher lactate levels, in tendons with painful tendinosis. However, it is yet to be investigated whether ischemia precedes the start of tendinosis, or whether the tendinotic tendon changes cause ischemia.

Microdialysis can also be performed outside (peritendineously) the Achilles tendon, and Michael Kjaer's excellent research group at the Bispebjerg Hospital in Copenhagen, Danemark, have demonstrated that the method can be used to study collagen synthesis and oxygen demand during exercise (Boushel *et al.* 2000; Kjaer *et al.* 2005).

IMMUNOHISTOCHEMICAL ANALYSES OF BIOPSIES

Immunohistochemical analyses and enzyme histochemistry were used to investigate the occurrence of glutamate NMDA receptors in Achilles tendon tissue (Alfredson *et al.* 2001). The results showed, for the first time, the occurrence of glutamate NMDAR1 receptors in Achilles tendon tissue. Furthermore, the NMDAR1 immunoreaction was confined to acetylcholinesterase-positive structures, implying that the receptors were localized in association with nerves.

Studies on biopsies taken from the area with tendinosis have shown nerve structures in close relation to vessels (Bjur *et al.* 2005). Furthermore,

SP nerves and the neurokinin-1 receptor (NK-1R) (known to have a high affinity for SP) were found in the vascular wall, and CGRP nerves were found close to the vascular wall (Forsgren *et al.* 2005). The findings of neuropeptides indicate that there still might be an inflammation in the tendon; however, not a chemical inflammation (PGE_2 mediated), but instead a neurogenic inflammation mediated via neuropeptides such as SP.

SONOGRAPHY

Another method to study possible differences between Achilles tendons with painful tendinosis and normal pain-free tendons is to use US and CD. In a study on patients with painful mid-portion Achilles tendinosis, the results showed that in 28 tendons with painful tendinosis, there was neovascularization inside, and outside, the ventral part of the area with tendon changes (Fig. 12.2) (Öhberg *et al.* 2001). Theoretically, these findings might have implications for the pathogenesis of chronic mid-portion Achilles tendinosis, and/or the pain symptoms that often are associated with this condition. Gray scale US and CD are methods that are well suited for prospective studies of the normal and injured tendon.

GENE TECHNOLOGY

The rapidly growing area of gene technology has created possibilities to study the expression of genes involved in pathologic and normal conditions in different tissues. The cDNA array technique allows the study of large amounts of gene expression and

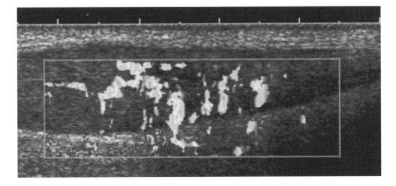

Fig. 12.2 Longitudinal ultrasound scan illustrating neovascularization in chronic mid-portion Achilles tendinosis. The tendon is thickened, with an irregular structure, and hypoechoic areas. Color Doppler is presented, and the neovessels are the pale gray structures inside and at the ventral side of the Achilles tendon.

by using the real-time polymerase chain reaction (PCR) technique more precise measurements of mRNA expression levels can be obtained. Ireland *et al.* (2001) have found a downregulation of matrix metalloproteinase-3 (MMP-3) and an upregulation of type I and III collagen in tendons from patients with chronic Achilles tendinopathy compared with normal tendons from autopsies. Very recently, in a study where tendinosis tissue was compared with control tissue from the same Achilles tendon, we found an upregulation of MMP-2 (destructive enzyme), fibronectin receptor involved in healing processes (FNRB), and vascular endothelial growth factor (VEGF) in painful tendinosis tissue (Alfredson *et al.* 2003). Also, in our study, there was no major regulation of the genes for a variety of different cytokines known to be involved in inflammatory processes. This finding further supports the view that there is no PGE_2-mediated inflammation in the chronic stage of Achilles tendinosis.

Unfortunately, tendon tissue specimens taken through biopsies are needed to use these gene technology methods, and to take multiple biopsies from the same tendon is unethical. The risks for complications have to be taken in account.

Treatment

There is a large variety of proposed treatment regimens for chronic painful conditions in the Achilles tendon. It is important to know that there is sparse scientific evidence for most of the conservative and surgical treatments. The few scientific prospective studies, and the absence of studies comparing different types of conservative and surgical treatment regimens in a randomized manner, are major disadvantages when evaluating the effects of specific treatment regimens.

Non-operative treatment

A non-operative (conservative) treatment regimen is recommended as the initial strategy by most authors (Welsh & Clodman 1980; Curwin & Stanish 1984; Kvist 1994; Kannus & Józsa 1997; Sandmeier & Renström 1997; Alfredson *et al.* 1998b; Khan *et al.* 1999). This strategy includes identification and

correction of possible etiologic factors, and also a symptom-related approach.

Biomechanical "abnormalities" (Welsh & Clodman 1980; Clement *et al.* 1984; Hess *et al.* 1989; Kvist 1991), training errors (James & Bates 1978; Welsh & Clodman 1980; Brody 1987), muscle weakness (Curwin & Stanish 1984; Appel 1986; Renström 1988; Nicol *et al.* 1991; Kannus & Józsa 1997), decreased flexibility (Welsh & Clodman 1980; Curwin & Stanish 1984; Wallin *et al.* 1985; Kvist 1991; Kannus & Józsa 1997), and poor equipment (Brody 1987; Jörgensen & Ekstrand 1988) have all been proposed as possible etiologic factors. However, it is important to know that these proposals rest on poor scientific grounds, and are to be characterized as non-proven theories. Åström (1997) demonstrated that biomechanical "abnormalities" were not important in chronic Achilles tendinopathy, and the value of orthotics in the treatment of chronic tendinopathy has been questioned.

NSAIDs have been used as part of the initial treatment (Welsh & Clodman 1980; Leppilahti *et al.* 1991; Weiler 1992; Leadbetter 1995; Teitz *et al.* 1997; Saltzman & Tearse 1998; Myerson & McGarvey 1999) despite the absence of scientific evidence for an ongoing chemical inflammation (Åström & Westlin 1992; Åström 1997). Also, the use of corticosteroid injections is considered controversial (Leadbetter 1995; Schrier *et al.* 1996; Kannus & Józsa 1997). Inspite of the fact that several authors found frequent partial ruptures after steroid injections in the treatment of chronic painful conditions in the Achilles tendon (Ljungkvist 1968; Williams 1986; Galloway *et al.* 1992; Åström 1998), corticosteroid injections are still being used. However, with the research findings in mind (Movin 1998; Khan *et al.* 1999; Alfredson *et al.* 1999, 2003), in my opinion it cannot be scientifically justified to use anti-inflammatory medication (NSAIDs, corticosteroid injections, etc.) with the purpose of treating a prostaglandin mediated inflammation in this condition.

Surgical treatment

It has been the general opinion that in approximately 25% of patients with chronic painful conditions located in the Achilles tendon, non-surgical treatment is not successful and surgical treatment is needed. Frequency of surgery has been shown to increase with patient age, duration of symptoms, and occurrence of tendinopathic changes (Kvist 1994).

Various surgical techniques are used. Most commonly, macroscopically hypertrophic parts of the paratenon are excised (Williams 1986; Schepsis & Leach 1987; Nelen *et al.* 1989; Leadbetter *et al.* 1992, Alfredson *et al.* 1996, 1998a; Morberg *et al.* 1997) and through a central longitudinal tenotomy, the tendon area with tendinosis is visualized and the "macroscopic abnormal" tissue is excised (Denstad & Roaas 1979; Schepsis & Leach 1987; Nelen *et al.* 1989; Leadbetter *et al.* 1992; Alfredson *et al.* 1996, 1998a; Morberg *et al.* 1997). Another method includes percutaneous multiple longitudinal incisions in the area with tendinosis (Maffuli *et al.* 1997).

Most authors suggest that the effect achieved with these types of surgery is an improvement of the local circulation, and thereby a return to a normal biochemistry in the tendon (Leadbetter *et al.* 1992). However, importantly, the scientific proofs are lacking, and these suggestions are to be considered as theories. In fact, there is no knowledge about where the pain comes from in this condition; consequently, it is difficult to know where to address the surgery and what effect to expect after the surgical treatment. Recent research (Alfredson *et al.* 2003) indicates that the source of pain might be the area with vasculoneural ingrowth localized ventral to the tendon.

Treatment with eccentric calf-muscle training

Curwin and Stanish (1984) stressed the importance of eccentric training as a part of the rehabilitation of tendon injuries. Influenced by their theories, we designed a special type of eccentric calf-muscle training regimen to be used in patients with a strictly defined diagnosis. The group of patients we decided to study had been diagnosed with chronic, painful mid-portion Achilles tendinosis. The mid-portion of the Achilles tendon is an area that is relatively easy to examine clinically and visualize with US or MRI. The patients performed their eccentric exercises (Fig. 12.3) 3 × 15 repetitions, twice daily, 7 days per week, for 12 weeks (Alfredson *et al.* 1998b). It needs to be mentioned that this type of tendon loading is painful, and patients were told to continue their exercises despite experiencing pain or discomfort from the tendon. In fact, the exercises were supposed to be painful, and when there was no tendon pain during exercise, the load was gradually increased to reach a new level of "painful training."

In a prospective pilot study on recreational athletes, we reported good clinical results with treatment consisting of heavy load, eccentric muscle training (Alfredson *et al.* 1998b). All 15 patients in that study had localized changes in the mid-portion of the tendon (at the 2–6 cm level from the insertion into the calcaneus) corresponding to the painful area (verified with US). In all patients, conventional treatment (rest, NSAIDs, change of shoes, orthoses, physical therapy, ordinary training programs) had been tried without any effect on the Achilles tendon pain, and all patients were on the waiting list for surgical treatment. The results showed that after the 12-week training regimen, all 15 patients were satisfied and back to their previous (before injury) activity level. No patient underwent surgery. The pain score (visual analog scale [VAS]) during activity (running) decreased from an average of 81.2 before the eccentric training regimen, to 4.8 after the 12 weeks of treatment. We have now followed this group of patients for 4 years or more (non-published data), and surgical treatment has been needed in only one patient because of the reoccurrence of Achilles tendon pain. All other 14 patients are still satisfied with the result of treatment. At our clinic, we have routinely used this type of painful treatment on patients with diagnosed chronic Achilles tendinosis (at the 2–6 cm level) and, out of 100 consecutive tendons, only 10 tendons have needed surgical treatment (unpublished data).

To determine if treatment with painful concentric calf-muscle training could result in a similar good clinical result, we performed a randomized, prospective, multicenter study where patients with chronic painful, Achilles tendinosis at the 2–6 cm level in the tendon were randomized to either concentric or eccentric training (Mafi *et al.* 2001).

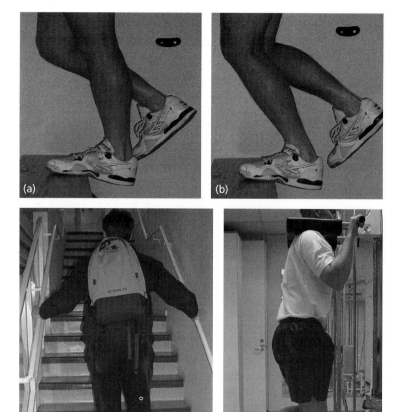

Fig. 12.3 Eccentric exercises. We recommend that patients start to do the exercises standing on a staircase. Start position: The patient is standing in an upright body position with all body weight on the ventral half part of the foot. The ankle joint is in slight plantar flexion or neutral position, lifted to that position by the non-injured leg. The calf muscle is loaded eccentrically by having the patient lower the heel beneath the lever. (a) Eccentric calf-muscle loading with the knee straight. (b) Eccentric calf-muscle loading with the knee bent. (c) Elevating the load by adding weight in a back-pack. (d) Elevating the load by adding weight in a weight machine.

The eccentric training program was as previously described (Alfredson *et al.* 1998b), while the concentric training program was designed to include exercises consisting of mainly concentric calf-muscle action. For both types of programs, training was encouraged despite experiencing pain or discomfort in the tendon. The results showed that the eccentric training regimen produced significantly better clinical results (81% of patients satisfied and back to previous activity level) than the concentric training regimen (38% satisfied patients).

To find out what happens in the tendon when subjected to eccentric training, we have performed clinical and sonographic (gray scale) follow-ups (Öhberg & Alfredson 2003). The results showed that in the successfully treated patients, the tendon thickness had decreased significantly after treatment, and the tendon structure looked more normal in most patients.

There could be several explanations for the good clinical results achieved with painful eccentric calf-muscle training. Theoretically, it could be the effects of loading-induced hypertrophy and increased tensile strength in the tendon, or, maybe, an effect of stretching, with a "lengthening" of the muscle tendon unit and consequently less strain during ankle joint motion. Also, the eccentric training regimen is painful to perform, and maybe this type of painful loading is associated with some kind of alteration of the pain perception from the tendon.

Findings in very recent studies have indicated possible effects on vasculoneural ingrowth with this type of treatment. A recent study using US and CD demonstrated that in Achilles tendons with chronic painful tendinosis, but not in normal pain-free tendons, there is a neovascularization both outside and inside the ventral part of the area with tendon changes (Öhberg *et al.* 2001). By using US and CD during eccentric calf-muscle contraction, we observed that the flow in the neovessels disappeared with the ankle joint in dorsiflexion. As we have demonstrated that there are nerves in close relation to the vascular wall, these observations raised the question as to whether the neovessels and accompanying nerves were the main source of pain and whether this could be an explanation of the good clinical effects demonstrated with eccentric training (Fig. 12.4) (Alfredson *et al.* 2001). Theoretically, during eccentric loading (the program includes 180 repetitions per day) the action on the neovessels and accompanying nerves could cause a vasculoneural injury leading to a dennervation of the painful area. Causing a nerve injury would fit with the fact that most of these patients complained of having severe tendon pain especially during the first 1–2 weeks of the eccentric training regimen. Further indications that the eccentric training regimen has effects on the area with neovascularization come from follow-ups of these patients. Results from follow-ups have shown that in most patients with a good clinical result after treatment, the neovessels demonstrated before instituted treatment had disappeared at follow-up (Öhberg & Alfredson 2004). In patients with poor results of treatment, there were remaining neovessels after treatment.

In a subsequent experiment, we injected local anesthesic into the area with neovessels outside (ventral side) the tendon. This resulted in a temporarily pain-free tendon and the patient could load their Achilles tendon without experiencing any pain. These findings raised the hypothesis that the neovessels and accompanying nerves were responsible for the pain in the area with tendinosis.

Sclerosing therapy

CHRONIC PAINFUL MID-PORTION TENDINOSIS

To test the hypothesis that the neovessels (demonstrated with US and CD) and accompanying nerves (immnuohistochemical analyses) were responsible for the pain in the area with tendinosis, in a non-controlled pilot study we injected a sclerosing agent in the area with neovessels on the ventral side of the tendon (Fig. 12.5). The purpose of this was to destroy the neovessels and accompanying nerves. Sclerosing therapy is widely used for treating varicose veins as well as teleangiectases (Guexx 1993; Conrad *et al.* 1995; Winter *et al.* 2000). We chose the sclerosing agent polidocanol, which is a registered medical pharmaceutical. Polidocanol was first developed as a local anesthetic, and is now widely used as a sclerosing agent with very few side-effects (Guexx 1993; Conrad *et al.* 1995). Polidocanol has a selective effect in the vascular intima causing thrombosis of the vessel. The agent also has an effect if the injection is performed extravascularly. This is

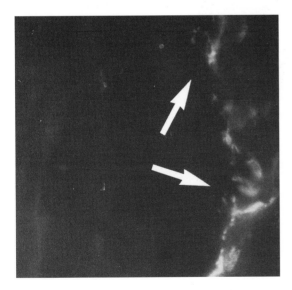

Fig. 12.4 Section of a specimen from a patient with chronic painful mid-portion Achilles tendinosis. There are immunoreactive nerve bundles in close relation to the vascular wall.

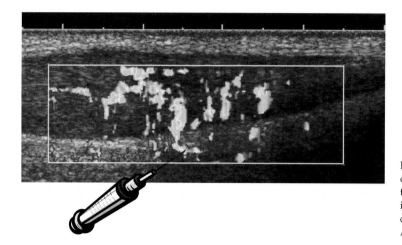

Fig. 12.5 Neovascularization in chronic painful mid-portion Achilles tendinosis. Sclerosing therapy with injection of polidocanol inside or close to the neovessels outside the Achilles tendon.

important when very small vessels are sclerosed. Theoretically, there might be an effect of polidocanol not only on the vessels, but also on nerves "traveling with the vessels." The sclerosing effect of polidocanol on the vessels might affect nerves adjacent to the neovessels, either directly (by destruction) or indirectly (by ischemia). In this pilot study, the short-term (6 months) results were very promising, and 8 out of 10 patients were pain-free and satisfied with treatment after a mean of two treatments (injections) (Öhberg & Alfredson 2002). In the successfully treated patients, there were no neovessels outside or inside the tendon, but neovessels remained in the two unsuccessfully treated patients (Fig. 12.6). A recent 2-year follow-up of these patients showed that the same eight patients

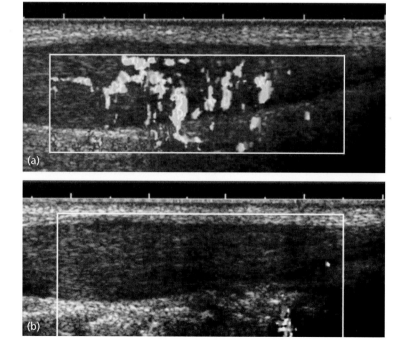

Fig. 12.6 (a) Neovascularization in chronic painful mid-portion Achilles tendinosis before sclerosing therapy. (b) The same tendon as in (a), after sclerosing therapy with injections of polidocanol. There is no remaining neovascularization.

were still satisfied and pain-free during Achilles tendon activity, the tendon structure looked more normal on US, and there were no remaining neovessels on CD (unpublished material). At our clinic, we have now treated more than 100 patients, from world class elite athletes to non-actives, and the clinical results continue to be very promising. These patients are followed closely, and there has only been one severe complication (a track and field athlete who 6 weeks after treatment sustained a total Achilles tendon rupture at the end of an 800-m race). Very recently, in a double-blind, randomized, controlled study, comparing the effects of injections of a sclerosing with a non-sclerosing substance to treat chronic painful mid-portion tendinosis, the importance of injecting the sclerosing substance was clearly demonstrated (Alfredson & Öhberg 2005).

Altogether, it seems very likely that the neovessels and accompanying nerves are responsible for the pain in this chronic condition (Alfredson et al. 2003). However, more research is needed to clarify this. We have ongoing studies on larger groups of patients with different tendon loading activity levels, and routinely perform follow-ups to evaluate the longer term effects of this treatment.

CHRONIC PAIN IN THE ACHILLES TENDON INSERTION

Painful conditions in the Achilles tendon insertion into the calcaneus, often referred to as insertion tendinopathy, are known to be more difficult to treat than painful conditions in the mid-portion of the tendon (Kvist 1991; Kannus & Józsa 1997). Conservative treatment is recommended in the acute phase, but with persisting (chronic) pain, surgery is often required (Kvist 1991, 1994; Järvinen et al. 1997). The origin of insertional pain has not been scientifically clarified, but is often considered to be multifactorial. The calcaneus, the superficial and retrocalcaneal bursae, and the Achilles tendon, separately or in combination, have all been suggested to be the origin of pain (Järvinen et al. 1997). It is well known that the retrocalcaneal bursae might be a focus for chronical inflammation, and consequently could be a source of nociceptive pain. Also, an impingement between a prominence of the upper posterior calcaneus and a thickened or normal tendon might mediate nociceptive pain from the bone and/or tendon (Vega et al. 1984). Furthermore, a partially or totally detached bone fragment, and possibly calcifications, may cause pain. These tissues alone, or together, might be responsible for the painful condition. Therefore, in clinical practice, it is often difficult to judge where to address the treatment. Importantly, the scientific evidence for the theories discussed above is unknown, and besides the calcaneus, bursae, and tendon, other sources might be responsible for the pain.

With the previously discussed promising clinical results using sclerosing therapy to destroy vasculoneural ingrowth in mind, we decided to study the importance of a neovascularization in patients with chronic insertional pain. The aim of the study was to test the hypothesis that destroying (sclerose) the area with neovascularization, but not addressing any treatment to the tendon, bursae, or bone itself, would affect chronic Achilles tendon insertional pain. Again, for this we chose polidocanol, a well-known and widely used sclerosing agent. In this pilot study, 11 patients with a long duration (mean 29 months) of chronic Achilles tendon insertional pain were included (Öhberg & Alfredson 2003). At sonography, all 11 patients had distal structural tendon changes and a local neovascularization inside and outside the distal tendon on the injured or painful side (Fig. 12.7), but not on the non-injured or pain-free side. In nine patients there was also a thickened retrocalcaneal bursae, and in four patients also bone pathology (calcification, spur, loose fragment) in the insertion. The sclerosing agent polidocanol was injected against the neovessels on the ventral side of the tendon insertion. At follow-up (mean 8 months), sclerosing of the area with neovessels had cured the pain in eight of the 11 patients, and in seven of the eight patients there was no remaining neovascularization. Pain during tendon-loading activity, recorded on a VAS scale, decreased from 82 before treatment to 14 after treatment in the successfully treated patients. In two patients with combination tendon, bone, and bursae pathology, there was remaining pain in the tendon insertion after treatment, and remaining neovessels.

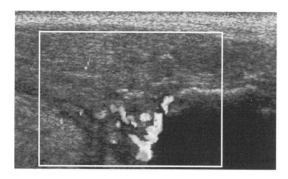

Fig. 12.7 Neovascularization in chronic painful Achilles tendon insertional pain. Longitudinal ultrasound scan. Thickened and irregular distal tendon, prominent cranial calcaneus, and minor calcifications. Color Doppler is presented in gray scale, and the neovessels are the pale gray structures.

In one patient with remaining pain after treatment, there were no remaining neovessels, but a loose bone fragment. Naturally, it is unlikely that this therapy would help patients with bone pathology such as large spurs or loose bone fragments that mechanically interfere with the tendon and skin, but studies on larger groups of patients are needed to be able to draw any conclusions as to what type of distal pathology this therapy is best suited. It is interesting that the absence of neovessels after treatment correlated well with reduced pain from the Achilles tendon insertion in seven out of eight patients. The findings support further studies, long-term follow-up, and preferably randomized studies on large groups of patients.

Clinical relevance and significance

Basic biology

• Histologic and gene technology analyses of tendon tissue biopsies, together with intratendinous *in vivo* microdialysis, have shown that there is no prostaglandin-mediated inflammation in the chronic stage of painful mid-portion Achilles tendinosis.

• Intratendinous *in vivo* microdialysis has shown, for the first time, that the neurotransmitter glutamate (a potent modulator of pain in the central nervous system) exists in the Achilles tendon. Also,

significantly higher concentrations of glutamate were found in chronic painful tendinosis tendons compared with normal pain-free tendons. The importance of these findings is currently not known. Furthermore, there were significantly higher concentrations of lactate in chronic painful tendinosis tendons compared with normal pain-free tendons.

• Immunohistochemical analyses of tendon tissue biopsies have shown that there are sensory nerves (SP and CGRP) in close relation to blood vessels, and glutamate NMDAR1 receptors in close relation to nerve structures in chronic painful tendinosis tissue.

• US and CD examinations have shown that in patients with chronic painful mid-portion Achilles tendinosis, there is an association between the occurrence of a neovascularization in the area with structural tendon changes, and Achilles tendon pain during tendon loading activities.

Treatment

• For patients with chronic painful mid-portion Achilles tendinosis, treatment with 12 weeks of painful eccentric calf-muscle training have, in different studies, resulted in good short- and mid-term clinical results. In a randomized study, painful eccentric training has been shown to give superior clinical results to painful concentric calf-muscle training.

• After treatment with painful eccentric training, US has shown that in most patients the tendon thickness had decreased significantly, and the tendon structure appeared sonographically more normal.

• Injections of local anesthesia in the area with neovessels outside the ventral side of the tendon, temporarily cured the pain during tendon loading activity.

• Sclerosing polidocanol injections, focusing on destroying the area with neovessels and accompanying nerves outside the tendon, has shown very promising short-term clinical results on patients (non-actives to elite athletes) with chronic painful mid-portion tendinosis.

• Short-term clinical results of a small pilot-study on patients with chronic pain in the Achilles tendon insertion have indicated that sclerosing polidocanol injections in the area with neovascularization outside the tendon might be effective.

• Very few complications have been seen after treatment with sclerosing polidocanol injections.

In summary, there is no prostaglandin-mediated inflammation inside the chronic painful Achilles tendon mid-portion. However, there might well be a so-called neurogenic inflammation mediated through neuropeptides such as SP and CGRP. Neovessels and sensory nerves on the ventral side of the chronic painful Achilles tendon mid-portion have been shown to be correlated with pain, and treatment with sclerosing polidocanol injections, targeting the neovessels (and nerves) outside the tendon, has shown good short-term clinical results and very few complications.

Future directions

Basic biology

More knowledge is needed about the intratendinous milieu in the chronic painful tendinosis tendon and normal pain-free tendon. It is important to determine what types of pain-related substances, such as neurotransmitters and neuropeptides, are associated with the tendinosis tendon, and what their roles are. In addition, the role of cytokines, growth factors, hormones, and lipids need to be investigated. Furthermore, investigations need to be undertaken to determine the effect of certain treatment regimens on the intratendinous milieu. Most likely, *in vivo* investigations such as intratendinous microdialysis would be helpful to obtain that information. Also, expanded immunohistochemical analyses of tendon tissue specimens together with US and CD examination, will most likely expand our knowledge about the tendon. Furthermore, a new technique—MRI spectroscopy— might give additional information.

Clinical treatment

There is a need for more knowledge about the effects of different treatment methods. Both clinical and radiologic (US and CD, MRI) effects should be studied in the short, medium, and long term perspective. In addition, the effect of treatment on tendon vascularity, thickness, and structure needs to be examined. It will also be important to determine if there are any side-effects associated with eccentric training and sclerosing therapy. Other factors to investigate include whether or not an early return to full Achilles tendon loading activity after treatment with sclerosing therapy can be achieved, and if there is a critical time limit. Finally, it may be possible to develop new treatment methods based on the recent findings about tendon pain, neovessels, and nerves. Proper clinical and radiologic (US and CD, MRI) follow-up, together with carefully planned scientific studies, can help us to obtain this information.

References

Alfredson, H. & Lorentzon, R. (2000) Chronic Achilles tendinosis. Recommendations for treatment and prevention. *Sports Medicine* **29**, 135–146.

Alfredson, H. & Öhberg, L. (2005) Sclerosing injections to areas of neovascularisation reduce pain in chronic Achilles tendinopathy: A double-blind randomized controlled trial. *Knee Surgery, Sports Traumatology, Arthroscopy* **13**, 338–344.

Alfredson, H., Bjur, D., Thorsen, K. & Lorentzon, R. (2002) High intratendinous lactate levels in painful chronic Achilles tendinosis. An investigation using microdialysis technique. *Journal of Orthopaedic Research* **20**, 934–938.

Alfredson, H., Forsgren, S., Thorsen, K., Johansson, H. & Lorentzon, R. (2001) Glutamate NMDAR1 receptors localised to nerves in human Achilles tendons. Implications for treatment? *Knee Surgery, Sports Traumatology, Arthroscopy* **9**, 123–126.

Alfredson, H., Lorentzon, M., Bäckman, S., Bäckman, A. & Lerner, U.H. (2003) cDNA-arrays and real-time quantitative PCR techniques in the investigation of chronic Achilles tendinosis. *Journal of Orthopaedic Research* **21**, 970–975.

Alfredson, H., Öhberg, L. & Forsgren, S. (2003) Is vasculo-neural ingrowth the cause of pain in chronic Achilles tendinosis? An investigation using ultrasonogrphy and colour Doppler, immunohistochemistry, and diagnostic injections. *Knee Surgery, Sports Traumatology, Arthroscopy* **11**, 334–338.

Alfredson, H., Pietilä, T., Jonsson, P. & Lorentzon, R. (1998b) Heavy-load eccentric calf muscle training for the treatment of chronic Achilles tendinosis. *American Journal of Sports Medicine* **26**, 360–366.

Alfredson, H., Pietilä, T. & Lorentzon, R. (1996) Chronic Achilles tendinitis and calf muscle strength. *American Journal of Sports Medicine* **24**, 829–833.

Alfredson, H., Pietilä, T., Öhberg, L. & Lorentzon, R. (1998a) Achilles tendinosis and calf muscle strength. The effect of short-term immobilization after surgical treatment. *American Journal of Sports Medicine* 26, 166–171.

Alfredson, H., Thorsen, K. & Lorentzon, R. (1999) *In situ* microdialysis in tendon tissue: high levels of glutamate, but not prostaglandin E_2 in chronic Achilles tendon pain. *Knee Surgery, Sports Traumatology, Arthroscopy* 7, 378–381.

Appel, H-J. (1986) Skeletal muscle atrophy during immobilization. *International Journal of Sports Medicine* 7, 1–5.

Archambault, J.M., Wiley, P. & Bray, R.C. (1995) Exercise loading of tendons and the development of overuse injuries. A review. *Sports Medicine* 20, 77–89.

Åström, M. (1997) On the nature and etiology of chronic Achilles tendinopathy [dissertation]. University of Lund, Lund.

Åström, M. (1998) Partial rupture in chronic Achilles tendinopathy: A retrospective analysis of 342 cases. *Acta Orthopaedica Scandinavica* 69, 404–407.

Åström, M. & Westlin, N. (1992) No effect of piroxicam on Achilles tendinopathy. A randomized study of 70 patients. *Acta Orthopaedica Scandinavica* 63, 631–634.

Bjur, D., Alfredson, H. & Forsgren, S. (2005) The innervation pattern of the human Achilles tendon studies on the normal and tendinosis tendon using markers for general, sensory and sympathetic innervations. *Cell Tissue Research* 320, 201–206.

Boushel, R., Langberg, H., Green, S., Skovgaard, D., Bulow, J. & Kjaer, M. (2000) Blood flow and oxygenation in peritendinous tissue and calf muscle during dynamic exercise in humans. *Journal of Physiology* 525, 305–313.

Brody, D.M. (1987) Running injuries. Prevention and management. *Clinical Symposia* 39, 1–36.

Clement, D.B., Taunton, J.E. & Smart, G.W. (1984) Achilles tendinitis and peritendinitis: etiology and treatment. *American Journal of Sports Medicine* 12, 179–184.

Coggeshall, R.E. & Carlton, S.M. (1998) Ultrastructural analysis of NMDA, AMPA and kainate receptors on unmyelinated and myelinated axons in the perifery. *Journal of Comparative Neurology* 391, 78–86.

Conrad, P., Malouf, G.M. & Stacey, M.C. (1995) The Australian polidocanol (aethoxysklerol) study. Results at 2 years. *Dermatological Surgery* 21, 334–336.

Curvin, S. & Stanish, W.D. (1984) *Tendinitis: its Etiology and Treatment.* Collamore Press, Lexington, DC.

Darimont, C., Vassaux, G., Gaillard, D., Ailhaud, G. & Négrel, R. (1994) *In situ* microdialysis of prostaglandins in adipose tissue: stimulation of prostacyclin release by angiotensin II. *International Journal of Obesity* 18, 783–788.

Davidson, E.M., Coggeshall, R.E. & Carlton, S.M. (1997) Peripheral NMDA and non-NMDA glutamate receptors contribute to nociceptive behaviors in the rat formalin test. *Neuroreport* 8, 941–946.

Denstad, T.F. & Roaas, A. (1979) Surgical treatment of partial Achilles tendon ruptures. *American Journal of Sports Medicine* 7, 15–17.

Dickenson, A.H., Chapman, V. & Green, G.M. (1997) The pharmacology of excitatory and inhibitory amino acid-mediated events in the transmission and modulation of pain in the spinal cord. A review. *General Pharmacology* 28, 633–638.

Forsgren, S., Danielsson, P. & Alfredson, H. (2005) Vascular NK-1R receptor occurrence in normal and chronic painful Achilles and patellar tendons. Studies on chemically unfixed as well as fixed specimens. *Regular Peptides* 126, 173–181.

Galloway, M.T., Jokl, P. & Dayton, O.W. (1992) Achilles tendon overuse injuries. *Clinical Sports Medicine* 11, 771–782.

Guex, J.J. (1993) Indications for the sclerosing agent polidocanol. *Journal of Dermatological Surgery and Oncology* 19, 959–961.

Hess, G.P., Capiello, W.L. & Poole, R.M. (1989) Prevention and treatment of overuse tendon injuries. *Sports Medicine* 8, 371–384.

Ireland, D., Harrall, R., Curry, V., Holloway, G., Hackney, R. & Hazleman, B. (2001) Multiple changes in gene expression in chronic human Achilles tendinopathy. *Matrix Biology* 20, 159–169.

James, S.L. & Bates, B.T. (1978) Osternig LR. Injuries to runners. *American Journal of Sports Medicine* 6, 40–50.

Järvinen, M., Józsa, L., Kannus, P., Järvinen, T.L.N., Kvist, M. & Leadbetter, W. (1997) Histopathological findings in chronic tendon disorders. *Scandinavian Journal of Medicine and Science in Sports* 7, 86–95.

Jörgensen, U., Ekstrand, J. (1988) Significance of heel pad confinement for the shock absorption at heel strike.

International Journal of Sports Medicine 9, 468–473.

Kannus, P. & Józsa, L. (1997) *Human Tendons: Anatomy, Physiology and Pathology.* Human Kinetics, New York.

Khan, K.M., Cook, J.L., Bonar, F., Harcourt, P. & Åström, M. (1999) Histopathology of common tendinopathies. Update and implications for clinical management. *Sports Medicine* 27, 393–408.

Kjaer, M., Langberg, H., Miller, B.F., *et al.* (2005) Metabolic activity and collagen turnover in human tendon in response to physical activity. *Journal of Musculoskeletal Neuronal Interactions* 5, 41–52.

Kvist, M. (1991) Achilles tendon injuries in athletes. *Annual Chirurgica Gynaecologica* 80, 188–201.

Kvist, M. (1994) Achilles tendon injuries in athletes. *Sports Medicine* 18, 173–201.

Leadbetter, W.B. (1995) Anti-inflammatory therapy and sports injury: The role of non-steroidal drugs and corticosteroid injection. *Clinical Sports Medicine* 14, 353–410.

Leadbetter, W.B., Mooar, P.A. & Lane, G.J. (1992) The surgical treatment of tendinitis. Clinical rationale and biologic basis. *Clinical Sports Medicine* 11, 679–712.

Leppilahti, J., Orava, S., Karpakka, J. & Takala, T. (1991) Overuse injuries of the Achilles tendon. *Annual Chirurgica Gynaecologica* 80, 202–207.

Ljungqvist, R. (1968) Subcutaneous partial rupture of the Axhilles tendon. *Acta Orthopaedica Scandinavica Supplement* 113, 1–86.

Maffuli, N., Testa, V., Capasso, G., Bifulco, G. & Binfield, P. (1997) Results of percutaneous longitudinal tenotomy for Achilles tendinopathy in middle- and long-distance runners. *American Journal of Sports Medicine* 25, 835–840.

Mafi, N., Lorentzon, R. & Alfredson, H. (2001) Superior results with eccentric calf-muscle training compared to concentric training in a randomized prospective multi-center study on patients with chronic Achilles tendinosis. *Knee Surgery, Sports Traumatology, Arthroscopy* 9, 42–47.

Morberg, P., Jerre, R., Swärd, L. & Karlsoon, J. (1997) Long-term results after surgical management of partial Achilles tendon ruptures. *Scandinavian Journal of Medicine and Science in Sports* 7, 299–303.

Movin, T. (1998) Aspects of aetiology, pathoanatomy and diagnostic methods in chronic mid-portion Achillodynia [dissertation]. Karolinska Institute Stockholm, Stockholm.

Movin, T., Gad, A. & Reinholt, F.P. (1997) Tendon pathology in long-standing Achillodynia. Biopsy findings in 40 patients. *Acta Orthopadica Scandinavica* **68**, 170–175.

Myerson, M.S. & McGarvey, W. (1999) Disorders of the insertion of the Achilles tendon and Achilles tendinitis. American Academy of Orthopaedic Surgeons. *Instructional Course Lectures* **48**, 1814–1824.

Nelen, G., Martens, M. & Burssens, A. (1989) Surgical treatment of chronic Achilles tendinitis. *American Journal of Sports Medicine* **17**, 754–759.

Nichols, A.W. (1989) Achilles tendinitis in running athletes. *Journal of the American Board of Family Practice* **2**, 196–203.

Nicol, C., Komi, P.V. & Marconnet, F. (1991) Fatigue effects of marathon running on neuromuscular performance. II: Changes in force, integrated electromyographic activity and endurance capacity. *Scandinavian Journal of Medicine and Science in Sports* **1**, 10–17.

Öhberg, L. & Alfredson, H. (2002) Ultrasound guided sclerosis of neovessels in painful chronic Achilles tendinosis: pilot study of a new treatment. *British Journal of Sports Medicine* **36**, 173–177.

Öhberg, L. & Alfredson, H. (2003) Sclerosing therapy in chronic Achilles tendon insertional pain-results of a pilot study. *Knee Surgery, Sports Traumatology, Arthroscopy* **11**, 339–343.

Öhberg, L. & Alfredson, H. (2004) Effects on neovascularization behind the good results with eccentric training in chronic mid-portion Achilles tendinosis. *Knee Surgery, Sports Traumatology, Arthroscopy* **12**, 465–470.

Öhberg, L., Lorentzon, R. & Alfredson, H. (2001) Neovascularization in Achilles tendons with painful tendinosis but not in normal tendons: an ultrasonographic investigation. *Knee Surgery, Sports Traumatology, Arthroscopy* **9**, 233–238.

Öhberg, L., Lorentzon, R. & Alfredson, H. (2004) Eccentric training in patients with chronic Achilles tendinosis: normalized tendon structure and decreased thickness at follow-up. *British Journal of Sports Medicine* **38**, 8–11.

Puddu, G., Ippolito, E. & Postacchini, F. (1976) A classification of Achilles tendon disease. *American Journal of Sports Medicine* **4**, 146–150.

Renström, P.A.F.H. (1988) Diagnosis and management of overuse injuries. In: *The Olympic Book of Sports Medicine* (Dirix A., Knuttgen H.G., Tiitel K., eds.) Vol. 1. Blackwell Scientific Publications, Oxford: 446–468.

Saltzman, C.L. & Tearse, D.S. (1998) Achilles tendon injuries. *Journal of American Academy Orthopaedic Surgery* **6**, 316–325.

Sandmeier, R. & Renström, P.A.F.H. (1997) Diagnosis and treatment of chronic tendon disorders in sports. *Scandinavian Journal of Medicine and Science in Sports* **7**, 96–106.

Schepsis, A.A. & Leach, R.E. (1987) Surgical treatment of Achilles tendinitis. *American Journal of Sports Medicine* **15**, 308–315.

Schrier, I., Matheson, G.O. & Kohl, H.W. III (1996) Achilles tendonitis: Are corticosteroid injections useful or harmful? *Clinical Journal of Sports Medicine* **6**, 245–250.

Solomon, L.M., Juhlin, L. & Kirchenbaum, M.B. (1968) Prostaglandins on cutaneous vasculature. *Journal of Investigation Dermatology* **51**, 280–282.

Teitz, C.C., Garrett, W.E. Jr. & Miniaci, A. (1997) Tendon problems in athletic individuals. *Journal of Bone and Joint Surgery. American volume* **79**, 138–152.

Thorsen, K., Kristoffersson, A.O., Lerner, U.H. & Lorentzon, R.P. (1996) *In situ* microdialysis in bone tissue. Stimulation of prostaglandin E_2 release by weight-bearing mechanical loading. *Journal of Clinical Investigation* **98**, 2446–2449.

Vega, M.R., Cavolo, D.J., Green, R.M. & Cohen, R.S. (1984) Haglund's deformity. *Journal of American Podiatry Association* **74**, 129–135.

Wallin, D., Ekblom, B. & Grahn, R. (1985) Improvement of muscle flexibility. A comparison between two techniques. *American Journal of Sports Medicine* **13**, 263–268.

Weiler, J.M. (1992) Medical modifiers of sports injury. The use of nonsteroidal anti-inflammatory drugs (NSAIDs) in sports soft-tissue injury. *Clinical Sports Medicine* **11**, 625–644.

Welsh, R.P. & Clodman, J. (1980) Clinical survey of Achilles tendinitis in athletes. *Canadian Medical Association Journal* **122**, 193–195.

Williams, J.G.P. (1986) Achilles tendon lesions in sport. *Sports Medicine* **3**, 114–135.

Winter, H., Drager, E. & Sterry, W. (2000) Sclerotherapy for treatment of hemangiomas. *Dermatological Surgery* **26**, 105–108.

Chapter 13

Hindfoot Tendinopathies in Athletes

FRANCESCO BENAZZO, MARIO MOSCONI, ALBERTO PIO, AND FRANCO
COMBI

Tendinopathies in the hindfoot are a major issue in
sport traumatology because of the biomechanical
importance of this region in the basic actions of
running, jumping, and walking. Various factors are
involved in the pathogenesis of tendon dysfunctions,
most of these are either mechanical (as a result of
athletic activities) or anatomic (ligamentous laxity,
articular hypermobilities, or bony abnormalities).
The structures involved include the Achilles,
peroneal tendons, tibialis posterior, flexor hallucis
longus tendons, and the plantaris fascia. Some of
these structures are tightly connected. This connection can be anatomic as in medial retromalleolar
syndrome, which involves the structures passing
through the bony fibrous tunnel posterior to the
medial malleolus (tibialis posterior tendon and
nerve, and flexor hallucis longus tendon). The connection can also be biomechanical if the pathogenetic role of failure of the plantaris fascia and
tibialis posterior tendon (the main static and
dynamic supports of the of longitudinal plantaris
arch) in traction injury of posterior tibial nerve is
considered. Anatomicopathologic lesions can be
inflammatory or degenerative in any area, leading
to different clinical patterns (peritendinitis, tendinosis, micro-tears, insertional tendinopathies, and
association of inflammatory and degenerative features). In addition, acute and chronic changes can
be seen. The aim of this chapter is to recognize
pathogenetic and clinical patterns of injury in this
anatomic region in order to result in a correct diagnosis. Accuracy in the diagnosis and detection of
anatomicopathologic patterns of the lesion is mandatory for both conservative and surgical treatment.

Introduction

The anatomic region referred to as the "hindfoot"
presents many different pathologies in athletes,
mainly resulting from functional overload and
less frequently from macro-traumas. The overload
pathologies of the hindfoot have been enlisted in
the so-called posterior carrefour syndrome (PCS)
(Ledoux & Morvan 1991). The syndrome includes
pathologies of bony, tendinous, capsular, and nervous structures:

- posterior portion of the talus (tuberculum, os
trigonum);
- posterior malleolus;
- posterior portion of the calcaneus;
- Achilles tendon;
- peroneal tendons
(longus and brevis); ⎫
- tibialis posterior tendon   being part of the
and/or nerve;   so-called medial
- flexor digitorum and flexor   retromalleolar
hallucis tendons;   syndrome
- plantar fascia. ⎭

  In this chapter, we take into consideration the
tendinopathies of this region, exposing the actual
knowledge, and look at the further developments of
research needed in this field.

Functional anatomy, biomechanics, and pathogenesis of the hindfoot

From the functional point of view, the hindfoot can
be ideally defined by a coronal plane passing through
the neck of the talus (Fig. 13.1): all the structures

184

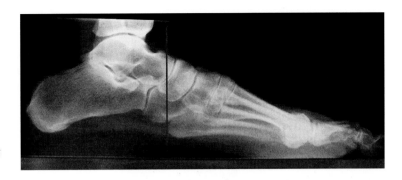

Fig. 13.1 The line indicates the coronal plane in the foot. The structures to the left of the plane can be considered the posterior region of the foot.

lying behind this plane can be considered part of the posterior region of the foot. The posterior portion of the subfascial layer contains the Achilles tendon and the specialized insertional area with its bursae. The peroneal tendons, longus and brevis, are located laterally, while the flexor tendons (tibialis posterior, hallucis longus, and digitorum longus) are placed medially. The plantar fascia is below and always contained by the prolongation of the crural fascia onto the calcaneal body. Notwithstanding, the medial and lateral tendons also run beyond these limits and will be considered as a whole. The rearfoot cannot be regarded as an isolated structure from the point of view of functional anatomy but must be considered as a whole with the leg, the midfoot, and forefoot.

The function of the foot is to absorb impact at the time of initial ground contact and to provide a rigid lever for toe off. All of these functions occur because of the ability of the rearfoot (ankle and subtalar joint) to transmit and translate the vertical and rotational forces passing through it.

Ankle joint

The talocrural joint is peculiar because the troclea is wider anteriorly than posteriorly. The concave distal tibial articular surface closely fits the talar troclea. Seventy percent of the rotation about the vertical axis is restricted by soft tissue constraints and 30% by the shape of the joint. The main function of the talocrural joint is the execution of dorsolateral flexion. In the early studies, it was seen as a pure hinge joint with an axis assumed to be fixed in the frontal plane (Inman 1976). However, Barnett and Napier (1965) noticed the tendency of the joint axis

to change inclination close to neutral position between plantar and dorsiflexion. On the contrary, the latest analysis (Langelaan 1983; Lundberg 1988) suggests that the ankle joint bears some resemblance to an ellipsoid joint with two degrees of freedom due to the variation of the rotational axis. The range of motion of the ankle joint varies from 13° to 33° of dorsiflexion and from 23° to 56° of plantar flexion.

Subtalar joint

The subtalar joint is formed by the inferior surface of the talus and the superior surface of the calcaneus. It is believed that its axis of motion passes from the dorsomedial face of the navicular bone and exits from the lateral plantar face of the calcaneus (Inman 1976). The motion that occurs in the subtalar joint consists of inversion, which is the movement of the calcaneus medially, and eversion, which is the deviation of the calcaneus laterally. The extent of this motion has been quantified to be 6° during level walking in the normal foot, 5° of movement in the sense of inversion–eversion, and 9° in flatfooted individuals (Wright et al. 1964) (Fig. 13.2).

The associated motion of the ankle–subtalar joint has been likened to that of a universal joint (Inman 1976). The importance of this analogy lies in the fact the degree of inclination of the axis of the two joints are intermittently related. This interrelationship permits compensation between the joints, while failure of this compensatory mechanism results in increased stress on the adjacent joints and structures such as tendons. Many studies (Langelaan 1983; Lundberg 1988) suggest that the motion in the rearfoot between the talus and the calcaneus can be

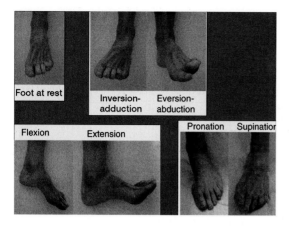

Fig. 13.2 Motions of the foot.

represented by means of a cone-shaped bundle of discrete axes representing the successive positions of a moving axis. This conditions even the function of the muscles crossing the two joints. The movements of the rearfoot is determined by six muscles that possess a stable moment arm during the coupled motion of the two joints (Klein *et al.* 1999). This is associated with the behavior of the triceps surae, which holds an inversion moment arm in eversion and the reverse with rearfoot inversion (Klein *et al.* 1999). This feature suggests a switch of joint axis to the opposite site of the line of action of this muscle.

The tibialis posterior is also the muscle with the wider moment arm at the subtalar joint in order to counteract the body weight and should be considered the major muscle maintaining the arch of the foot. Therefore, it is involved in every movement of the rearfoot, and can be easily overloaded on its tendinous end.

From the functional point of view, all muscles whose tendons run in this region have a role in the stance phase and in the toe-off phase. The muscles contract in the first phase of contact as soon as the forefoot touches the ground; primarily, the tibialis posterior but also the flexor tendons counteract against the subtalar pronation and the internal rotation of the leg according to a myotactic reflex which begins 25–35 ms after the initial contact (Novacheck 1994). The contraction is mainly eccentric in this phase. Any condition decreasing the efficiency of these muscles, such as fatigue or ligament failure, may cause an increased pronation with possible overload of all the tendons of the subtalar joint (Root *et al.* 1977) and the plantar fascia. Immediately after the stance phase, the muscles of the calf (triceps surae including the tibialis posterior) contract and shorten isotonically to provide the push off phase. The contraction is mainly concentric in this phase.

The peroneal tendons work differently. The brevis tendon acts by everting the foot, while the longus tendon everts the foot and lowers the first metatarsal bone. Therefore, they work in the swing phase of running, after the push off of the foot.

The presence of the os trigonum, which is an accessory center of ossification of the talus (Turner 1882) and not a fracture of the posterolateral tubercle (Shepard 1882) or of a hypertrophied tubercle, can be the cause of an impingement with the tibialis posterior and/or flexor tendons themselves with a consequent degenerative pathology of these tendons. These syndromes are mainly the result of jumping activities, but have also been seen in athletes who participate in hurdle events (110 m, 400 m, and steeplechase), when the foot hits the ground in equinism in a forced plantar flexion with eccentric contraction of the calf muscles. It then extends dorsally in the stance phase and returns immediately to equine position in the toe-off phase. It is possible that an excessive dorsiflexion after impact descending from the hurdle (and this is repeated many times in each training session and competition) can cause a sudden strain in the os trigonum via the bifurcate ligament but above all in the tendons (Achilles insertion, peroneal, or tibialis posterior). An excessive pronation (either real, or functional resulting from muscle exertion) can increase the contact time with the ground, decrease the buffering action of the myotendinous unit, and consequently place a high level of strain on tendons.

The jumping mechanism is another example of how overload of the hindfoot can be initiated. In the high jump event there are two phases that can damage the hindfoot: the run-up in the final phase and the take-off phase. The purpose of the run-up is to enable the athlete to gain enough linear speed to be transformed into vertical translation of his or her center of gravity. The length of the run-up is usually 9–13 steps. In the first three-quarters of the run-up, the athlete's position is perpendicular to the axis of the bar, while during the last 3–4 steps of accelera-

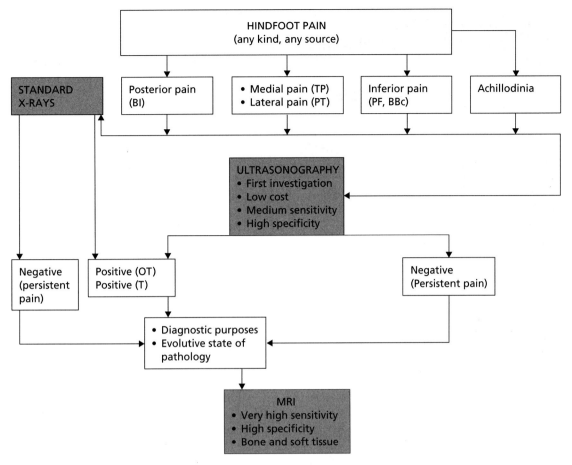

Fig. 13.3 Algorithm of diagnosis of the hindfoot pain. Ultrasounds are able to diagnose the soft tissue derangement, but in athletes the investigation must be completed with magnetic resonance imaging (MRI), which is able to rule out the bone involvement. BBc, bone bruise calcaneus; BI, bony impingement; OT, os trigonum; PF, plantar fasciitis; PT, peroneal tendons; T, tendons; TP, tibialis posterior.

tion the athlete runs parallel to the bar. In this phase, the athlete's chest must bend inwards to the curve so he or she can gain centrifugal power, and while the foot of the push-off leg maintains contact with the inner portion, the foot of the take-off leg stays in contact with the lateral border so there is increased supination on ground contact. Errors in performing this phase can lead to lesions of the hindfoot. If the rhythm of acceleration is limited to the final last 2 run-up steps instead of the last 3–4, there is an excessive abrupt pronation of the take-off foot, with the possible consequence of excessive strain to the tibialis posterior tendon at the insertion and along the pulley, excessive twisting of the Achilles tendon and strain at the junctions, and strain at the insertion and along the pulley of the peroneus longus. A high level of strain can also be reached during the recovery phase of this abnormal pronation.

If excessive lowering of the center of gravity occurs, the limb is pushed too far forward in the last step, resulting in increased plantar flexion of the ankle with bony impingement of the posterior talus. In the take-off phase, the contact time should be as brief as possible. If the starting position is an excessive pronation, strain applied to the tendons can be high. A high number of injuries are caused by any one of these mechanisms. The diagnostic algorithm for hindfoot pain is shown in Fig. 13.3.

Peroneal tendon pathology

Peroneal tendon pathology has been neglected because these tendons are often damaged by an ankle sprain in up to 50% of cases (Alanen *et al.* 2001), which represents the most evident source of pain and is therefore treated first. For the same reason, epidemiologic data can be biased by a late or failed diagnosis. Fallat *et al.* (1998) stated that in ankle sprains, "frequently other structures are also injured." In a series of 639 consecutive patients, the peroneal tendons were involved in 83 cases and the Achilles in 67 cases. However, with the wide use of magnetic resonance imaging (MRI), damaged tendons or sheaths can be easily diagnosed, even if asymptomatic.

From the anatomic point of view, the peroneal tendons (longus and brevis) originate from the corresponding muscles attached to the upper portion of the fibula, run posterior to the lateral malleolus, and are contained by the superior and inferior retinaculae within the fibular groove and the lateral surface of the calcaneus. The peroneus brevis inserts in the base of the fifth metatarsal, while the longus (passing deep to the brevis) inserts medially at the base of the first metatarsal and of the first cuneiform. Therefore, they have quite different functions. The brevis is responsible for eversion of the foot while the longus is responsible for depression of the first metatarsal together with eversion of the foot.

Anatomic factors such as the presence of three fixed pulleys are involved in the pathogenesis of tendon dysfunction. These factors include the location posterior to the lateral malleolus in the peroneal sulcus (brevis), the peroneal throclea of the calcaneus where the peroneal longus runs, and the inferior edge of the cuboid bone (longus). Mechanical factors involved include lateral malleolar fractures, calcaneal fractures, and peroneal osteosynthesis with plate and screws.

The peroneal tendinopathies can be classified as follows:
• Acute tenosynovitis (but more often chronic and therefore stenosing);
• Chronic tenosynovitis with tendon degeneration;
• Partial ruptures (longitudinal split—often associated with and/or consequence of an ankle sprain);

• Total ruptures;
• Subluxation/luxation conditions (often associated with tenosynovitis, and involves partial splits more often then a total rupture of the tendons) (Gunn 1959; Sobel *et al.* 1990); and
• Accessory muscle belly (simulating and/or causing tendon pathology).

Tenosynovitis is rare in the general population but occurs quite frequently in athletes and dancers as a consequence of an iterative overload resulting from the friction against bony surfaces and within fibrous retinaculae. Stenosis can occur in the areas mentioned above. Furthermore, trauma causing fractures of the lateral malleolus and/or calcaneus, osteosynthesis with plates and screws of the fibula, may cause or exacerbate an increased friction with unavoidable inflammation of the sheaths. Chronic inflammation is accompanied by tendon degeneration, and at that stage a minor ankle injury can cause splitting of the tendon(s). From the objective point of view, pain and tenderness are caused by palpation behind and below the malleolus, with edema and local swelling, and by active maneuvers such as forced inversion, adduction and plantar flexion, or active eversion against resistance especially starting from an inverted position.

Partial rupture of the tendon(s) (both longus and brevis) is frequently associated with or caused by a chronic ankle laxity (Bonnin *et al.* 1997). A longitudinal split of the tendon is often associated with an ankle sprain. Pain is exacerbated by local palpation and by the maneuvers listed above, which reveals an enlarged tendon. Total rupture is very rare and occurs more frequently in rheumatoid patients than in athletes. The diagnosis of partial rupture can be easily carried out with axial MRI, while sonography can reveal the amount of peritendinous swelling.

While the incidence of peroneal tendon instability is quite high when compared with the other pathologies described, it can be the initiating moment of inflammations and splits. Subluxation or full dislocation occurs when the inverted foot is forcefully dorsiflexed with simultaneous contraction of the peroneal muscles, causing a tear of the superior retinaculum or a periosteum avulsion. This maneuver can happen when the tip of the ski is caught in the snow, the skier falls forward, the foot is inverted, and the peroneal muscles contract forcefully. The superior retinaculum strips the periosteum out from the bone, and the tendon dislocates.

The treatment of such peroneal tendon pathology can be differentiated. Conservative treatment of tenosynovitis consists of reduction of activity, non-steroidal anti-inflammatory drugs (NSAIDs), orthotics with lateral wedge, and casting to prevent weight bearing. However, local steroid injections must be avoided because they have little or no benefit and may be dangerous for tendon integrity. On the other hand, these treatments may not be successful if the main cause of pathology is stenosis. In this situation, surgery with ablation of the inflamed and thickened sheaths is mandatory, as well as careful reconstruction of the retinaculae.

If instability is the cause of dislocation, 50% of patients treated conservatively tend to have chronic redislocation of the tendons (Ferran *et al.* 2006), while acute surgical repair has a 75% success rate (Safran *et al.* 1999). The subluxation can be left untreated as long as no secondary tendinopathies occur. In chronic dislocations, many different procedures have been described including bone block procedures, creation of an Achilles sling, transferring the tendons under the calcaneofibular ligament, fibular grooving, and reefing of the superior peroneal retinaculum.

Medial retromalleolar syndrome

The bony fibrous tunnel beside the medial malleolus contains vascular, nervous, and tendinous structures that can be compressed as the tunnel is inextensible. Symptoms resulting from dysfunction of these structures are closely connected from an anatomic point of view and their pathologies are often difficult to distinguish clinically. As a result, a syndrome resulting from a combination of tibialis posterior dysfunction, plantar fascitis, and tarsal tunnel syndrome has been recently described. Failure of the main static (plantar fascia) and dynamic (posterior tibialis tendon) supports of the longitudinal arch of the foot has resulted in traction injury to the posterior tibial nerve (i.e. tarsal tunnel syndrome). This syndrome has also been called heel pain triad

(HPT) (Labib *et al.* 2002). Accuracy in clinical assessment and radiology is mandatory in order to identify the structures involved and plan treatment.

Tibialis posterior pathology

Tibialis posterior pathologies and valgus flatfoot pronation deformities are closely related. Repeated excessive pronation, such as that found in runners, leads to tibialis posterior overuse syndrome. On the other hand, tibialis posterior dysfunction results in eversion of the hindfoot and fall of the medial longitudinal plantar arch resulting in a pronated valgus flatfoot. Consequently, posterior tibialis pathology (including tenosynovitis, chronic degeneration, rupture) is mainly based upon this kind of dysfunction.

The tibialis posterior arises from the posterior surface of proximal tibia and fibula and inserts on the inferomedial face of navicula and the inferior face of cuneiform bones as well as occasionally on the II, III, and IV metatarsals. It is the most anterior structure under flexor retinaculum beneath the medial malleolus and just 4 cm distally before the navicula insertion, as well as the less vascularized zone of the tendon (Frey *et al.* 1990). The tibialis posterior tendon is the main dynamic foot stabilizer against eversion and the main dynamic support of the longitudinal arch. Its action inverts the midfoot and locks the talonavicular and the calcaneocuboid joints (transverse tarsal joints).

Therefore it is clear that dysfunction of the tibialis posterior is the most important cause of painful acquired flatfoot in adulthood (Johnson & Strom 1989; Mosier *et al.* 1999; Geidemann & Johnson 2000). Dysfunction develops progressively together with the collapse of the medial longitudinal arch, valgus hindfoot, and forefoot deformities (forefoot abduction demonstrated by the "too many toes sign").

At the time of surgery, many anatomicopathologic patterns can be found, such as acute tenosynovitis of inflammatory origin, as well as a true degenerative tendinosis. In particular, degeneration changes lead to a non-specific response to tissue injury showing fibroblast hypercellularity, chondroid metaplasia, mucinous degeneration, and neovascularization (Mosier *et al.* 1999). Collagen bundle structure and orientation are therefore disrupted and the tendon compromised and predisposed to rupture under physiologic loads.

Numerous factors have been proposed to explain the pathophysiology of posterior tibialis tendon dysfunction. Mechanical factors include ligamentous laxity, articular hypermobility, shallow retromalleolar groove, tight flexor retinaculum, and navicular bone abnormalities (accessory navicula, prominent navicular tubercle) (Cozen 1965; Langeskiold 1967). The action of tendons around the ankle seems to have an important role in progression of posterior tibialis tendon pathology. As the medial arch falls, the unopposed action of peroneus brevis pulls the hindfoot in valgus. As a result, actions of the Achilles tendon and the tibialis anterior become eccentric and misdirected, consequently amplifying the deformity. Meanwhile, the peroneus longus pulls the forefoot in abduction.

Ischemic factors include the zone of hypovascularity immediately posterior to medial malleolus due to normal anatomy and/or traumatic factors. In the physical examination for posterior tibialis tendon dysfunction, the examiner looks for an insufficiency of this tendon. The patient is evaluated seated and weight bearing. In the standing position, the examiner looks for flatfoot, valgus hindfoot, and abduction of the forefoot. An unilateral flatfoot is appreciated with loss of longitudinal medial arch as well as fullness in the posteromedial aspect of the ankle. When examining the limb from the back, a valgus hindfoot is evident and a great number of lateral toes can be seen because of the abduction of of the forefoot ("too many toes sign").

A dynamic test must be performed to show if the patient is able to do a double heel-rise test or a single heel-rise test. Subtle signs of tibialis posterior dysfunction are detectable by asking the patient to perform a repetitive heel-rise test. During this test it is very important to check the position of the calcaneum. In the normal foot it is inverted, whereas in the presence of tibialis posterior dysfunction the hindfoot remains neutral or valgus and asymmetric to the unaffected limb. In the sitting position, edema and tenderness of posteromedial aspect of the ankle, around the posterior tibialis tendon or

at its insertion on the navicular bone are found. Flexion and inversion of the hindfoot against resistance are assessed and compared with unaffected limb. Range of motion of the ankle, hindfoot, and midfoot must be assessed. Mobility of the subtalar joint can be markedly limited and an Achilles tendon retraction can be associated (see also the pathogenesis of Achilles tendinopathy). In further steps of disease, when valgus deformity is fixed, failure of the deltoid ligament and degeneration of the lateral side of the ankle could be present. At this time, a supination deformity of the forefoot can occur, in order to keep the foot plantigrade in presence of a fixed valgus hindfoot.

There are no laboratory tests helpful in diagnosing posterior tibialis tendon dysfunction if it is not secondary to a systemic disease. Ultrasound and MRI are normally used in radiologic assessment to provide information about the extent of disease and the degree of tendon pathology. More precisely, ultrasound positively identifies peritendinitis and tendinosis, but has more difficulty with partial tears of the posterior tibialis tendon. MRI is a more sensitive test than either clinical or ultrasound evaluation for diagnosis of a posterior tibialis tendon tear.

Ultrasound and MRI are the preferred diagnostic tools for monitoring tendon pathology in athletes, while diagnosis of posterior tibialis tendon dysfunction in older patients can be formulated on X-ray (Myerson 1997). The radiographic features that must be noted in the anteroposterior view include partial uncovering of talar head, increased talus-I metatarsal angle, and divergence of the talus-calcaneus. In the lateral view, it is important to note flattening of longitudinal arch, increased talus-I metatarsal angle, divergence of the talus-calcaneus and sag in the talonavicular, naviculo-cuneiform, or tarsometatarsal joints. While different clinical forms can be described, most of them could be considered as different steps of the same pathology.

Acute and chronic tenosynovitis

In acute and chronic tenosynovitis, the synovium surrounding the tendon can be redundant and edematous while the tendon tissue itself is minimally or not involved. Generally, symptom onset is gradual and relatively non-specific, but may include symptoms of tibialis posterior tendon dysfunction, pain that is worsened by prolonged weight bearing, and deambulation. Pain is also elicited by retro-malleolar compression, passive eversion, and abduction, as well as active inversion and adduction. Local swelling is often present, particularly in the postero-inferior portion of the retromalleolar sulcus. Rarely, in chronic forms, intratendinous calcifications can be found on ultrasound or MRI, but cannot be detected clinically. The involvement of tendineous tissue is thought to lead to rupture of the tendon passing through the classic pathway of inflammation, degeneration, partial tears, and rupture.

Partial and complete closed rupture

Posterior tibialis tendon rupture is often missed in sports-related injuries. Unlike the Achilles tendon, ruptures of this tendon are relatively uncommon in sport traumatology. Partial tears are more frequently found in young athletes whereas total ruptures are more typical of middle-aged or former athletes (Porter *et al.* 1998). In the zone where the tendon wraps around the medial malleolus, histologic structure changes from dense connective tissue to fibrocartilaginous tissue. This transformation is probably caused, according to the biomechanics of this area, by compressive and shear stresses that act around this pulley, which determine the amount and the quality of the cells and of the extracellular matrix. In addition, the fibrocartilage is avascularized and relatively more vulnerable to tensile forces. For these reasons, degenerative changes and ruptures of tendon are relatively frequent in this region. From a clinical point of view, however, the diagnosis can be difficult.

History of a twisting ankle injury, especially in the setting of high-impact loading, is frequent. The patient presents with a pronated forefoot and an asymmetric flatfoot, which is more pronounced on the affected side. Pain and swelling are generalized on the medial side of the ankle, the function of tibialis posterior is absent at the manual test, and the patient is usually unable to perform single leg heel rise. Clinical signs of tendon failure are absent but local pain and swelling, pain revealed with forced eversion and inversion against resistance, and an enlarged tendon can lead to diagnosis.

Avulsion of accessory navicular or degeneration of the accessory navicular synchondrosis

In middle-aged patients, avulsion of the accessory navicula and of tendon can be seen as well as partial or total separation through the synchondrosis (Chen *et al.* 1997). We have had experience of this partial detachment in soccer players. The clinical signs and symptoms of a partial detachment are the same as total rupture. Treatment of tenosynovitis of tibialis posterior is with rest, NSAIDs, and orthotics with a longitudinal arch support, which avoids eversion. When the main cause of this pathology is friction or stenosis, surgery is the treatment of choice and involves removal of the thickened inflamed sheets, longitudinal incisions of the tendon, and reconstruction of retinaculum. For total rupture and avulsion of the tendon, surgical treatment is mandatory.

Plantar fasciitis

Plantar fasciitis does not affect a tendon but rather an aponeurotic fascia. It is very similar to insertional tendinopathies. Plantar fascia starts proximally as a fibrous band of thick, dense connective tissue from the anterior calcaneal tuberosity. Distally, it becomes wider and thinner, and, close to metatarsal heads, it divides into five processes, one for each toe. The function of this fascia is to maintain the longitudinal arch with its tension, improving the pushing power during running and jumping. Excessive and iterative strain of the fascia for higher speeds, longer distances, or stronger jumps are the cause of micro-tears and the inflammatory process on the insertional portion of the fascia near the calcaneum. Calcifications, often found at the insertion in asymptomatic adult patients, can be the result of either periosteum irritation (Doxey 1987) or of bleeding resulting from micro-tears (Warren 1990).

Etiologic factors involved in plantar fascia pathology in athletes can include anatomic as well as mechanical factors. Anatomic factors can include flatfoot or pes cavus as well as a short Achilles tendon. Mechanical factors include overtraining, excessive pronation, calf tightness, hard surface, or shoes with a tender or worn-out sole. However, the most important risk factor in the pathophysiology of plantar fasciitis seems to be the range of ankle dorsiflexion. In fact, risk of plantar fasciitis increases as the ankle dorsiflexion decreases (Riddle *et al.* 2003). Other important risk factors are the amount of time spent weight bearing and being overweight. Recent studies have shown that patients with plantar fasciitis respond with a gait adjustment with reduced force beneath the rear foot and the forefoot. Furthermore, digital function has been seen to have an important role as a protective factor in plantar fasciitis (Wearing *et al.* 2003).

From a histologic point of view, fibrous tissue at the insertion of the calcaneum in plantar fasciitis is thicker than usual and has lost its organization. Sometimes, a granulomatous tissue area can be found (Schepsis *et al.* 1991). Jarde *et al.* (2003) revised 38 cases of plantar fasciitis that underwent surgical treatment. Histologic examination showed inflammation in all cases, and calcifications of aponeurosis, cartilaginous metaplasia, and fibromatosis. Based upon anatomicopathologic findings at the time of surgery, other recent studies suggest that plantar fascitiis is a "degenerative fasciosis" without inflammation and therefore not a fasciitis. Mixoid degeneration, fragmentation of the plantar fascia, and bone marrow vascular ectasia of the calcaneum were found (Lemont *et al.* 2003).

Plantar fasciitis is common in non-athletes and middle-aged patients, but is also typical in middle and long distance runners, gymnasts, tennis, volleyball and basketball players, as well as triple jumpers. Middle-aged athletes are more affected than young athletes. Patients usually complain of a gradual onset of pain at the plantar side of the calcaneum, and in particular on the medial aspect of the tuberosity. The onset can be sudden in the case of failed jumps with wrong contact with the ground. Sometimes, the pain spreads along all the medial plantar side. Differential diagnosis includes calcaneum stress fractures, bursitis between the calcaneum and plantar fat pad, fat pad syndrome, tarsal tunnel syndrome, tenosynovitis of the posterior tibialis, flexor allucis longus and flexor digitorum tendons, rheumatoid entesitis, and trauma (Furey 1975; Glazer & Hosey 2004).

Treatment of plantar fasciitis is usually conservative. The main goal of rest, and systemic NSAIDs, is to improve clinical symptoms resulting from inflammation but orthoses with longitudinal arch supports are recommended in order to discharge the tension of the fascia during activity. Dorsiflexion splints have been proposed to stretch the fascia passively during rest (Powell *et al.* 1998). Although often used, local injections of steroids should be re-evaluated because of their potential to induce fascial rupture in the absence of inflammation (Lemont *et al.* 2003). Extracorporeal shock wave treatment is a controversial issue, and evidence of a true positive action is still lacking (Haake *et al.* 2003).

Specific treatment of plantar fasciitis includes ultrasound, laser therapy, electroantalgic and bioelectric stimulation, and electromagnetic or microwave therapy. These modalities must be employed to reduce the inflammation and to create conditioning of the pathologic tissue which facilitates the biologic times of recovery. A custom-made orthosis or strapping may be prescribed, but only after careful examination of the footwear to ensure a firm, well-fitting heel counter, good heel cushioning, a neutral subtalar joint, and adequate longitudinal arch support. Local relief of the area of damage and a bilateral heel lift (5–10 mm) may relieve the strain on the plantar fascia.

A taping procedure may be useful in the first days after lesion and when the athlete enters the advanced rehabilitation program with running and sport activity. In the first case, taping has the main purpose of contention with traction in rotation and supination of the foot, in order to decrease tension on the fascia. The taping has to be kept in place all day long. Later, its only function is to protect the structure and to correct the lines of force. Therefore, during rehabilitation the foot needs to be dressed only during running and specific sport activity.

A rehabilitation program includes water cardiocirculatory activity, swimming, and running on a flat surface. Once healing has begun, increased stepping and more difficult exercises are performed. Rehabilitation begins with progressive mobilization of the fascia and activation of the intrinsic muscles. The calf muscles have to be activated with correct stretching to prevent Achilles tendon retraction and excessive fascia tension. Stretching has to be performed progressively, cooling the fascia, and with progressive flexor muscle activation with stretch and spray methods. During these exercises, the triceps muscle needs to relax, such as with the use of a hot pillow. Increasing activation of intrinsic and extrinsic muscles must be obtained. At the beginning, the foot needs to be maintained in a medial rotation until the complete range of motion has been restored. Isometric assisted contractions are prescribed first, followed by isotonic contractions with manual resistance and with progressive resistance rubber bands. At the same time, progressive weight bearing must be regained with foot flexor muscle improvement. The restoration of footing and rehabilitation must be totally pain free and checked by ultrasound, which monitors the correct healing of the tissue. The presence of retractions or adherences may lead to chronic fasciitis, which is difficult to heal. Surgical treatment should be performed for resection of calcification and degeneration areas, partial release of the medial insertion, and in the resection of the calcaneal branch of the tibialis posterior nerve.

Flexor hallucis longus syndrome

Whereas the relation between flexor hallucis longus (FHL) tendon injuries and dancers is well known, disorders of this tendon are often overlooked in other individuals. FHL syndrome is considered an overuse tendinopathy usually presenting either as tenosynovitis or tendon tears. Sometimes, pseudocysts can also be present. FHL begins from the posterior surface of the fibular diathesis and inserts at the distal phalanx of hallux. Along its pathway three main stenosis zones are usually spotted.

The first zone is alongside the medial malleolus, where the tendon runs between the talus and the medial malleolus, in the bony fibrous tunnel that contains the posterior tibial neurovascular bundle, the tibialis posterior and flexor digitorum tendons. This tunnel acts as a pulley and at this level the tendon may be compressed and thus its synovium irritated. The presence of an accessory tendon or muscle

belly has been described as a cause of compression in the tunnel (Eberle *et al.* 2002). Furthermore, enlarged os trigonum tarsi, calcaneal fracture, and soft tissue scars can entrap the FHL at this level (Lo *et al.* 2001). The second zone is in the Henry node, where the flexor digitorum longus passes besides the FHL at the plantar side of the I metatarsal bone.

The third zone is between the two sesamoid bones at the plantar side of the head of the I metatarsal (Sanhudo 2002).

In dancers, often in point-position, the FHL acts as the Achilles tendon. This kind of position stresses the tendon as dynamic stabilizer of ankle and foot. Furthermore, in dance as well as in other sports, hyperpronation strains the tendons beside the retinaculum, leading to inflammation and predisposing them to tendinosis.

Anatomicopathologic features do not differ from other tendinopathies. Macroscopic aspects of pathology depend on the structures involved. For instance, the synovium may be thicker than normal, and may form a true cyst (Fig. 13.4) while effusion and inflammation are present. When the tendon is involved, it is thinner. Micro-tears are frequently the result of chronic degeneration while pseudocysts or calcified nodules and fibrosis may be seen. Microscopically, the patterns of normal aspecific tenosynovitis and tendinosis are detectable by inflammation and edema, disarrangement of fibers, mucoidocystic degeneration, and scar nodules.

Clinical features include pain and discomfort in the medial retromalleolar region of fibro-osseous tunnel elicited by flexion of toes and sometimes hyperesthesia or crepitation can be present. Fullness between the Achilles tendon and the tibia may be a result of edema and inflammation of the synovia within the tunnel. Other symptoms that can reveal tendon involvement include stiffness of the hallux with limited dosiflexion of hallux at the metatarsophalangeal joint when the ankle is dorsiflexed or nodules that can be palpated or a snap felt as the nodule passes under the retinaculum. Dislocation of the FHL may also occur. In this case, a snap will be triggered by maximal ankle dorsiflexion combined with plantar flexion of the hallux at the metatarsophalangeal joint.

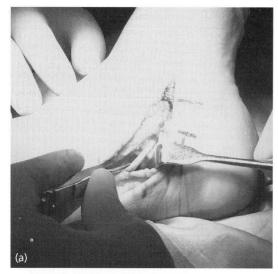

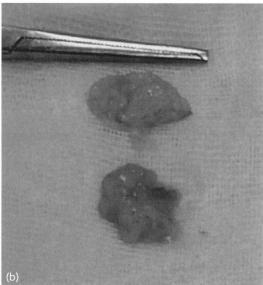

Fig. 13.4 The flexor hallucis longus (FHL) tendon may be involved in a cystic formation developed from the sheath.

MRI is the radiologic examination of choice for the diagnosis. Patterns of tenosynovitis, images of pseudocysts, degeneration, tears or micro-tears of tendon as well as an abnormal position (i.e. in case of dislocation) will be detectable. While the ultrasound diagnosis of some pathologic conditions of the hindfoot such as FHL pathology can be quite difficult, it can be readily detected with high reso-

lution ultrasonography. Early recognition of the tendinopathy is important for successful treatment.

In acute phases, rest, NSAIDs and avoidance of posture in plantar flexion can be helpful. Surgical treatment is a controversial issue. Some authors (Hamilton 1988) prefer a conservative approach for as long as possible, the theory being that scar tissue caused by intervention will lead to persistent pain. When conservative treatment has failed, intervention must be carried out in order to remove the cause of stenosis, free the tendon from the inflamed sheets, even ablating them, and removing degenerated areas of tendon.

Achilles tendon pathology

The Achilles tendon is the strongest tendon in the human body. Achilles tendinopathy is one of the most common overuse injuries sustained by running athletes. Less frequently, it may occur after a trauma, or as a part of a systemic enthesopathy. The number of clinical presentations of Achilles tendinopathy is high and can be classified as insertional, non-insertional, degenerative, or inflammatory in nature. In addition, ruptures represent another chapter presenting different clinical features, treatment options, and outcomes.

Anatomy and function

The Achilles tendon runs from the musculotendinous junction of the gastrocnemius and soleus down to the posterosuperior margin of the calcaneus. It consists of type I collagen fibrils held in parallel bundles by small proteoglycan molecules of dermatan sulfate organized in uniform groups. Being the strongest tendon in the body, the collagen fibrils are of large dimension, but another group of smaller diameter also exists. The two groups are mixed like logs stacked in a wood-pile (Fig. 13.5) in order to optimize the architecture of the tendon from the functional point of view. The uniform groups are primary fascicles which are grouped in secondary fascicles of 0.125–0.375 mm^2 and then further organized in tertiary bundles. The tendon is enveloped by a thin sheath of connective tissue (epitenon) in contact with the endotenon (the elastin-

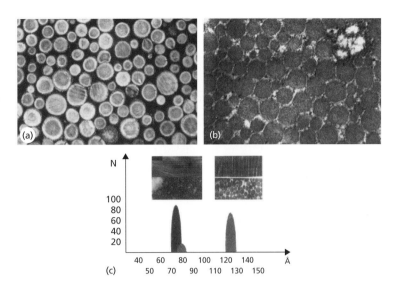

Fig. 13.5 The collagen fibrils in transverse section (a) are stacked like logs in a wood-pile (b), in order to increase the side contact between the fibrils and consequently the mechanical strength of the tendon. The fibrils can be separated in two different groups according to the diameter, in order to favor interdigitation with the above described structure; the differentiation in two different groups is given by exercise and maturation of the tissue, as shown in (c).

rich connective tissue surrounding the fascicles, containing blood and lymph vessels), and covered with the paratenon outside which is an areolar soft tissue. The paratenon is divided into two layers: a deeper layer in contact with the epitenon, and a superficial layer, the peritenon, connected with the deeper layer via the mesotenon which carries blood and lymph vessels. The paratenon is externally in contact with the fascia cruris. This complicated structure of collagen fibrils and sheaths is necessary for the correct function of the Achilles tendon.

The role of collagen is to resist tensile forces while the elastin provides flexibility. Normally, the tendon can stretch without damage up to 4–5% of its original length. However, beyond this point a plastic deformation takes place instead of elastic deformation and the links between fibrils fail. Once a tendon has been stretched to approximately 8% of its original length, rupture can occur. However, many other factors are involved, such as aging, with its unavoidable changes in cell viability and collagen organization, as well as the previous condition of the collagen structure such as the presence and duration of tendinosis and peritendinitis.

Epidemiology

The incidence of the different forms of Achilles tendinopathy is difficult to ascertain because of the high number of clinical entities and the unclear classifications utilized by different authors. In addition, different clinical scenarios can occur together (e.g. insertional tendinopathy with peritenditis). More epidemiologic data are available for Achilles tendon ruptures, which are easily detected as they cause an almost complete invalidity. Complete data have been presented for badminton players, indicating that among elite players in Sweden (66 players), 32% have had a disabling painful condition of the Achilles tendon during the last 5 years, while 17% had an ongoing problem. Furthermore, 57% of the injuires involved the mid-portion of the tendon (Fahlstrom *et al.* 2002). In a middle-aged group of badminton players, 44% complained of Achilles tendon problems, and a positive correlation was found between symptoms and age (Fahlstrom *et al.* 2002). Another study found 95 out of 1405 recruits (6.8%) with Achilles tendinopathy (peritendinitis in 94% of the cases) had a statistically significant difference between incidence in winter (9.4%) and in summer (3.6%) (Milgrom *et al.* 2003). The prevalence of Achilles tendinopathy in runners is approximately 6–11%, while 16% of the running population was forced to give up the sport indefinitely. As far as the ruptures are concerned, black people are more prone to this type of injury compared with non-black people (Davis *et al.* 1999), while the incidence of ruptures in Scotland has increased from 4.7/100.000 in 1981 to 6/100.000 in 1996, and in women more then in men (Maffulli *et al.* 1999), even if men outnumber women as much as 7 : 1.

Etiology and pathology

The Achilles tendon is poorly vascularized and can therefore withstand long periods of relative ischemia during activity, but it also has a low healing capacity. The ability of the Achilles tendon to adapt to training is therefore different from that of muscle, which quickly responds with hypertrophy and acquisition of specific metabolic properties to mechanical stimuli. Imbalance between the force that a muscle can exert and the force a tendon is able to transmit safely can arise. Excessive training is still the main cause of Achilles tendinopathy, but the term excessive is relative to a given individual, and to his or her structural limit. Training means that the physiologic threshold of the amount necessary to imply a reparative response has to be overcome which leads to a strengthening of the tissue. If this equilibrium is not maintained by the athlete, the pathologic response is bigger then the reparative reaction.

During running, jumping, and other ballistic activities, the Achilles tendon is subjected to tension, torsion, and vibration, reduction of the blood flow in the least vascular intermediate portion of the tendon, and heat generation. Furthermore, the tendon is pulled along its axis during the stance phase of running, and at the precise moment of contact of the foot with the ground (eccentric contraction of the gastrocnemius unit), a further tension is applied with the concentric contraction for the take off. In addition to this, at the moment of full contact of the foot, a whiplash effect takes place that induces vibrations, which are directly related to the type of ground (artificial turf above all), and the shoe. The whiplash effect and vibrations are also related to the torsion of the Achilles tendon during the stance phase, which is in turn connected to the amount of pronation of the midfoot. Both hyperpronation and hypopronation can be involved. In the case of subtalar hypomobility, a greater shock is transmitted through the tendon, while in the case of

hypermobility a greater torque is applied. In the first scenario, micro-tearing can occur, while in the second the blood supply can be impaired by squeezing of the vessels.

Another attractive, but still not fully demonstrated theory concerning Achilles tendon alteration involves heat production during exercise. When heat, especially in hot environment, is not dispersed, the temperature in the core of the tendon can reach a value as high as 42.5°C, which is not compatible with a full cell viability (Wilson & Goodship 1994).

The Achilles tendon responds to these negative stimuli in two ways: inflammation of its sheaths, and degeneration of its main body. However, this distinction can be artificial, because the closeness of the tendon and its sheaths, and the Kager's triangle fat pad, can result in a combination of the two stimuli. The alteration of the mid-substance of the tendon is not merely degenerative, as we have demonstrated the production of different amounts and quality of glycosaminoglycans (GAGs) (Benazzo *et al.* 1996). The GAGs reached 0.57% of the dry weight (0.066% being the normal value), and chondroitin sulfate (ChS) was much more represented than the normal dermatan sulfate, causing water retention with fibril organization disruption (Fig. 13.6), and the typical hypoechogenic and hyperintense appearance in ultrasonography and MRI. Investigations are currently underway to determine if ChS is also responsible for pain (Khan & Cook 2000). Furthermore, *in vitro* experiments have shown tenocytes from ruptured as well as from tendinopathic Achilles tendons produce type III collagen in larger amounts than normal tenocytes, instead of type I collagen. The different type of collagen produced as a result of an abnormal healing response could also be responsible for tissue failure (Maffulli *et al.* 2000).

The mid-substance of the Achilles tendon, together with the corresponding portion of the sheath, is the most susceptible to changes because it is the least perfused area, and the spiraling configuration of the fibers tends to "wring out" this region (OKU, Sports Medicine, 1994) and to increase ischemia especially in an abnormally pronating foot. It is still an open question as to whether degenerative or inflammatory changes prevail, but clinical

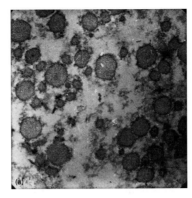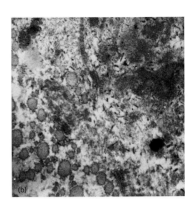

Fig. 13.6 The collagen fibrils packaging is disrupted, and the fibrils are indented and irregular in transverse section.

experience and diagnostic tools clearly indicate that tendinosis rather then tendinitis occurs in the chronic phases.

In disorders affecting the calcaneal insertion, a true inflammation of the bursa is usually found, with resulting formation of painful adherences around the tendon and its bony attachment. The bursa is usually enlarged with inflammatory synovial fluid, and the internal wall shows true synovial villi as in synovitis. The entire insertional area is therefore involved and painful because of the increased volume of the bursa, its inflammatory content, and the impingement with the Achilles tendon both in flexion and extension of the foot.

The presence of a clinically detectable inflammation of the sheaths and of the bursa can be easily understood from the pathogenetic point of view as caused by overload in altered biomechanics of the lower leg, and consequently as a source of pain because these structures are highly innervated. It is more difficult to understand the alterations of the connective tissue, which is caused by an iterative overload that does not overcome the intrinsic mechanical resistance of the tendon and does not cause tears of the connective tissue but is a source of pain without inflammation.

Bestwick and Maffulli (2000) hypothesized that the production of reactive oxygen species within and around the tendons as a consequence of hyperthermia and repetitive ischemia and reperfusion can interfere negatively, if not neutralize, tissue remodeling and cause tissue degeneration by acting on gene transcription and modulation. Khan and Cook (2000) hypothesized that the pain can derive from biochemical mediators such as glutamate produced in excess within the tendon and/or in the surrounding tissues. ChS is another potential candidate. Alfredson and Lorentzon (2002) also indicate that glutamate could be responsible for tendon pain, and hypothesized a possible drug treatment.

Classification (Table 13.1)

The classification of the Achilles tendon disorders should be based upon histopathologic proven conditions (Table 13.1). Therefore, the term Achilles tendinitis, which is still frequently used, is not really correct as the tendon mid-substance involved undergoes degenerative changes more than inflamma-

Table 13.1 Classification of Achilles tendinopathy.

Achillodinia (the term is equivalent to pubalgia and refers to symptoms more than to a specific pathologic condition)
Peritendinitis
- Acute (crackling)
- Chronic (fibrotic)

Tendinosis (pure degeneration of the tendon usually localized at the middle third)
Peritendinitis with tendinosis (usually fibrotic in nature)
Insertional tendinopathy
- With bursitis (pre-achilles and/or retro-achilles insertion)
- With peritendinitis (usually fibrotic thickening of the sheaths)
- Pseudo Haglund and Haglund deformities (acquired more often than congenital hypertrophy of the calcaneal superior border)

Partial tear (either insertional or middle third substance)
Rupture (usually at the middle third)

tory changes. The term achillodynia refers simply to an unspecific condition of pain in the region of the Achilles tendon, and is a purely descriptive term. We should therefore consider the term tendinopathy as the correct word indicating a condition of tendon pathology with impaired performance, specified by terms such as peritendinitis if the sheaths are involved, tendinosis if the tendon itself is degenerated, peritendinitis with tendinosis if the two conditions are combined, or insertional tendinopathy with bursitis in disorders of the calcaneal region.

The deformity of the posterior border of the calcaneum can be acquired as a consequence of chronic over-pulling on the bony insertion, and by the persisting inflammation of the region, and is referred to as pseudo-Haglund, or congenital, where the bone prominence is remarkable, and impinges the ventral face of the tendon in dorsiflexion. The latter is a true Haglund deformity. The term partial tear indicates a condition of subcutaneous acute lesion where an interruption of some fibers is demonstrated. The tear can be located in any portion of the tendon, in the mid-substance as well as in the distal portion, where an Haglund deformity can facilitate the fiber's disruption. Rupture of the tendon is the interruption of the whole substance of the tendon.

Physical examination, clinical features, and imaging

The physical examination and subjective symptoms are of paramount importance in leading to the diagnosis. However, imaging is also fundamental in order to describe the amount and distribution of the pathology, and to monitor progress to healing or to deterioration. Starting from the distal insertion, in the case of insertional tendinopathy with bursitis, athletes have tenderness at palpation and signs of inflammation with a palpable pre-Achilles bursa, and an enlarged bony prominence in the chronic cases. Subjectively, the athlete complains of pain when he or she starts exercising, and typically the pain worsens during warming up, jumping, and running uphill more than downhill. Uphill running and jumping increase the impingement with the tendon ventrally, while dorsally the tendon is compressed by heel counter.

Acute peritendinitis is characterized by crepitus while moving the foot, palpable and audible subjectively (like walking in fresh, icy snow), with diffuse swelling of the tendon. Ankle motion is difficult especially after a short rest, and in the morning. The condition is not compatible with sport participation. A chronic form is more common, where pain is elicited by palpation with two fingers of the tendon during active motion, swelling is localized on either part (medial and/or lateral) of the tendon, and chronic adhesions are recognized as an extended nodule which does not move with the tendon itself. Pain decreases with warm-up and with activity, and reappears after a cool-down. Peritendinitis can be associated with tendinosis with similar subjective symptoms and objective signs.

When pure tendinosis occurs, an increase of the tendon dimensions can be detected, or a fusiform nodule can be palpated within the tendon. Subjectively, pain can be surprisingly mild. More frequently in the Achilles tendon than in other tendons, there is a discrepancy between the degree of pathology and the symptoms the athlete complains of. Heavily degenerated tendons are almost asymptomatic (with worrying sonograms and MRI), while microscopic tears at the osteotendinous junctions, and/or involvement of the sheaths and bursa (with scarcely positive sonograms and MRI) may be responsible for aching pain that interferes with sports participation. Tendinosis can be complicated by partial tears, characterized by a sudden increase of pain and swelling. Tears are rare distally, but are more frequent in the mid-substance of the tendon (Haims et al. 2000).

In general, symptoms can appear after a change in the training routine such as an increase in mileage, a different training surface, a worn-out or a new shoe. Symptoms may also be accompanied by other concomitant factors such as an inadequate warm-up, cool-down, or stretching program, change in the time of training (too early in the morning when flexibility is poor; training immediately after a long flight which causes venous blood retention), cold or hot weather, and imperfect health conditions (flu, infections) (Clement et al. 1984; Rosenbaum & Hennig 1995).

Plain films are able to show bony spurs of the

insertion, and calcification in the distal extent of the tendon, as well as bony overgrowth consistent with chronic inflammation. They must not be considered in other Achilles tendon injuries, ruptures included. Ultrasound can be performed dynamically, showing the impingement of the tendon with the bursa and with the bone, and the dimensions of the bursa itself. This is extremely important in the diagnosis of peritenditis, both acute and chronic, and in tendinosis. The presence of fluid around the tendon is easily detected, as well as areas of hypoechogenicity within the tendon, indicating nodular or diffuse degeneration and possibly partial tears. The dynamic examination can reveal if the thickening of the sheaths is accompanied by nodular degeneration of the tissue. MRI can show the same areas as hyperintense if the water content is higher then normal with a better three-dimensional resolution than ultrasound and it helps in diagnosing the extent of bony reaction to an insertional tendinopathy. The peritendinitis can be easily detected, but non-dynamic examination should also be performed (Dunfee et al. 2002).

Treatment

The treatment of all kinds of Achilles tendinopathies can be conservative or surgical. If the tendinopathy is not severe, reduction of sports participation, revision of the training program, change in footwear, analysis of the athlete's alignments, and an inflammatory therapy with ultrasound may lead to correct healing. When tendonitis is severe, sport activity needs to be suspended for several weeks and a tendon lifter used. Resting splints or casting may be used for 3–6 weeks. Physical therapy includes ice, ultrasound, laser therapy, and tecar therapy to reduce inflammation. In addition, it is very important in the subacute phase to prevent new inflammation and to stimulate regeneration. Peritendineous infiltration in acute and subacute phases is controversial.

In crackling tendonitis, low molecular weight heparin may be used to decrease inflammation and consequent adhesions. Some authors have suggested infiltration of the peritendinous sheaths with polysulfate glycosaminoglican in order to increase tissue regeneration. Local injection of autologous serum with platelets and their growth factors seems to reduce inflammation and to increase healing but further results are needed for this procedure (Aspenberg & Virchenko 2004).

When the acute phase is reduced, rehabilitation has a very important role. Progressive active and passive mobilization helps in reducing peritendineous adhesions while isometric exercises, submaximal at the beginning and maximal successively, keep good muscle activity. When inflammation decreases, concentric isotonic exercises with manual resistance and with bands are encouraged. Manual eccentric contractions and, later, eccentric exercises which are also known as Stanish exercises should be performed. Eccentric contractions are an important stimulus in generating tendon hypertrophy (Stanish et al. 1986; LaStayo et al. 2003).

Specific exercises for tendon regeneration should be added to exercises as necessary for the maintainance and the improvment of the strength of the leg muscles. Muscles are inhibited by the inflammation of these tendons and reduce their tropism immediately. The greatest problem in the treatment of these tendinopathies is to correctly evaluate the exercise progression, running and sport activity while avoiding other episodes of inflammation. Sometimes, acute inflammation is a consequence of functional overload, may last for a long time, and involves the whole tendon. Therefore, any error in the rehabilitation progression may lead to acute inflammation. Extreme caution is urged in the rehabilitation progression and increasing activity without pain is suggested.

Surgical indication is based upon the following criteria: recalcitrant symptoms and/or persisting pathology in Achilles tendinopathies that are not responsive to a previous, well-conducted conservative treatment, and remarkable tissue alterations such as chronic, thick, peritendinous adhesions, wide areas of degeneration, large inflamed bursa, and marked bony impingement, all occuring without previous treatment.

Nowadays, Achilles tendon surgery should follow the criteria of minimal invasivity, and with endoscopy playing an increased part. The skin incision should be reduced as much as possible, while skin mobility allows for the detection of a large portion of the tendon with the further advantage of placing scars in different planes when removing the sheaths. In this sense, multiple subcutaneous tenotomy has been advocated, but its validity on a large scale has not been demonstrated. The skin may not be sutured with stitches, but only with sterile adhesive strips.

Conservative treatment is similar for all conditions of Achilles pathology and includes rest (concerning the specific activity and/or the exercise causing most of the pain), heel lift, orthotics to correct anatomic and/or functional abnormalities of the foot and ankle, NSAIDs (systemic and locally applied), physical modalities such as ultrasound, iontophoresis, laser, electric stimulation, tecar, hyperthermia, O^3 injections, steroid injections in the inflamed bursa, and injections of sclerosing substances (Alfredson & Lorentzon 2002). The clinical use of autologous growth factors injected around the tendon is currently under investigation and no reliable clinical data have yet been collected.

Once the acute symptoms resolve, strengthening of the gastrocnemius unit is advocated, and strong eccentric training has been suggested. In chronic recalcitrant peritendinitis, surgery begins with opening the thickened crural fascia with underskin incision extended to the lower third of the calf. However, there is a chance of damage to the crossing vein with postoperative bleeding. Therefore, the fascia must be left open. Next, excise the thickened sheaths, and avoid leaving the cutting edges transversely placed to the tendon. The ventral portion of the sheaths, which contain vessels, should be left alone. The excision of this highly innervated tissue can relieve pain dramatically. Activity must be resumed quickly.

In chronic tendinosis, different options are available. The skin incision must be placed over the most involved area. Then débridement and excision of degenerated and/or necrotic tissue should be performed. Tendon transfer can be used as a mechanical or biologic augmentation if the amount of tissue excised is significant. If this is the case, the plantaris gracilis or the FHL can be used with the advantage of putting its muscle belly in proximity to the unhealthy vascular Achilles tendon. Because this technique is demanding both in harvesting the

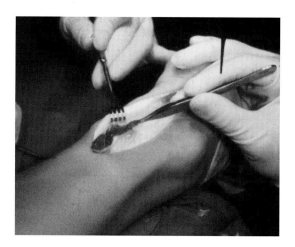

Fig. 13.7 The soleus muscle bundle is grafted into the Achilles tendon for a better and quicker regeneration of the tissue.

graft and in tensioning the tendon, a pure muscle fiber transplant can be adopted (Benazzo *et al.* 1997, 2000, 2001). A cylindrical bundle of the soleus muscle that is long enough to reach the degenerated area can be isolated and remain attached distally. The bundle is then turned 180° and placed inside an incision in the degenerated tendon (Fig. 13.7). A double transfer can be performed according to the extension of the degeneration.

For insertional tendinopathy, the incidence of which is increasing, the following surgical steps can be adopted. First, endoscopic débridement of the pre-Achilles bursa and excision of the fibrotic scars in the fat pad and regularization of the bony prominence of the calcaneum should be performed with an abrader. Then, if an open treatment is chosen, a skin incision can be placed laterally or medially. However, some authors advocate an incision in the median line, with longitudinal tendon splitting, débridement of the degenerated areas, and regularization of the bone through the split. The lateral incision allows a good approach to the bursa, and an optimal visualization of the ventral and dorsal aspects of the tendon in order to remove the diseased portions and the thickened inflamed peritendinous tissue. However, the medial corner of the insertion is hard to reach and regularization of the medial border of the calcaneum may be difficult. The same is true for the medial incision in the opposite corner. However, the median incision carries a higher chance of painful scarring, while the other approaches are generally preferred.

Future directions

When many different tendons are contained in a small space, with different functions and biomechanical properties, athletes may easily suffer from an inflammatory and/or degenerative pathology. It is well known that the basic pathology of the tendons is almost the same and consists of degeneration of the tendon with splitting in the long medial tendons or with intratendinous ruptures of different sizes in the Achilles tendon, and inflammation of the sheaths with true tenosynovitis in the long medial tendons, and peritendinitis in the Achilles tendon.

While all these differences are well known,

the source and cause of the pain is still not clear. Currently, ChS, glutamate, and substance P are under investigation. Microdialysis and other techniques have been applied to investigate this field. The role of the temperature in tendon degeneration has yet to be elucidated and experiments are currently under development to clarify the problem.

As far as conservative treatment is concerned, injections of sclerosing substances around the tendon is the obvious answer to the discovery of an increased vascularization of the sheaths. However, it is still not clear if this is the cause or the consequence of pain and tissue pathology. Techniques such as grafting of tendon and muscle within the Achilles tendon are being demonstrated to be valid with reliable and quick results. In the near future, the role of growth factors and stem cells in the treatment of tendon degeneration will need to be investigated.

References

Alfredson, H. & Lorentzon, R. (2002) Chronic tendon pain: no signs of chemical inflammation but high concentrations of the neurotransmitter glutamate. Implications for treatment? *Current Drug Targets* 3, 43–54.

Alanen, J., Orava, S., Heinonen, O.J., Ikonen, J., Kvist, M. (2001) Peroneal tendon injuries. Report of 38 operated cases. *Ann Chir Gynaecol* 90 (1), 43–46.

Aspenberg, P., Virchenko, O. (2004) Platelet concentrate injection improves Achilles tendon repair in rats. *Acta Orthopaedic Scandinavia* 75 (1), 93–99.

Barnett, C.H. & Napier, J.R. (1965) The axis of rotation of the ankle joint in man. *Journal of Anatomy* 86, 1–9.

Benazzo, F., Stennardo, G. & Valli, M. (1996) Achilles and patellar tendinopathies in athletes: pathogenesis and surgical treatment. *Bulletin of the Hospital for Joint Diseases* 54, 236–240.

Benazzo, F., Todesca, A. & Ceciliani, L. (1997) Achilles tendon tendonitis and heel pain. *Operative Techniques in Sports Medicine* 5, 179–188.

Benazzo, F., Zanon, G. & Maffulli, N. (2000) An operative approach to Achilles tendinopathy. *Sports Medicine Arthroscopy Review* 8, 96–101.

Benazzo, F., Stennardo, G., Mosconi, M., Zanon, G., Maffulli, N. (2001) Muscle transplant in the rabbit's Achilles tendon. *Med Sci Sports Exercise* 33 (5), 696–701.

Bestwick, C.S. & Maffulli, N. (2000) Reactive oxygen species and tendon problems: review and hypothesis. *Sports Medicine Arthroscopy Review* 8, 6–16.

Bonnin, M., Tavernier, T. & Bouysset, M. (1997) Split lesions of the peroneus brevis tendon in chronic ankle laxity. *American Journal of Sports Medicine* 25, 699–703.

Chen, Y.J., Hsu, R.W. & Liang, S.C. (1997) Degeneration of the accessory navicular synchondrosis presenting as rupture of the posterior tibial tendon. *Journal of Bone and Joint Surgery, American volume* 79, 1791–1798.

Clement, D.B., Taunton, J.E., Smart, G.W. (1984) Achilles tendinitis and peritendinitis: etiology and treatment. *American Journal of Sports Medicine* 12(3), 179–184.

Cozen, L. (1965) Posterior tibialis synovitis secondary to foot strain. *Clinical Orthopaedics* 42, 101–107.

Davis, J.J., Mason, K.T. & Clark, D.A. (1999) Achilles tendon ruptures stratified by age, race, and cause of injury among active duty U.S. Military members. *Military Medicine* 164, 872–873.

Doxey, G.E. (1987) Calcaneal pain: a review of various disorders. *Journal of Orthopaedic and Sports Physical Therapy* 9, 25–32.

Dunfee, W.R., Dalinka, M.K., Kneeland, J.B. (2002) Imaging of athletic injuries to

the ankle and foot. *Radiology Clinics of North America* 40 (2), 289–312.

Eberle, C.F., Moran, B. & Gleason, T. (2002) The accessory flexor digitorum longus as a cause of flexor hallucis syndrome. *Foot and Ankle International* 23, 51–55.

Fahlstrom, M., Lorentzon, R. & Alfredson, H. (2002) Painful conditions in the Achilles tendon region in elite badminton players. *American Journal of Sports Medicine* 30, 51–54.

Fallat, L., Grimm, D.J. & Saracco, J.A. (1998) Sprained ankle sundrome: prevalence and analysis of 639 acute injuries. *Journal of Foot and Ankle Surgery* 37, 280–285.

Ferran, N.A., Oliva, F., Maffulli, N. (2006) Recurrent subluxation of peroneal tendon. *Sports Medicine* 36 (10), 839–846.

Furey, J.G. (1975) Plantar fasciitis. The painful heel. *Journal of Bone and Joint Surgery, American volume* 57, 672–673.

Frey, C., Shereff, M. & Greenidge, N. (1990) Vascularity of posterior tibialis tendon. *Journal of Bone and Joint Surgery, American volume* 72, 884–888.

Geideman, W.M. & Johnson, J.E. (2000) Posterior tibial dysfunction. *Journal of Orthopaedic and Sports Physical Therapy* 30, 68–77.

Glazer, J.L., Hosey, R.G. (2004) Soft-tissue injuries of the lower extremity. *Primary Care* 31 (4), 1005–1024.

Gunn, D.R. (1959) Stenosing tenosynovitis of the common peroneal tendon sheath. *British Medical Journal* **5123**, 691–2.

Haake, M., Buch, M., Schoellner, C., *et al.* (2003) Extracorporeal shock wave therapy for plantar fasciitis: randomised controlled multicenter trial. *British Medical Journal* **12**, 327–375.

Haims, A.H., Schweitzer, M.E., Patel, R.S., Hect, P., Wapner, K.L. (2000) MR Imaging of the Achilles tendon: overlap of findings in symptomatic and asymptomatic individuals. *Skeletal Radiology* **29** (11), 640–645.

Hamilton, W.G. (1988) Foot and ankle injuries in dancers. *Clinics in Sports Medicine* **7**, 143–173.

Inman, V.T. (1976) *The Joints of the Ankle*. Williams & Wilkins, Baltimore.

Jarde, O., Diebold, P., Havet, E., Boulu, G. & Vernois, J. (2003) Degenerative lesions of the plantar fascia: surgical treatment fasciectomy and excision of the heel spur. A report of 38 cases. *Acta Orthopaedica Belgica* **69**, 267–274.

Johnson, K.A. & Strom, D.E. (1989) Tibialis posterior dysfunction. *Clinical Orthopaedics* **239**, 196–206.

Khan, K. & Cook, J.L. (2000) Overuse tendon injuries: where the pain come from? *Sports Medicine Arthroscopy Review* **8**, 17–31.

Klein, S., Mathy, S. & Roose, M. (1999) Moment arm lenght variation of selected muscles acting on talo crural and subtalar joint during movement. *Journal of Biomechanics* **29**, 21–30.

Labib, S.A., Gould, J.S., Rodriguez-del-Rio, F.A. & Lyman, S. (2002) Heel pain triad (HPT): the combination of plantar fasciitis, posterior tibial tendon dysfunction and tarsal tunnel syndrome. *Foot and Ankle International* **23**, 1054.

Langelaan, E.J. (1983) A kinematical analysis of tarsal joints. Thesis. University of Leiden. *Acta Orthopaedic Scandinavica Supplement* **54**, 204.

Langenskiold, A. (1967) Chronic non-specific tenosynovitis of the tibialis posterior tendon. *Acta Orthopaedic Scandinavica* **38**, 301–305.

LaStayo, P.C., Woolf, J.M., Lewek, M.D., Snyder-Mackler, L., Reich, T., Lindstedt, S.L. (2003) Eccentric muscle contractions; their contribution to injury, prevention, rehabilitation, and sport, *J Orthop Sports Phys Ther* **33**(10), 557–571.

Ledoux, A. & Morvan, G. (1991) Syndrome du carrefour posterior (SCP). In: *Tomodensitométrie du Pied et de la Cheville* (Morvan, G., Busson, J., Wyber, M., eds.) Masson: 150–159.

Lemont, H., Ammirati, K.M. & Usen, N. (2003) Plantar fasciitis: a degenerative process (fasciosis) without inflammation. *Journal of the American Podiatric Medical Association* **93**, 234–237.

Lo, L.D., Schweitzer, M.E., Fan, J.K., Wapner, K.L. & Hect, P.J. (2001) MR imaging findings of entrapment of the flexor hallucis longus tendon. *American Journal of Roentgenology* **176**, 1145–1148.

Lundberg, E. (1988) Pattern of motion of the ankle/foot complex. Thesis. Department of Orthopaedics, Karolinska Hospital, S-104 01 Stockholm.

Maffulli, N., Ewen, S.W., Waterstone, S.W., Reaper, J. & Barrass, V. (2000) Tenocyets from ruptured and tendinopathic achilles tendons produce greater quantities of type III collagen than tenocytes from normal tendons. An *in vitro* model of human tendon healing. *American Journal of Sports Medicine* **28**, 499–505.

Maffulli, N., Waterston, S.W., Squair, J., Reaper, J. & Douglas, A.S. (1999) Changing incidence of Achilles tendon rupture in Scotland: a year study. *Clinical Journal of Sport Medicine* **9**, 157–160.

Milgrom, C., Finestone, A., Zin, D., Mandel, D. & Novack, V. (2003) Cold weather training: a risk factor for Achilles paratendinitis among recruits. *Foot and Ankle International* **24**, 398–401.

Mosier, S.M., Pommeroy, G. & Manoli, A. (1999) Pathoanatomy and ethiology of posterior tibial tendon dysfunction. *Clinical Orthopaedics* **365**, 12–22.

Myerson, M.S. (1997) Adult acquired flatfoot deformity: Treatment of dysfunction of the posterior tibial tendon. *Instructional Course Lecture* **46**, 393–405.

Novacheck, T.F. (1994) Implications for training and injury. Instructional Course, American Academy of Orthopaedic Surgeons, 61st Annual Meeting, New Orleans, Louisiana.

Porter, D.A., Baxter, D.E., Clanton, T.O. & Klootwyk, T.E. (1998) Posterior tibial tendon tears in young competitive athletes: two case reports. *Foot and Ankle International* **19**, 627–630.

Powell, M., Post, W.R., Keener, J. & Wearden, S. (1998) Effective treatment of chronic plantar fasciitis with dorsiflexion night splints: a crossover prospective randomized outcome study. *Foot and Ankle International* **19**, 10–18.

Riddle, D.L., Pulisc, M., Pidcoe, P. & Johnson, R.E. (2003) Risk factors in plantar fasciitis: a matched case–control study. *Journal of Bone and Joint Surgery. American volume* **85**, 872–877.

Root, M.L., Orien, W.P. & Weed, J.H. (1977) Functions of the muscles of the foot. In: *Normal and Abnormal Function of the Foot* (Root, M.L., Orien, W.P. & Weed, J.H., eds.). Clinical Biomechanics Corporation, Los Angeles, CA.

Rosenbaum, D., Hennig, E.M. (1995) The influence of stretching and warm-up exercises on Achilles tendon reflex activity. *Journal of Sports Science* **13**(6), 481–490.

Safran, M.R., O'Malley, D. Jr., Fu, F.H. (1999) Personeal tendon subluxation in athletes; new exam technique, case reports, and review. *Med Sci Sports Exercise* **31** (7 Suppl), S487–492.

Sanhudo, J.A. (2002) Stenosing tenosynovitis of the flexor hallucis longus tendon at the sesamoid area. *Foot and Ankle International* **23**, 801–803.

Schepsis, A.A., Leach, R.E. & Gorzyca, J. (1991) Plantar fasciitis. *Clinical Orthopaedics* **266**, 185–196.

Shepard, F.J. (1882) A hitherto undescribed fracture of the astragalus. *Journal of Anatomy and Physiology* **17**, 79–81.

Sobel, M., Leavy, M.E. & Bohne, W.H.O. (1990) Longitudinal attrition of the peroneus brevis tendon in the fibular groove: an anatomic study. *Foot and Ankle International* **11**, 124–128.

Stanish, W.D., Rubinowich, M., Curwin, S. (1986) Eccentric exercise in chronic tendinitis. *Clinical Orthopaedics and Related Research* **208**, 65–68.

Turner, W. (1882) A secondary astragalus in the human foot. *Journal of Anatomy and Physiology* **17**, 82–83.

Warren, J.J.P. (1990) Plantar fasciitis in runners. *Sports Medicine* **10**, 338–345.

Wearing, S.C., Smeathers, J.E. & Urry, S.R. (2003) The effect o plantar fasciitis on vertical foot–ground reaction force. *Clinical Orthopaedics* **409**, 175–185.

Wilson, A.M. & Goodship, A.E. (1994) Exercise-induced hypertermia as a possible mechanism for tendon degeneration. *Journal of Biochemisty* **27**, 899–905.

Wright, D.G., Desai, S.H. & Hendersson, W.H. (1964) Action of the subtalar and ankle joint complex during stance phase of walking. *Journal of Bone and Joint Surgery* **46A**, 361–372.

Chapter 14

Alternative Approaches in the Management of Tendinopathies—Traditional Chinese Medicine: From Basic Science to Clinical Perspective

Tendinopathy is an intriguing problem. To date, there is still a lack of clear understanding of the pathogenesis of tendinopathy. The inconsistent outcome of many treatment modalities has led to a proliferation of a number of approaches. In many Asian countries, traditional Chinese medicine, which emphasizes "a holistic approach to life equilibrium between the mind, body and their environment, and an emphasis on health rather than on disease", has been an accepted treatment methodology. Its clinical paradigm consists of four main strategies: herbal medicine, acupuncture, manipulative therapy, and general restorative exercise such as Tai Chi.

The clinical spectrum on tendinopathies includes pain, mechanical weakness leading to rupture in certain regions, functional loss, and tendon adhesion. There is now a consensus that tendinopathy is a form of inadequate healing leading to matrix disturbance, tenocyte death, increased vulnerability to injury, and then a final stage of non-healing. Based on scientific analysis, traditional Chinese medicine modalities have defined the possible sites of action in the process of tendinosis. While traditional Chinese medicine is widely practiced, we encourage an effective dialog between the athletes, coaches, scientists, and practitioners to look at the various scientific pathways of utilizing this time-honored alternative approach in the management of tendinopathies. In the future, we envision that traditional Chinese medicine treatment modalities will receive worldwide acceptance.

Introduction

Intriguing tendinopathies—an alternative approach to a diversified clinical spectrum

Tendinosis is a common medical condition that has been described with many names in the literature. It is a mysterious chronic tendon disorder with a confusing picture. The pathogenesis of tendinosis remains unresolved with micro-trauma, overuse, and degenerative changes all claiming direct or indirect links. Research efforts have been made to correlate why athletes of all ages sometimes present with gradual onset of pain localized to the Achilles tendon, patellar tendon, or rotator cuff tendons. Initially, these conditions were considered as totally different entities resulting from uncontrolled training habits, overuse, or degeneration in athletes. When conservative treatments of these sports injuries failed, surgical approaches were used. However, we soon recognized that the tissues excised from these various locations during surgery looked remarkably similar to normal under both macroscopic and microscope examination. Comparing data and initiating experimental studies, we observed that the ongoing process in all these tendons resembles a halt in an early healing process. If caused by initial overuse, why does the damage look permanent as this injury is not healed after months of rest, anti-inflammatory treatment, and avoidance of the triggering factors that are supposed to cause the injury? If caused by degeneration, why is it also found in young and fit athletes?

The clinical manifestation of tendinosis includes a gradually increasing activity-related localized pain and dysfunction. Typical patients are recreational athletes in sports such as long distance running, basketball, golf, or tennis. However, this disorder may also be found in manual workers or recreational weekend warriors.

It has been postulated, but not demonstrated, that a gradual deterioration of tendinosis may lead to rupture of the tendon, with well-known clinical consequences. From the evidence base, we still do not know whether or not these conditions are closely linked. However, the disorganized collagen in tendinosis tissues is no doubt related to a reduced tensile strength. Management of tendinosis often, by routine, involves anti-inflammatory drugs or cortisone injections, neither of which is efficient nor indicated. Tendinosis is typically not associated with inflammation, as defined from the absence of inflammatory cells in the tissues. Physiotherapy including temporal avoidance of triggering activities, controlled eccentric strength exercises and flexibility training are standard initial treatments and may help in some cases, as supported by a few clinical studies. If no improvement is observed after 2–3 months, surgical excision of macroscopically pathologic tissue will be advocated.

Definition of "alternative medicine"

In response to a rapid increase in the use of alternative medicine over the past decade, the World Health Organization (WHO) has created the first 5-year global strategy for traditional medicine, the "WHO Traditional Medicine Strategy 2002–2005" issued in May 2002. The WHO has delineated a working definition of traditional medicine as "including diverse health practices, approaches, knowledge and beliefs incorporating plant, animal, and/or mineral based medicines, spiritual therapies, manual techniques and exercises applied singularly or in combination to maintain well-being, as well as to treat, diagnose or prevent illness" (WHO 2002). Traditional medicine is based on "a holistic approach to life, equilibrium between

the mind, body and their environment, and an emphasis on health rather than on disease." It is also referred to as complementary or alternative medicine and includes diverse practices such as acupuncture, yoga, shiatsu massage, and aromatherapy.

Such a unique vision, which is not at all common in the Western "scientific" approach to health, is in the pathway designed by the constitutional definition of health, which goes beyond the mere absence of disease and introduces a state of complete physical, mental, and social well-being. Traditional medicine has been used for millennia in the developing world and remains widespread. According to the WHO, 80% of the population in Africa use traditional therapies, and more than 70 countries have already regulated the use of herbal medicine. Moreover, the use of traditional medicine as a response to primary health care needs amongst some of the less developed and privileged countries with the poorest population, makes it to be one of the most useful means to reach the Health for All objective.

Traditional Chinese medicine—a holistic approach to tendinopathy

In the clinical paradigm of traditional Chinese medicine (TCM), there are generally four main strategies that can be utilized in the management of tendinopathies (Fig. 14.1). It should be noted that all four parameters interact with one another to provide a synergistic effort. When we analyze the possible specific targets of action of the four

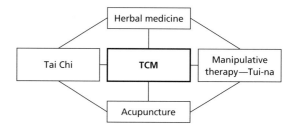

Fig. 14.1 Four main strategies in the holistic management of tendinopathy. TCM, traditional Chinese medicine.

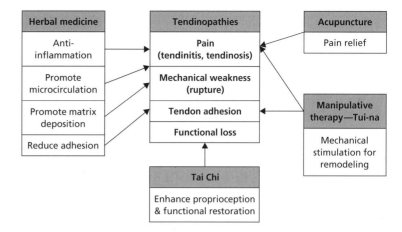

Fig. 14.2 Schematic representations of possible specific targets of actions of the four main strategies in the management of tendinopathy.

main parameters in tendinopathies, we postulate the schematic representations seen in Fig. 14.2.

Herbal medicine explores bioactive substances from natural products to restore balance of body functions that are disturbed during disease processes. Tendon healing is composed of three different stages: inflammation, proliferation and granulation, and remodeling. In the inflammatory phase, pain is the main symptom that requires treatment. Recruitment of reparative tenoblasts as well as the resumption of disrupted microcirculation are the important events in this stage. In the proliferation and granulation phase, the reparative tenoblasts increase in numbers and start to repair the wound by active synthesis of extracellular matrix proteins. In the final stage of remodeling, the newly deposited matrix proteins are reorganized to meet the biomechanical needs of the tendons. Different kinds of herbal medicine exhibit modulatory activities in these processes. With a timely application according to the time course of healing, tendon healing can be optimized.

Apart from pharmacologic interventions, TCM also develops characteristic biophysical interventions that are beneficial to analgesic aspects and rehabilitation. Acupuncture is one of the most well-known means for pain management. It explores the modulatory responses of specialized regions in the surface of the body called acupoints. In the case of tendon injuries and tendinopathies, acupuncture is effective in relieving pain, as well as stimulating

the restoration of local somatosensory functions. The modulatory roles of acupoints can also be explored by acupressure, also known as Tui-na, which provides proper mechanical stimulation to tendons and enhances the remodeling process. In fact, the modern ideas of rehabilitation have an ancient root, manifested by the restoration exercise in TCM such as Tai Chi. Tai Chi can promote the proprioception of musculoskeletal units, thus the functional restoration of tendons from tendinopathies can be fortified.

The four main strategies in the management of tendinopathies

The four main strategies in the holistic management of tendinopathies include herbal medicine, acupuncture, manipulative therapy (Tui-na), and Tai Chi.

HERBAL MEDICINE

Tendon healing consists of three phases: inflammation phase, proliferation and granulation phase, and remodeling phase. The strategies of applying herbal medicine can specifically target on these three phases. Herbal medicine can be administered either topically or orally. Topical application of herbal medicine includes the use of an ointment, stupe, alcohol-based concoction, medicinal washing, patch, or iontophoresis.

ACUPUNCTURE

Acupuncture has been practiced in China for more than 5000 years. Acupuncture was particularly valued by the practitioners of martial art who dealt mainly with acute injuries and overuse chronic painful conditions. With this tradition, acupuncture has an overwhelming role in the armamentarium of healers who deal with sports injuries that require instantaneous and quick recovery.

The practical value of acupuncture is so obvious that it has been included into the broad area of alternative medical practice on an international level. In 1984, the WHO interregional seminar drew up a provisional list of 47 diseases and conditions that lend themselves to acupuncture treatment (Chung 1984). Amongst them, 16 are musculoskeletal and neurologic disorders.

MANIPULATIVE THERAPY—TUI-NA

Tui-na is an oriental bodywork therapy that has been used in China for 2000 years. According to Beal (2000), the current form of traditional Chinese manipulative therapy is Tui-na, which appeared in texts written in the Ming Dynasty (1368–1644 CE). Tui means "push" and na means "squeeze and lift." Tui-na uses the traditional Chinese medical theory of the flow of Qi through the meridians as its basic therapeutic orientation. Through the application of massage and manipulation techniques, Tui-na seeks to establish a more harmonious flow of Qi through the system of channels and collaterals, allowing the body to naturally heal itself.

TAI CHI

Athletes recovering from the acute phase of tendinopathies will need to go through an appropriate phase of rehabilitation. The traditional Chinese Tai Chi offers an excellent option (Fig. 14.3). Tai Chi is a low weight bearing exercise with muscle strengthening elements, especially for the lower extremities. It is best characterized by its closed kinetic chain, sports specificity, weight bearing, and proprioceptional properties. It is essentially a generative restorative exercise to enhance body functions

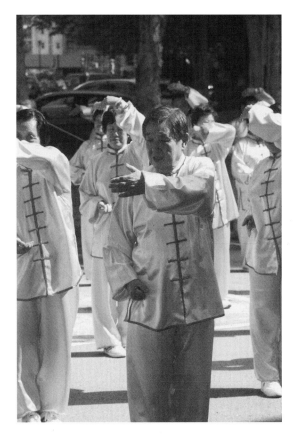

Fig. 14.3 Tai Chi exercise.

in promoting muscle performance, increasing flexibility and proprioception while the weight bearing nature stimulates bone and soft tissue. It is therefore recommended as an option of rehabilitation for athletes during their acute phase of tendinopathy.

In summary, to date, there is still a lack of understanding of the exact pathogenesis of tendinosis. The outcome of all the current treatment modalities is certainly not outstanding. This is precisely the background of the inclination of some clinicians to tackle this intriguing problem with an alternative approach.

Materials and methods

Scientific concept of tendon "non-healing" in tendinopathy

Tendinopathies are often described as a "non-healing" status in tendons, chiefly manifested as failed responses to conservative treatments and characterized by histopathologic changes as tendinosis. A theoretical model for the tendinosis cycle was proposed by Leadbetter (1992) and modified by Khan (1999):

Inadequate healing → matrix disturbance → tenocyte death → increased vulnerability to injury → non-healing

This model emphasizes "inadequate" healing which can cause progressive matrix disturbances in a vicious cycle. Overuse and degeneration can be conceived as possible extrinsic factors for the inadequate healing. It follows that the key determinants for the development of non-healing status are the interactions of extrinsic factors and the cells in tendons that might bifurcate the end points of healing.

Therefore, we postulate a model of pathogenesis of tendinosis that primarily stems from the concept of non-healing (Fig. 14.4). Normally, active tenoblasts undergo proliferation, matrix deposition, and apoptosis and differentiation into tenocytes at the end of tendon healing. This process is not 100% guaranteed and several factors may block or deviate the progress of active tenoblasts to its normal destination. For example, persistent inflammatory responses may result in tendinitis. Accumulation of active tenoblasts at the expense of extracellular matrix may lead to a long-standing status of tendinosis. On the other hand, if reparative tenoblasts from peritendinous tissues become too active or fail to revert to tenocytes, excessive fibrotic responses will result in tendon adhesion. Disturbances at different stages of tendon healing may therefore result in different kinds of non-healing tendinopathies. Thus, further studies should focus on the effects of various risk factors on the fate of tendon cells during the healing process. Treatment for tendinopathy should also aim at optimizing the healing process at different stages.

The four main strategies in the management of tendinopathy

There are four main strategies in the holistic management of tendinopathy: herbal medicine, acupuncture, manipulative therapy (Tui-na), and Tai Chi.

HERBAL MEDICINE

There are two major ways of administrating herbal medicine: topical application and parenteral application. While parenteral application essentially refers to orally taking the solution that is obtained by boiling the herbs with water for 1–2 hours, topical application may include ointment, stupe, alcohol-based concoction, medicinal washing, patch and iontophoresis.

In order to create the ointment, the herbs are ground to powder form and dissolved in ointment for application. This medicated ointment is replaced each day and the treatment lasts for approximately 1 week. For stupe, herbs are mixed and heated. The mixture is then allowed to cool until it has reached a temperature that can be tolerated by the patient. Then, the mixture is applied to the affected area for 1 hour two to three times a day for 1 week. An

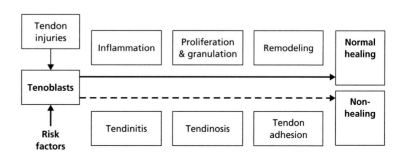

Fig. 14.4 Proposed model of pathogenesis of tendinosis based on the concept of "non-healing."

alcohol-based concoction refers to the process in which herbs are added to alcohol or vinegar and allowed to dissolve in the solvent. Then, the solution is applied to the trauma and heated with infrared. In medicinal washing, the herbs are heated in water for a period of time. The mixture is strained and the herbs discarded. The remaining solution may then be used either hot or cold for bathing or washing the treated area. A patch is a way of administering herbs in which the active ingredients of the drugs are added to a patch and adhered to the treated area.

Iontophoresis, the electrical driving of charged molecules into tissue, passes a small direct current (approximately 0.5 mA·cm^2) through a drug-containing electrode in contact with the skin. A grounding electrode elsewhere on the body completes the circuit. Three main mechanisms enhance molecular transport:

1 Charged species are driven primarily by electrical repulsion from the driving electrode;

2 The flow of electric current may increase the permeability of skin; and

3 Electro-osmosis may affect uncharged molecules and large polar peptides.

Efficiency of transport depends mainly on polarity, valency, and mobility of the charged species, as well as electrical duty cycles and formulation components (Naik *et al*. 2000).

ACUPUNCTURE

Acupuncture is akin to physical medicine, like physical therapy, chiropractic, and massage. Acupuncture has been demonstrated to have very specific anti-inflammatory properties. The insertion of the fine, hair-like acupuncture needle into the acupoints draws out inflammation from the local tissues around the needle by "depolarizing" the inflamed tissue. Acupoints are identified by standard anatomic landmarks supplemented by the measurement with the subject's own hand or finger called the "own body scale." In 1950, Nakatani found that the electric impedance at some acupoints was 1/20 to its surrounding skin area. Impedance detector might therefore further confirm the acupoints (Richardson & Vincent 1986).

Physiologic mechanisms of acupuncture

The two main theories about the physiologic mechanisms of acupuncture are neural and humoral.

Neural The acupunctural points connected together or the channel formed by a series of acupoints is called a meridian. The meridian is closely related to but independent of the peripheral nerves. Anatomically, some acupunctural points are found to have a high concentration of proprioceptive receptors, capillary network, and mast cells. Biophysical studies also demonstrate significant changes in electrophysiologic characteristics such as the impedance. The mechanism of acupuncture has long been the subject of intensive research. It is suggested that neurophysiologic changes related to acupoints are produced by stimulating different receptors around the acupoints.

The characteristic sensation of acupuncture needling, which is called "de qi," is a prerequisite for being effective. It can be evoked only by puncturing and twirling at the acupoint. In general, manual needling evokes activities in Type II and III fibers. Electrical acupuncture stimulation mainly excites Type II fibers while Type III and IV fibers might be excited when needling is applied so strongly that even pain sensation is evoked (Wu 1990).

An alternative neurologic explanation to the mechanism of acupuncture is the process of physiologic learning, which may induce permanent physiologic changes and physiologic memory. The repetitive stimulation on the acupoints by needling causes repetitive firing of neurons. This may alter the anatomic, physiologic, and chemical components of the synaptic junctions, thus creating neuronal memory circuits (Bensoussan 1990).

Humoral Acupuncture has also been found to operate through the hypothalamus–pituitary–adrenal axis through which a number of hormones such as vasopressin (ADH), β-endorphin, adrenocorticotrophin (ACTH) and melanotrophin-stimulating hormone (MSH) may be released to give analgesic effects (Bensoussan 1990). Some other pain relief substances, such as spinal cord enkephalin and dynorphin, midbrain enkephalin, raphemagnus, and reticular para-gigantocellularis, pituitary–hypothalamus β-endorphin, may also be released.

There has been a question of whether meridian mapping is a fact or a myth, as acupoints do not work alone. Acupuncture bears the concept of integrating the whole body by connecting the acupoints to different parts of the body. Generally speaking, the acupoints located at various anatomic regions of our body oversee these regions and form the channels (meridians). Moreover, the points and meridians are anatomically, electrically, and functionally connected (Bensoussan 1990).

In another study of meridians, out of 324 acupoints examined, most were related with a superficial cutaneous nerve, half with a deep cutaneous nerve, and some with both (Zhang 1974). A newer concept of the relationship between meridian distribution and the segmental nerve distribution involving the dermatomes is available. However, channels are not restricted to a single anatomic dermatome and are only partially associated with the functional dermatomes (Bensoussan 1990).

When the acupoint is needled, a sensory stimulus is generated along the meridians called propagated channel sensation. It is debatable whether this propagated channel sensation is a peripheral or a central one. The physiologic changes induced by needling may be explained by the bioelectrical theory of acupuncture which stated that the acupoints and channels are electromagnetic in nature. Needling may alter their electromagnetic properties so as to induce the physiologic changes (Bensoussan 1990).

Last but not the least, more attention should be paid to the integrative physiologic functions of meridian channels but not restrained by its anatomic structure because the nature of meridian is a combination of the peripheral and central nervous systems, circulatory system, and humoral passage.

TUI-NA

Tui-na includes the use of hand techniques to massage the soft tissues (muscles and tendons) of the body, acupressure techniques to directly affect the flow of Qi, and manipulation techniques to realign the musculoskeletal and ligamentous relationships

(bone-setting). Manipulative techniques include stretching and rotation of body parts, and use of the thumbs, hands, elbows, and knees of the practitioner on the client's body. External herbal poultices, compresses, liniments, and salves are also used to enhance other therapeutic methods.

TAI CHI

When compared with high impact exercise, low weight bearing Tai Chi exercise is a unique form of physical activity that involves neuromuscular coordination, low velocity of muscle contraction, and low impact. It involves no jumping and is therefore recommended for people with chronic musculoskeletal conditions, such as elderly people, and is also a good candidate for rehabilitation of athletes during their acute phase of tendinopathy. There are several Tai Chi styles practiced in the Asian culture, such as Chen, Wu, Sun, and Yang. Each style has its own unique features, although they share common kinematics with regard to musculoskeletal function. In general, Tai Chi is a low impact, weight bearing exercise characterized by gentle movements designed to dissipate force throughout the body while the subject changes poses, with well-coordinated sequences of both isometric and isotonic segmental movements in the trunk and four extremities.

Clinical relevance

Herbal medicine

The treatment of herbal medicine on tendon healing is based on several mechanisms, which include the inflammation phase and the proliferation and remodeling phases. The inflammation phase refers to the process in which herbal medicine helps to stop both external and internal bleeding, reduce edema, and provide analgesic effect, facilitate the anti-inflammatory effect as well as remove blood clots, stasis, dead cells, and necrotic tissue.

Recent studies have shown a number of important findings that illustrate the clinical significance of herbal medicine in treating tendinopathy. For example, a complex formula containing *Phellodendron amourense*, *Cacumen Platycladi Orientalis* and

Rheum palmatum L. can reduce pain, swelling, and blood stasis in acute soft tissue injury (Cheng *et al.* 2003). This combination also suppresses non-infective inflammation and enhances proliferation. Yanginhua ointment is another effective herbal medicine for the treatment of acute soft tissue injury. It contains two major herbal medicines: Yangginhua and Zijingpi. Traditionally, Yangginhua has an analgesic effect whereas Zijingpi is a strong anti-inflammatory drug that can reduce edema (Wang & Li 2000).

The proliferation and remodeling phases refer to the process in which herbs might help to promote cell proliferation and matrix deposition, stimulate the growth of new blood vessels (angiogenesis), act as an antioxidant to scavenge free radicals produced by inflammatory cells and ischemia reperfusion injuries, increase uptake of nutrients to target organ by promoting circulation, and decrease the tendon cell growth in a disorganized form and hence reduce the adhesion of tendon.

A number of promising research findings from recent studies have also illustrated that herbal medicine promotes the proliferation and remodeling phases. For example, *Hippophae rhamnoides* (Sea buckthorn, Shaji) has an antioxidant and anti-ulcerogenic effect on wound healing. It has been used for patients with thrombosis because of its suppression on platelet aggregation (Cheng *et al.* 2003). It promotes microcirculation and has a beneficial effect in the healing of connective tissue. Our studies show that the total flavone of *Hippophae rhamnoides* (TFH) may suppress inflammation and promote angiogenesis in tendon healing in animal models. Figure 14.5 shows a well-established gap wound in patellar tendon in animal model to investigate the effect of TFH on healing tendon. The results demonstrated an increase in mean ultimate stress of healing tendon (shown as percentage of healing/sham) from 15.38% to 30.26% at postoperative day 14 with TFH injection after the surgery (Fu *et al.* 2005). However, this medicine had no effect on gene expression of procollagen type I and III on tendon fibroblasts in our studies (Fu *et al.* 2005). TFH can promote the early restoration of tensile strength in healing tendon. While it may not directly act on tendon fibroblasts, TFH may act on other

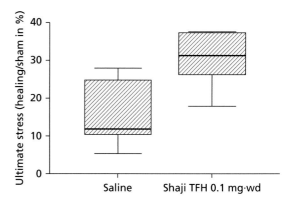

Fig. 14.5 The effect of postoperative total flavone of *Hippophae rhamnoides* (TFH) on ultimate stress of healing tendon.

indirect factors such as mediation of cytokine or angiogenesis to stimulate matrix deposition.

Traditionally, *Dipsacus asperoides* (Xuduan) can help to strengthen the connective tissue, as explained by its Chinese name, "re-union the ruptured." It also acts as an anti-inflammatory or analgesic agent. It has been reported that Xuduan administered intrathecally has a dose-dependent anti-nociceptive effect (Gao *et al.* 2002). *In vitro* studies demonstrated that Xuduan can significantly upregulate the gene expression of procollagen I, III, and decorin in rat tendon fibroblast which may accelerate proliferation and matrix deposition (Fig. 14.6) (Chan *et al.*, unpublished data). In animal

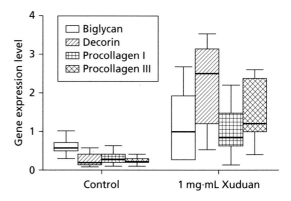

Fig. 14.6 The effect of Xuduan on gene expression level in rat tendon fibroblast.

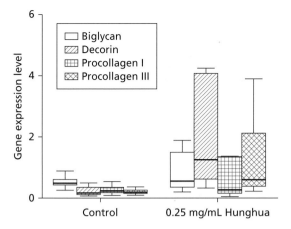

Fig. 14.7 The effect of Hunghua on gene expression level in tendon fibroblast.

studies, we injected Xuduan on healing tendon after the induction of a gap wound in patellar tendon in the rat. The results showed that ultimate stress of tendon at 2 weeks post-injury had been improved.

In Chinese medicine, *Carthamus tinctorius L.* (Honghua) can promote the removal of blood clot and microcirculation. It is useful in the treatment of cardiovascular disease and thrombosis. It acts as a scavenger of oxygen-derived free radicals to reduce the cellular damage induced by cerebral ischemia in rats (Leung *et al.* 1991). The effect of Hunghua on tendon fibroblast is illustrated in Fig. 14.7 (unpublished observation), and the results demonstrated that the gene expression of decorin, biglycan, and procollagen type III of tendon fibroblast was increased by Honghua and implies it may enhance the collagen and proteoglycan deposition.

The topical application of *Cnidium offcinale* (Chuenxiong) gelatin can decrease the adhesion in flexor tendon in chicken (Wei *et al.* 2000). Histologic studies showed that at day 28 after injury, a better alignment of collagen fibers was found in the healing site of the treatment group.

Acupuncture

Sports injuries are associated with pain and swelling. According to the ancient concept of traditional Chinese medicine, pain is within the rank of *Bi* syndrome. It is caused by trauma, "humid"

pathogens, "cold" and "wind." *Bi* syndrome leads to stagnation of *Qi* and blood, and obstructs channels of *Qi*. Manipulation of the acupoints may relieve pain and induce cold sensation, improve circulation and immunity as well as relieve other symptoms such as swelling and hotness. Under most circumstances, the treatment procedure for a diagnosed disease is composed of a number of acupoints. For instance, LIV5 (li gou) on the foot terminal yin involving liver meridian is needled in combination with KID3 (tai xi) on the left ankle, in treatment of Achilles tendinitis (Bensky 1997). A report for treatment of tennis elbow used more than 10 acupoints located at the shoulder and the swollen hands (Wang 1992).

Clinically, positive effects of acupuncture have included an analgesic effect, improvement of circulation and an immunologic response. The analgesic effects of acupuncture were demonstrated as the growth and decline of acupuncture-induced analgesia (Bensoussan 1990). It may be mediated through various neurotransmitters (Bensoussan 1990) such as β-endorphin. The mechanism is not dissimilar to the use of transcutaneous electrical nerve stimulation (TENS). One of the hypotheses for the understanding of the analgesic effects of acupuncture is the gate control theory (Lee & Cheung 1978). Some small nerve fibers send pain impulse to the central nervous system which, in turn, triggers counter impulse down spinal cord to close the gate and decline pain.

Alternatively, the analgesia of acupuncture may be a result of hyperstimulation (Melzack *et al.* 1977). There are some brainstem areas that are known to exert a powerful inhibitory control over transmission in the pain signaling system. These areas, which may be considered to be a "central biasing mechanism," receive inputs from widespread parts of the spinal cord and brain. It is thus conceivable that the relief of pain by stimulation of acupoints may be a result of hyperstimulation. The stimulation through needling could bring about increased inputs to the central biasing mechanism, which may help to close the gates to sensory inputs from selected body areas. The cells of reticular formation area in the mid-brain are known to have large receptive fields and the stimulation of points within the reticular formation can produce analgesia in discrete areas of the body. It is then possible that particular body areas may be projected strongly to some reticular areas, and these, in turn, could completely block the inputs from related parts of the body. In addition, there are other mechanistic explanations of acupuncture-induced analgesia such as muscle spasms, joint problems, and trauma, which also cause blockade of the channels.

Acupuncture has also been demonstrated to improve the elasticity of blood vessels and enlarge capillary networks. This may be influential to the inflammatory process associating with soft tissue injuries and to the resolution of hematoma. Finally, acupuncture may elicit an immunologic response as it alters activities in cell mediated and humoral immunity (Bensoussan 1990).

Recent studies combining acupuncture with the use of a laser may offer new promises. Mester *et al.* (1985) found that under the $0.5-5 \text{ J/cm}^3$ power range, laser radiation stimulates cellular function of the whole tissue irradiated in 15 experimental biologic models. At a higher and non-damaging power, it reduces or even stops biologic functions of the tissue. Bolognani *et al.* (1994) used an infrared laser (904 nm) both *in vitro* and *in vivo* and found an increase in adenosine triphosphate (ATP), Na^+, K^+, and activated ATPase levels after irradiation. Kudoh *et al.* (1988) observed a change in $Na - K$ ATPase in the rat saphenous nerve after treatment with a GaAIAs diode laser (830 nm). The authors emphasized that this phenomenon may be very important for the control of pain because this has the additional advantages of being non-invasive and having better patient tolerance.

On the whole, electricalor LASER (cold LASER) acupuncture is very suitable for the treatment of athletic injuries. With the assistance of an acupoint detector, the application of acupuncture in musculoskeletal injuries could be further simplified and made more effective in the management of the acute or subacute soft tissue injuries.

Tui-na

Tui-na is well suited for the treatment of specific musculoskeletal disorders and chronic stress-related disorders of the digestive, respiratory, and reproductive systems. Therapeutic massage is effective for persistent low back pain, apparently providing long-lasting benefits. Massage was prone to be an effective alternative to conventional medical care for persistent back pain (Cherkin *et al.* 2001). From December 1990 to December 1993, 278 cases of cervical spondylopathy were treated with electroacupuncture and massotherapy. The cure rate was 82.7% in the treated group but only 61% in the control group, indicating that electroacupuncture and massotherapy may enhance the cure rate ($P <0.05$). Of the 278 cases treated in 3–5 sessions, the pain and numbness disappeared in approximately 96% of patients.

Tai Chi

Tai Chi is considered to be a suitable form of exercise for rehabilitating sporting injuries. It promotes integrated improvement in skeletal alignment, tendon function, and joint flexibility. Because of its low impact loading and low velocity nature, and emphasis on proprioceptive and internal sense of body position and motion, Tai Chi helps to reduce the load on the lower limbs joints, particularly in knee and ankle, which are often sites of degeneration in the athletes. Kristeins *et al.* (1991) also did not find any adverse effects on the active range of motion or weight bearing joint integrity of patients with rheumatoid arthritis. From the standpoint of exercise prescription, Tai Chi offers great value for rehabilitation treatment in elderly patients with mild chronic diseases and musculoskeletal disorders. Indeed, Tai Chi is also becoming increasingly popular in health promotion among the geriatric population.

Future directions

Future scientific studies are needed to identify the active ingredients in herbal medicine with regard to its purification and chemical analysis as well as the biologic and pharmacologic activities. Randomized controlled trials are needed to demonstrate the effectiveness of herbal preparation in the systematic diagnosis of indicated cases for treatment and the identification of guidance for adjustments for individual variations.

In managing tendinopathy using herbal medicine, technical advances of drug delivery of herbal preparation will be required for efficient administration. Examples might include industrial preparation of dehydrated granules of herbal preparation and iontophoresis to enhance topical administration of herbal preparation. It is also advisable to merge herbal medicine treatment with modern clinical practice, so that they can complement each other for optimal treatment of tendinopathy.

Acupuncture is an effective ancient Chinese therapy. It is based on symptomatic rather than disease-oriented treatment, and has been interpreted and verified by its own theoretical model. The clinical use of acupuncture is obviously anecdotal. On one hand, we have a wealth of clinical experience well documented in the traditional medicine literature. On the other hand, when scrutinized under the Western medicine discipline such as the exact anatomic structure, physiologic mechanism, and pharmacokinetics, there are still conflicting views. This is precisely why further research should be directed towards the possible mechanism of action by scientific methodology.

Electrical and laser acupuncture are very suitable for treatment of athletic injuries. However, unsatisfactory results in the management of myofascial pain or fibromyalgia were reported (Levin & Huan-Chan 1993). Therefore, further investigations on the application of electrical and laser acupuncture are necessary.

Newer means of acupuncture can be further developed. Osteopuncture is a technique to needle the bone, where rich nerve plexus exist and synapse with nerves to central nervous system. The aim of this therapy is primarily relief of pain in the upper and lower extremities as well as the lower back and the head (Lee & Cheung 1978).

Complications of acupuncture have been well documented. The systemic complication chiefly involves vasovagal syncope as a result of needle stimulation. This is a potential hazard that should be properly recognized and resuscitative measures should be made available. The use of invasive needles is obviously a concern of disease transmission. Strict aseptic technique with the use of disposable needles should be enforced. However, the lack of legislation and control on the use of acupuncture is well reflected by the frequent occurrence of significant infection problems culminating in fat necrosis, scarring, and even functional disabilities. In order to ensure that acupuncture can enjoy a time-honored efficacy, it should be performed with the same respect as any invasive procedure with the utmost precaution and care.

A uniform international legislation concerning the practice of acupuncture should be established, including the syllabus of didactic and clinical training in this field, as there is currently no such legislation. Future development of the scientific basis of acupuncture should make use of the quantifiable nature of electroacupuncture. It has been used to evaluate the effect of other traditional Chinese medicinal treatments such as qigong.

Alternative medicine is gaining recognition in the overall health care delivery system, in particular, the major concern on cost containment and outcome studies. It is therefore timely that acupuncture and other traditional Chinese medicine treatment modalities should be put under the same degree of vigorous assessment to define its future role in the management of soft tissue injuries.

References

Beal, M.W. (2000) Acupuncture and Oriental body work: traditional and biomedical concepts in holistic care: history and basic concepts. *Holistic Nursing Practice* **14**, 69–78.

Bensky, D. (1997) An Achilles heel. In: *Acupuncture in Practice: Case History Insights from the West* (MacPherson, H. & Kaptchuk, T.J., eds) Churchill Livingston, New York.

Bensoussan, A. (1990) Accupuncture as learning. In: *The Vital Meridian: A Modern Exploration of Acupuncture* (Bensoussan, A., ed.) Churchill Livingstone, London: 51–76, 127–132.

Bolognani, L., Bolognani Fantin, A.M., Franchini, A., Volpi, N., Venturelli, T.,

Conti, A.M. (1994) Effects of low-power 632 nm radiation (HeNe laser) on a human cell line: influence on adenyluncleotides and cytoskeletal structures. *Journal of Photochemistry Photobiology B* **26**, 257–264.

Cheng, J., Kondo, K., Suzuki, Y., Ikeda, Y., Meng, X. & Umemura, K. (2003) Inhibitory effects of total flavones of

Hippophae Rhamnoides L on thrombosis in mouse femoral artery and *in vitro* platelet aggregation. *Life Sciences* **4**, 2263–2271.

Cherkin, D.C., Eisenberg, D., Sherman, K.J., *et al*. (2001) Randomized trial comparing traditional Chinese medical acupuncture, therapeutic massage, and self-care education for chronic low back pain. *Archives of Internal Medicine* **161**, 1081–1088.

Chung, F.S. (1984) Fundamentals of acupuncture and moxibustion. Taipei China Acupuncture Research Institute 1984, Dec 10–11. (In Chinese).

Fu, S.C., Hui, C.W.C., Li, L.C., *et al*. (2005) Shaji TFH promotes early restoration of mechanical properties in healing patella tendon. *Medical Engineering and Physics* **27**, 313–321.

Gao, Z., Zou, K. & Liao, Q.B. (2002) Scavenging effects of Dipsacus asper Wall on DPPH Radical group. *Journal of China Three Gorges University (Natural Sciences)* **24**, 366–368.

Khan, K.M., Cook, J.L., Bonar, F., Harcourt, P. & Astrom, M. (1999) Histopathology of common tendinopathies. Update and implications for clinical management. *Sports Medicine* **27**, 393–408.

Kristeins, A., Dietz, F. & Hwang, S. (1991) Evaluating the safety and potential use of a weight-bearing exercise, tai-chi chuan, for rheumatoid arthritis patients. *American Journal of Physical Medicine and Rehabilitation* **70**, 136–141.

Kudoh, Ch., Inomata, K., Okajima, K., Motegi, M., Ohshiro, T. (1988) Low level laser therapy pain attenuation mechanisms, 1: Histochemical and biochemical effects of 830 nm gallium aluminium arsenide diode laser radiation on rat saphenous nerve Na-K-ATPase activity. *Laser Therapy*, 3–6.

Leadbetter, W.B. (1992) Cell–matrix response in tendon injury. *Clinics in Sports Medicine* **11**, 533–578.

Lee, J.F. & Cheung, C.S. (1978) Osteopunture. In: *Current Accupunture Therapy* (Lee, J.F. & Cheung, C.S., eds) Medical Book Publications: 374–376.

Leung, A.W.N., Mo, Z.X. & Zheng, Y.S. (1991) Reduction of cellular damage induced by cerebral ischemia in rats. *Neurochemical Research* **16**, 687–692.

Levin, M.F. & Hui-Chan, C.W.Y. (1993) Conventional and acupuncture like transcutaneous electrical nerve stimulation excite similar afferent fibers. *Archives of Physical Medicine and Rehabilitation* **74**, 54–60.

Melzack, R., Stillwell, D.M., Fox, E.J. (1977) Trigger points and acupuncture points for pain: correlations and implications. *Pain* **3**, 3–23.

Mester, E., Mester, A.F., Mester, A. (1985) The biomedical effects of laser application. *Lasers in Surgery and Medicine* **5**, 31–9.

Naik, A., Kalia, Y.N. & Guy, R.H. (2000) Transdermal drug delivery: overcoming the skin's barrier function. *Pharmaceutical Science and Technology Today* **3**, 318–326.

Richardson, P.H. & Vincent, C.A. (1986) Acupuncture for the treatment of pain: A review of evaluative research. *Pain* **24**, 15–40.

Wang, K. (1992) A report of 22 cases of temporomandibular joint dysfunction syndrome treated with acupuncture and laser radiation. *Journal of Traditional Chinese Medicine* **12**, 116–118.

Wang, P.M. & Li, Z.W. (2000) Effect of Yanginhua ointment in the treatment of acute closed soft tissue injury. *China Journal of Orthopaedics and Traumatology* **13**, 209–210.

Wei, L., Zhu, F.W., Li, K. (2000) A study on the effect of tetramethylpyrazine topical gelatin dressing to prevent flexor tendon adhesion. *Journal of Guang Xi Chinese Medicine Academy* **17** (4): 57–58.

World Health Organization. WHO Traditional Medicine Strategy 2002–2005. Document WHO/EDM/TRM/2002.1. WHO, Geneva: 7.

Wu, D.Z. (1990) Acupuncture and neurophysiology. *Clinical Neurology and Neurosurgery* **92**, 13–25.

Zhang, X.J. (1974) A hypothesis on the relationship of Meridians, skin cortex and Zang/Fu Organs. In: *Acupuncture*, Ed. By Shanghai Chinese Medical School, People Healthcare Publishing, Beijing: p. 100. [Translated from Chinese]

Chapter 15

Surgery for Chronic Overuse Tendon Problems in Athletes

DEIARY KADER AND NICOLA MAFFULLI

Excessive loading of the musculotendinous unit during vigorous training activities is regarded as the main pathologic stimulus that leads to tendinopathy. When conservative management of tendinopathy is unsuccessful, surgery may be necessary. Although 85% of patients return to competitive sports following surgery, we do not know the physiologic, biochemical, and biologic bases of its effects. While there are several surgical techniques to deal with the same clinical problem, comparative studies are lacking and no randomized trial has ever been performed in the field of surgery for tendinopathy. Each tendon has peculiarities in terms of clinical presentation, specific aspects of conservative and surgical management, recovery, etc. The discussion that follows focuses on the Achilles and patella tendon, as they are the most studied and commonly encountered in clinical practice. Also, many of the technical and biologic considerations applied to those two tendons can be extrapolated to other tendons. However, it is acknowledged that not all tendons behave in the same fashion, and that different areas in the same tendon give rise to different pathologies (e.g. tendinopathy of the main body of the Achilles tendon, and insertional Achilles tendinopathy). Hence, different management strategies have to be implemented. While the patient's plans may dictate the timeline to return to a high level of training and competition, 6 months of rehabilitation is generally recommended after surgery. Even successful surgery for chronic overuse tendon conditions does not reconstitute a normal tendon. Usually, the result is functionally satisfactory despite morphologic differences and biomechanical weakness compared to a normal tendon. The therapeutic use of growth factors by gene transfer may produce a tendon that is biologically, biomechanically, biochemically, and physiologically more "normal."

Introduction

Overuse tendon injuries are a major problem in sports and occupational medicine. Up to 50% of all sports injuries are caused by overuse (Herring & Nilson 1987). Repetitive overload of the musculotendinous unit beyond the physiologic threshold, with inadequate time for tissue restoration, often leads to chronic overuse tendon injuries, which is best described by the term tendinopathy. We advocate the use of the term tendinopathy as a generic descriptor of the clinical conditions in and around tendons arising from overuse (Khan & Maffulli 1998; Maffulli et al. 1998b). The terms tendinosis and tendinitis should be used after histopathologic examination (Maffulli et al. 1998a).

Tendinosis is defined (Józsa & Kannus 1997) as intratendinous degeneration (i.e. hypoxic, mucoid or myxoid, hyaline, fatty, fibrinod, calcific, or some combination of these), resulting from a variety of causes (e.g. aging, microtrauma, vascular compromise) (Leadbetter 1992; Åstrom & Rausing 1995; Józsa & Kannus 1997; Movin et al. 1997; Khan & Maffulli 1998). It is a failure of cell matrix adaptation to trauma brought about by an imbalance between matrix degeneration and synthesis (Leadbetter 1992). Macroscopically, the affected portions of the tendon lose their normal glistening white appearance and become gray and amorphous. The thickening can be diffuse, fusiform, or nodular (Khan *et al.* 1999).

In athletes, upper extremity overuse tendon injuries affect mainly swimmers, tennis players, golfers, throwers, rowers, and weight lifters. The supraspinatus, with or without the biceps tendon, is mainly injured in swimmers, throwers, and weight lifters. Tennis players frequently have problems with the common origin of the wrist extensors (i.e. tennis elbow). Other upper extremity overuse syndromes include golfer's elbow, or tendinopathy of the flexor or pronator tendon, and cross-over tendinopathy of the adductor pollicis longus and extensor pollicis brevis tendons in rowers. In the lower extremity, overuse tendon injuries affect mainly football players, runners, ballet dancers, sprinters, and basketball and volleyball players. Achilles and posterior tibial tendons overuse injuries are often seen in football players and runners. Ballet dancers typically present with flexor hallucis longus tendinopathy, and sports involving jumping (e.g. basketball, volleyball) often cause symptoms in the patellar tendon.

Tendinopathy has been attributed to a variety of intrinsic and extrinsic factors including tendon vascularity, age, gender, body weight and height, changes in training pattern, poor technique, inadequate warm-up and stretching prior to training, previous injuries, and environmental factors (Kvist 1991a; Binfield & Maffulli 1997).

The source of pain in tendinopathy is still under investigation. Classically, pain was attributed to inflammatory processes. However, tendinopathies are degenerative, not inflammatory conditions. Tendon degeneration with mechanical breakdown of collagen could theoretically explain the pain mechanism, but clinical and surgical observations challenge this view (Khan *et al.* 2000a). Recently, the biochemical model has become more appealing because of the identification of many chemical irritant and neurotransmitters such as lactate, chondroitin sulfate, substance P and glutamate which may produce pain in tendinopathy (Khan *et al.* 2000b; Alfredson *et al.* 2002).

The main stay of tendinopathy treatment remains conservative. Over the years, various treatment programs have been tried: physical therapy, rest, training modification, splintage, taping, cryotherapy, electrotherapy, pharmaceutical agents such as non-steroidal anti-inflammatory drugs (NSAIDs), and various peritendinous injections. Most of these treatments essentially follow the same principles. However, very few randomized, prospective, placebo controlled trials exist to assist in choosing the best evidence-based treatment. Surgery, on the other hand, is only recommended to patients in whom conservative management has proved ineffective for at least 6 months. Studies have shown that 24–45.5% of patients with tendinopathy fail to respond to conservative treatment and eventually require surgical intervention (Kvist & Kvist 1980; Leppilahti *et al.* 1991; Paavola *et al.* 2002).

What do we know?

Primary tendon healing

As in other areas in the body, tendon healing occurs in three integrated phases:
1 Inflammatory phase;
2 Reparative or collagen-producing phase; and
3 Organization or remodeling phase.
Tendons possess intrinsic and extrinsic healing capabilities. The intrinsic model produces obliteration of the tendon and its tendon sheath. Extrinsic healing occurs through the migration of tenocytes into the defect from the ends of the tendon sheath (Wang 1998). Initially, the extrinsic response, which far outweighs the intrinsic one, results in rapid filling of the defect with granulation tissue, tissue debris, and haematoma (Sharma & Maffulli 2005). The migrating tenocytes have a phagocytic role, and are arranged in a radial fashion in relation to the direction of the fibers of the tendon (Maffulli & Benazzo 2000). In the inflammatory phase, 3–7 days after injury, cells migrate from the extrinsic peritendinous tissue such as the tendon sheath, periosteum, subcutaneous tissue, and fascicles, as well as from the epitenon and endotenon (Reddy *et al.* 1999).

The migrated tenocytes begin to synthesize collagen around day 5 and for the next 5 weeks. Initially, these collagen fibers are randomly oriented. During the fourth week, a noticeable increase in the proliferation of tenocytes of intrinsic origin, mainly from the endotenon, takes place. These cells take over the main role in the healing process, and both synthesize and reabsorb collagen. The newly formed tissue starts to mature, and the collagen fibers are increasingly oriented along the direction of force through the tendon. This phase of repair continues for about 8 weeks after the initial injury. Final stability is acquired during the remodeling induced by the normal physiologic use of the tendon. This further aligns the fibers along the direction of force. In addition, cross-linking between the collagen fibrils increases the tensile strength of the tendon. During the repair phase, the mechanically stronger type I collagen is produced in preference to type III collagen, thus slightly altering the initial ratio of these fibers to increase the strength of the repair.

Despite intensive remodeling over the following months, complete regeneration of the tendon is never achieved. The tissue replacing the defect remains hypercellular. In addition, the diameter of the collagen fibrils is altered, favoring thinner fibrils with reduction in the biomechanical strength of the tendon.

In tendinopathic and ruptured tendons, there is a reduction in the proportion of type I collagen, and a significant increase in the amount of type III collagen (Maffulli *et al.* 2000), responsible for the reduced tensile strength of the new tissue because of a reduced number of cross-links compared to type I collagen (Józsa *et al.* 1990). Recurring micro-injuries lead to the development of hypertrophied, biologically inferior tissue replacing the intact tendon.

Growth factors and other cytokines have a key role in the embryonic differentiation of tissue and in the healing of tissues (Grotendorst 1988). Growth factors stimulate cell proliferation and chemotaxis and aid angiogenesis, influencing cell differentiation. They regulate cellular synthetic and secretory activity of components of extracellular matrix. Finally, growth factors influence the process of healing.

In the normal flexor tendon of the dog, the levels of basic fibroblast growth factor (bFGF) are higher than the levels of platelet derived growth factor (PDGF). In injured tendons, the converse is true (Duffy *et al.* 1995). Under the influence of PDGF, chemotaxis and the rate of proliferation of fibroblasts and collagen synthesis are increased (Pierce *et al.* 1995). Fibroblasts of the patellar tendon show increased proliferation *in vitro* after the administration of bFGF (Chan *et al.* 1997). In addition, an angiogenic effect is evident (Gabra *et al.* 1994). During the embryogenesis of tendon, bone morphogenic proteins (BMP), especially BMP 12 and 13, cause increased expression of elastin and collagen type I. Also, BMP 12 exerts a positive effect on tendon healing (Enzura *et al.* 1996).

The growth factors of the transforming growth factor β superfamily induce an increase in mRNA expression of type I collagen and fibronectin in cell culture experiments (Ignotz & Massague 1986). High expression of type I collagen seems essential to achieve faster healing of tendons. Consequently, there should be a shift from the initial production of collagen type III to type I early in the healing process. The aforementioned growth factors could potentially be used to influence the processes of regeneration of tendons therapeutically. However, it is unlikely that a single growth factor will give a positive result. The interaction of many factors present in the right concentration at the right time will be necessary.

Operative management of tendinopathy

In overuse tendon disorders, surgery is recommended after exhausting conservative methods of management. Complete or modified rest from sport, NSAIDs, cryotherapy, deep frictional massage, ultrasound therapy, pulsed electromagnetic fields, laser therapy, orthoses, eccentric exercises (Blazina *et al.* 1973; Baker 1984), and local administration of sclerosing drug (Alfredson 2004) have all been described in the management of tendinopathy, together with local peritendinous injections of steroids or aprotinin for review (Kader *et al.* 2002; Maffulli & Kader 2002). If these measures fail, surgery is an option (Leadbetter *et al.* 1992; Khan *et al.* 2000b).

Treatment of chronic tendinopathy aims to allow patients to return to a normal level of physical activity (Leadbetter *et al.* 1992; Khan *et al.* 2000b). Percutaneous needling of the tendon for such purpose has been reported, even though no results have been published (Leadbetter *et al.* 1992), and open longitudinal tenotomy has been long established (Orava *et al.* 1986; Khan *et al.* 2000b). In the absence of frank tears, the traditional operation involves a longitudinal skin incision over the tendon (Martens *et al.* 1982; Phillips 1992), paratenon incision and stripping, multiple longitudinal tenotomies, and excision of the area of degeneration if present (Orava *et al.* 1986; Khan *et al.* 2000a). The goal of surgery is to promote wound repair induced by a modulation of the tendon cell–matrix environment (Leadbetter *et al.* 1992), but even in very experienced surgeons, the rate of complications can be high (Paavola *et al.* 2000a) and success is not guaranteed (Maffulli *et al.* 1999).

A variety of surgical methods for treatment of patella tendinopathy have been described. These include drilling of the inferior pole of the patella, realignment (Biedert *et al.* 1997), excision of macroscopic degenerated areas (Karlsson *et al.* 1991; Raatikainen *et al.* 1994), repair of macroscopic defects (Martens *et al.* 1982), longitudinal tenotomy (Puddu & Cipolla 1993), percutaneous needling (Leadbetter *et al.* 1992), percutaneous longitudinal tenotomy (Testa *et al.* 1999), and arthroscopic débridement (Coleman *et al.* 2000a).

Surgical treatment of Achilles tendinopathy can be broadly grouped in four categories:
1 Open tenotomy with removal of abnormal tissue without stripping the paratenon;
2 Open tenotomy with removal of abnormal tissue and stripping of the paratenon;
3 Open tenotomy with longitudinal tenotomy and removal of abnormal tissue with or without paratenon stripping; and
4 Percutaneous longitudinal tenotomy (Schepsis & Leach 1987; Nelen *et al.* 1989; Leach *et al.* 1992; Testa *et al.* 1996; Clancy & Heiden 1997; Rolf & Movin 1997).

The technical objective of surgery is to excise fibrotic adhesions, remove degenerated nodules and make multiple longitudinal incisions in the tendon to detect and excise intratendinous lesions. Reconstruction procedures may be required if large lesions are excised (Ljungqvist 1967). We use peroneus brevis tendon transfer when the tendinopathic process has required debulking of at least 50% of the main body of the Achilles tendon (Pintore *et al.* 2001). Other authors have used flexor hallucis longus (Den Hartog 2003).

The biologic objective of surgery is to restore appropriate vascularity and possibly stimulate the remaining viable cells to initiate cell–matrix response and healing (Clancy *et al.* 1976; Clancy & Heiden 1997; Rolf & Movin 1997; Benazzo & Maffulli 2000). It is still unclear as to why multiple longitudinal tenotomies work. Recent investigations show that the procedure triggers neoangiogenesis in the tendon, with increased blood flow (Friedrich *et al.* 2001). This would result in improved nutrition and a more favorable environment for healing.

OUTCOME OF SURGERY

The outcome of surgery for tendinopathy is entirely unpredictable. A review of 23 papers studying the outcome of surgical treatment of patella tendinopathy showed that the outcomes of surgery varied between 46% and 100% (Coleman *et al.* 2000b). In the three studies that had more than 40 patients, authors reported combined excellent and good results of 91%, 82%, and 80% in series of 78, 80, and 138 subjects, respectively. However, in Achilles tendinopathy, most authors report excellent or good result in up to 85% of cases, and most articles reporting surgical success rates have over 70% of successful results (Tallon *et al.* 2001). Schepsis and Leach (1987) report good results in patients with Achilles paratendinopathy and mucoid degeneration. Kvist (1991b) reports good and excellent results of both Achilles paratendinopathy and tendinopathy. However, this is not always observed in clinical practice (Maffulli *et al.* 1999). Recently, it was shown that the scientific methodology behind published articles on the outcome of tendinopathy after surgery is poor, and that the poorer the methodology the higher the success rate (Coleman *et al.* 2000b). Therefore, the long-term outcome of operative management is still not fully clarified.

After Achilles tendon surgery the limb is elevated on a Braun frame. Following review by a physiotherapist, the patient is generally discharged the day following surgery. A full below knee cast is applied with the ankle in natural equinus and retained for 2 weeks until outpatient review. Patients are allowed to bear weight on tip toes of the operated leg as tolerated, but are told to keep the leg elevated as much as possible until seen in the clinic, when the cast is removed. The lower limb is left free, and patients are encouraged to weight bear on the operated limb as soon as they feel comfortable, and to gradually progress to full weight bearing. The patients are taught to perform gentle mobilization exercises of the ankle, isometric contraction of the gastrosoleus complex, and gentle concentric contraction of the calf muscles. Patients are encouraged to perform mobilization of the involved ankle several times per day. Patients are given an appointment 6 weeks from the operation, when they are referred for more intensive physiotherapy. They are allowed to begin gentle exercise such as swimming and cycling at 8 weeks following surgery.

Insertional tendinopathy

Some patients may present with disorders at the osteotendinous junction. Acute insertional tendenopathy is rare. The mainstay of treatment in chronic insertional tendenopathy is again conservative: rest, modification of activities to promote healing, stretching, controlled exercise program, and acupuncture. Operative management should be considered as a last resort and be limited to patients who have failed 6–9 months trial of conservative management (Khan 2000). The seven goals of surgery are listed by Leadbetter et al. (1992): inducing scar tissue, removing aberrant tissue, encouraging healing, relieving extrinsic pressure, relieving tensile overload, repairing relevant tears, and replacing or augmenting injured tendon structure. These goals can be achieved by excising intratendinous or peritendinous abnormal tissue, decompression, bursectomy, synovectomy,

longitudinal tenotomy, and tendon repair or transfer (Sandmeier & Renstrom 1997).

Achilles insertional tendinopathy is a prime example of insertional tendinopathy. It is often associated with retrocalcaneal bursitis (Yodlowski et al. 2002), which can be treated (Alfredson et al. 1998; Baker 1984) by bursectomy, excision of the diseased tendon, and resection of the calcific deposit (Subotnick & Sisney 1986; Kolodziej et al. 1999). If necessary, the Achilles tendon surrounding the area of calcific tendinopathy is detached by sharp dissection. The area of calcific tendinopathy is excised from the calcaneus. The area of hyaline cartilage at the posterosuperior corner of the calcaneus is excised using an osteotome, and, if needed, its base paired off with bone nibblers. The tendon is reinserted in the calcaneus using 2–5 bone anchors. Postoperative care involves keeping the leg in a below knee, lightweight cast and mobilize with crutches under the guidance of a physiotherapist. Patients are allowed to bear weight on the operated leg as tolerated, but are told to keep the leg elevated as much as possible for the first 2 postoperative weeks. The cast is removed 2 weeks after the operation. A synthetic anterior below knee slab is applied, with the ankle in neutral. The synthetic slab is secured to the leg with three or four removable Velcro (Velcro USA Inc., Manchester, NH, USA) straps for 4 weeks. Patients are encouraged to continue to weight bear on the operated limb, and to gradually progress to full weight bearing, if they are not already doing so. Patients are taught gentle mobilization exercises of the ankle, isometric contraction of the gastrosoleus complex, and gentle concentric contraction of the calf muscles. Patients are encouraged to perform mobilization of the involved ankle several times per day after unstrapping the relevant Velcro strap(s). The anterior slab is removed 6 weeks from the operation. Stationary cycling and swimming is recommended from the second week after removal of the cast. We allow return to gentle training 6 weeks after removal of the cast. Gradual progression to full sports activity at 20–24 weeks from the operation is planned according to the patient's progress. Resumption of competition depends on the patient's plans, but is not recommended until 6 months after surgery.

Soft tissue endoscopy

Arthroscopy is now in the armamentarium of orthopaedic surgeon for the routine management of rotator cuff disorders (Bittar 2002). "Tendoscopy" has been used by several authors to approach in a minimally invasive fashion a variety of tendinopathic tendons, including tibialis anterior (Maquirriain *et al.* 2003), Achilles tendon, where the surgical endoscopic technique includes peritenon release and débridement, and longitudinal tenotomies (Maquirriain 1998; Maquirriain *et al.* 2002), patellar tendon (Romeo & Larson 1999), peroneal tendons (van Dijk & Kort 1998), tibialis posterior (van Dijk *et al.* 1997), and tennis elbow (Grifka *et al.* 1995), with encouraging results.

Some authors have used arthroscopic techniques for biceps tenodeses (Gartsman & Hammerman 2000). Given the limited field of vision that these techniques involve, care must be taken to avoid iatrogenic lesion of the surrounding tissues.

To our knowledge, only one study has compared arthroscopic techniques with classic open techniques (Coleman *et al.* 2000a). In that study, which focused on the patellar tendon, arthroscopic patellar tenotomy was as successful as the traditional open procedure, and both procedures provided virtually all subjects with symptomatic benefit. However, only about half of the subjects who underwent either open or arthroscopic patellar tenotomy were able to compete at their former sporting level at follow-up.

More recently, endoscopic techniques have been used to manage tibialis posterior and peroneal tendinopathy (van Dijk *et al.* 1997, van Dijk & Kort 1998; Chow *et al.* 2005), showing that it is effective in controlling stage I tibialis posterior tendon dysfunction, with small scars, little wound pain, and a short hospital stay.

Future directions

Gene therapy to provide growth factors

Growth factors have a limited biologic half-life. Given the complexity of the healing process of tendons, a single application of growth factors is unlikely to be successful. As there is no bioavailability of oral proteins, repeated local injections would be necessary to maintain levels in the therapeutic range. This can be technically difficult in operatively treated tendons. The transfer of genes for the relevant growth factors seems an elegant alternative (Moller *et al.* 1998). After cellular uptake and expression of genes, high levels of the mediators can be locally produced and secreted.

To achieve this goal, viral and non-viral vectors are used, enabling the uptake and expression of genes into target cells. Viral vectors are viruses deprived of their ability to replicate into which the required genetic material can be inserted. They are effective, as the introduction of their genetic material into host cells forms part of their normal life cycle. Non-viral vectors have specific characteristics that enable penetration of the nucleus (e.g. liposomal transport). The genes are released in the vicinity of the target cells without systemic dilution.

In vivo and *in vitro* strategies are employed for transfer using vectors. For *in vivo* transfer, the vectors are applied directly to the relevant tissue. *In vitro* transfer involves removal of cells from the body. The gene is then transferred *in vitro*, and these cells are cultured before being reintroduced into the target site. Direct transfer is less invasive and technically easier, and can be started during treatment of the acute phase of the injury. A disadvantage is the non-specific infection of cells during the injection process. In addition, because of the amount of extracellular matrix present, a vector with high transgenic activity is necessary to be able to transfer the gene to enough cells.

Indirect transfer of genes is safer. The relevant cell type is isolated and genetically modified. Prior to reintroduction into the body, cells can be selected and tested for quality. Because of the work involved in this technique, it would be more suitable for the treatment of degenerative processes instead of acute injuries. The first studies on the feasibility of this procedure have been conducted using marker genes (Lou *et al.* 1996). The main gene used, LacZ, codes for the bacterial beta galactosidase, which is not present in eukaryotic cells.

The addition of a suitable substrate changes the staining properties of the cells, which express the new gene, thus enabling to ascertain the effectiveness of transmission and the duration of expression of the foreign gene. With the vectors currently available, the gene is expressed for 6–8 weeks in tendon tissue. Using this strategy, the transfer and expression of PDGF gene into the patellar tendon of rats led to an increase in angiogenesis and collagen synthesis in the tendon over 4 weeks. Gene expression of this duration could influence the whole healing process of tendons and could be the start of an optimized healing process (Maffulli *et al.* 2002).

Summary

What do we know?

Conservative management of tendinopathy is often unsuccessful, and surgery is therefore necessary. Although surgery allows return to competitive sport in up to 85% of cases, we do not know the physiologic, biochemical, and biologic bases of its effects. Hence, new treatments are difficult to plan and execute.

What do we need to know?

How does surgery work? Is the same mechanism of action at work in different tendons and at different locations in the same tendon? What are the physiologic, biochemical, and biologic bases of the action of surgery?

How do we get there?

There are several surgical techniques to deal with the same clinical problem, but comparative studies are lacking, and no randomized trial has ever been performed in this field. From a biologic viewpoint, we need to ascertain whether tendon healing can be improved upon by the use of growth factors and gene therapy, or additional, better planned postoperative rehabilitation regimes.

Conclusions

Surgery for chronic overuse tendon conditions, even when successful, does not result in a normal tendon. Mostly, the result is functionally satisfactory despite morphologic differences and biomechanical weakness compared with a normal tendon. The therapeutic use of growth factors by gene transfer seems may produce a tendon that is biologically, biomechanically, biochemically, and physiologically more "normal."

References

Alfredson, H. (2004) Chronic tendon pain: implications for treatment: an update. *Current Drug Targets* **5**, 407–410.

Alfredson, H., Bjur, D., Thorsen, K., Lorentzon, R. & Sandstrom, P. (2002) High intratendinous lactate levels in painful chronic Achilles tendinosis. An investigation using microdialysis technique. *Journal of Orthopaedic Research* **20**, 934–938.

Alfredson, H., Pietila, T. & Jonsson, P. (1998) Heavy-load eccentric calf muscle training for the treatment of chronic Achilles tendinosis. *American Journal of Sports Medicine* **26**, 360–366.

Astrom, M. & Rausing, A. (1995) Chronic Achilles tendinopathy. A survey of surgical and histopathologic findings. *Clinical Orthopaedics and Related Research* 151–164.

Baker, B.E. (1984) Current concepts in the diagnosis and treatment of musculotendinous injuries. *Medical Science Sports Exercise* **16**, 323–327.

Benazzo, F. & Maffulli, N. (2000) An operative approach to Achilles tendinopathy. *Sports Medicine Arthroscopy Review* **8**, 96–101.

Biedert, R., Vogel, U. & Friedrichs, N.F. (1997) Chronic patellar tendinitis: a new surgical treatment. *Sports Exercise and Injury* **3**, 150–154.

Binfield, P.M. & Maffulli, N. (1997) Surgical management of common tendinopathies of the lower limb. *Sports Exercise and Injury* **3**, 116–122.

Bittar, E.S. (2002) Arthroscopic management of massive rotator cuff tears. *Arthroscopy* **18** (Suppl 2), 104–106.

Blazina, M.E., Kerlan, R.K., Jobe, F.W. & Carter, V.S. (1973) Jumper's knee. *Orthopaedic Clinics of North America* **4**, 665–672.

Chan, B.P., Chan, K.M., Maffulli, N., Webb, S. & Lee, K.K. (1997) Effect of basic fibroblast growth factor. An *in vitro* study of tendon healing. *Clinical Orthopaedics and Related Research* **342**, 239–247.

Chow, H.T., Chan, K.B. & Lui, T.H. (2005) Tendoscopic debridement for stage I posterior tibial tendon dysfunction. *Knee Surgery, Sports Traumatology, Arthroscopy* **13**, 695–698.

Clancy, W.G. & Heiden, E.A. (1997) Achilles tendinitis treatment in the athletes. Contemporary approaches to the Achilles Tendon. *Foot and Ankle Clinics* 1083–1095.

Clancy, W.G.J., Neidhart, D. & Brand, R.L. (1976) Achilles tendonitis in runners: a report of five cases. *American Journal of Sports Medicine* **4**, 46–57.

Coleman, B.D., Khan, K.M., Kiss, Z.S., Bartlett, J., Young, D.A. & Wark, J.D.

(2000a) Outcomes of open and arthroscopic patellar tenotomy for chronic patellar tendinopathy: a retrospective study. *American Journal of Sports Medicine* **28**, 183–190.

Coleman, B.D., Khan, K.M., Maffulli, N., Cook, J.L. & Wark, J.D. (2000b) Studies of surgical outcome after patellar tendinopathy: Clinical significance of methodological deficiencies and guidelines for future studies. *Scandinavian Journal of Medicine and Science in Sports* **10**, 2–11.

Den Hartog, B.D. (2003) Flexor hallucis longus transfer for chronic Achilles tendonosis. *Foot and Ankle International* **24**, 233–237.

Duffy, F.J. Jr, Seiler, J.G., Gelberman, R.H. & Hergrueter, C.A. (1995) Growth factors and canine flexor tendon healing: initial studies in uninjured and repair models. *Journal of Hand Surgery [American]* **20**, 645–649.

Enzura, Y., Rosen, V. & Nifuji, A. (1996) Induction of hypertrophy in healing patellar tendon by implantation of human recombinant BMP 12. *Journal of Bone and Mineral Research* **11**, 401.

Friedrich, T., Schmidt, W. & Jungmichel, D. (2001) Histopathology in rabbit Achilles tendon after operative tenolysis (longitudinal fiber incisions). *Scandinavian Journal of Medicine and Science in Sports* **11**, 4–8.

Gabra, N., Khayat, A., Calabresi, P. & Khayat, A. (1994) Detection of elevated basic fibroblast growth factor during early hours of *in vitro* angiogenesis using a fast ELISA immunoassay. *Biochemical and Biophysics Research Communications* **205**, 1423–1430.

Gartsman, G.M. & Hammerman, S.M. (2000) Arthroscopic biceps tenodesis: operative technique. *Arthroscopy* **16**, 550–552.

Grifka, J., Boenke, S. & Kramer, J. (1995) Endoscopic therapy in epicondylitis radialis humeri. *Arthroscopy* **11**, 743–748.

Grotendorst, G.R. (1988) Growth factors as regulators of wound repair. *International Journal of Tissue Reactions* **10**, 337–344.

Herring, S.A. & Nilson, K.L. (1987) Introduction to overuse injuries. *Clinics in Sports Medicine* **6**, 225–239.

Ignotz, R.A. & Massague, J. (1986) Transforming growth factor-beta stimulates the expression of fibronectin and collagen and their incorporation into the extracellular matrix. *Journal of Biological Chemistry* **25**, 4337–4345.

Józsa, L. & Kannus, P. (1997) *Human Tendon: Anatomy, Physiology and Pathology.* Human Kinetics, Champaign, IL.

Józsa, L., Reffy, A., Kannus, P., Demel, S. & Elek, E. (1990) Pathological alterations in human tendons. *Archives of Orthopaedic and Trauma Surgery* **110**, 15–21.

Kader, D., Saxena, A., Movin, T. & Maffulli, N. (2002) Achilles tendinopathy: some aspects of basic science and clinical management. *British Journal of Sports Medicine* **36**, 239–249.

Karlsson, J., Lundin, O., Lossing, I.W. & Peterson, L. (1991) Partial rupture of the patellar ligament. Results after operative treatment. *American Journal of Sports Medicine* **19**, 403–408.

Khan, K.M. (2000) Overuse tendinosis, not tendonitis. *Journal of Sports Medicine and Physical Fitness* **28**, 38–48.

Khan, K.M. & Maffulli, N. (1998) Tendinopathy: an Achilles heel for athletes and clinicians. *Clinical Journal of Sport Medicine* **8**, 151–154.

Khan, K.M., Cook, J.L. & Bonar, F. (1999) Histopathology of common tendinopathies. Update and implications for clinical management. *Sports Medicine* **27**, 393–408.

Khan, K.M., Cook, J.L. & Maffulli, N. (2000a) Where is the pain coming from in tendinopathy? It may be biochemical, not only structural, in origin. *British Journal of Sports Medicine* **34**, 81–83.

Khan, K., Jill, L. & Cook, P.T. (2000b) Overuse tendon injuries: where does the pain come from? *Sports Medicine Arthroscopy Review* **8**, 17–31.

Kolodziej, P., Glisson, R.R. & Nunley, J.A. (1999) Risk of avulsion of the Achilles tendon after partial excision for treatment of insertional tendonitis and Haglund's deformity: a biomechanical study. *Foot and Ankle International* **20**, 433–437.

Kvist, H. & Kvist, M. (1980) The operative treatment of chronic calcaneal paratenonitis. *Journal of Bone and Joint Surgery. British volume* **62**, 353–357.

Kvist, M. (1991a) Achilles tendon overuse injuries. University of Turku, Finland.

Kvist, M. (1991b) Achilles tendon injuries in athletes. *Annales Chirurgiae et Gynaecologiae* **80**, 188–201.

Leach, R.E., Schepsis, A.A., Takai, H. (1992) Long-term results of surgical management of Achilles tendinitis in runners. *Clinical Orthopaedics and Related Research* 208–212.

Leadbetter, W.B. (1992) Cell–matrix response in tendon injury. *Clinics in Sports Medicine* **11**, 533–578.

Leadbetter, W.B., Mooar, O.A., Lane, G.J. & Lee, S.J. (1992) The surgical treatment of tendinitis. Clinical rationale and biological basis. *Clinics in Sports Medicine* **11**, 679–712.

Leppilahti, J., Orava, S. & Karpakka, J. (1991) Overuse injuries of the Achilles tendon. *Annales Chirurgiae et Gynaecologiae* **80**, 202–207.

Ljungqvist, R. (1967) Subcutaneous partial rupture of the Achilles tendon. *Acta Orthopaedica Scandinavica Supplementum.*

Lou, J., Manske, P.R., Aoki, M. & Joyce, M.E. (1996) Adenovirus-mediated gene transfer into tendon and tendon sheath. *Journal of Orthopaedic Research* **14**, 513–517.

Maffulli, N. & Benazzo, F. (2000) Basic sciences of tendons. *Sports Medicine and Arthroscopy Review* **8**, 1–5.

Maffulli, N., Binfield, P.M. & King, J.B. (1998a) Tendon problems in athletic individuals. *Journal of Bone Joint Surgery. American volume* **80**, 142–143.

Maffulli, N., Binfield, P.M., Moore, D. & King, J.B. (1999) Surgical decompression of chronic central core lesions of the Achilles tendon. *American Journal of Sports Medicine* **27**, 747–752.

Maffulli, N., Ewen, S.W., Waterston, S.W., Reaper, J. & Barrass, V. (2000) Tenocytes from ruptured and tendinopathic achilles tendons produce greater quantities of type III collagen than tenocytes from normal achilles tendons. An *in vitro* model of human tendon healing. *American Journal of Sports Medicine* **28**, 499–505.

Maffulli, N. & Kader, D. (2002) Tendinopathy of tendo achillis [see comment]. *Journal of Bone and Joint Surgery. British volume* **84**, 1–8.

Maffulli, N., Khan, K.M. & Puddu, G. (1998b) Overuse tendon conditions: time to change a confusing terminology. *Arthroscopy* **14**, 840–843.

Maffulli, N., Moller, H.D. & Evans, C.H. (2002) Tendon healing: can it be optimised? *British Journal of Sports Medicine* **36**, 315 0150316.

Maffulli, N., Testa, V., Capasso, G., Bifulco, G. & Binfield, P.M. (1997) Results of percutaneous longitudinal tenotomy for Achilles tendinopathy in middle- and long-distance runners. *American Journal of Sports Medicine* **25**, 835–840.

Maquirriain, J. (1998) Endoscopic release of Achilles peritenon. *Arthroscopy* **14**, 182–185.

Maquirriain, J., Ayerza, M., Costa-Paz, M. & Muscolo, D.L. (2002) Endoscopic surgery in chronic achilles tendinopathies: A preliminary report. *Arthroscopy* **18**, 298–303.

Maquirriain, J., Sammartino, M., Ghisi, J.P. & Mazzuco, J. (2003) Tibialis anterior tenosynovitis: Avoiding extensor retinaculum damage during endoscopic débridement. *Arthroscopy* **19**, 9E.

Martens, M., Wouters, P., Burssens, A. & Mulier, J.C. (1982) Patellar tendinitis: pathology and results of treatment. *Acta Orthopaedica Scandinavica* **53**, 445–450.

Moller, H.D., Evans, C.D., Robins, P.D. & Fu, F.H. (1998) Gene therapy in orthopaedic sports medicine. In: *Controversies in Orthopaedic Sports Medicine* (Chan, K.M., Fu, F.H., Maffulli, N., Kurosaka, M., Rolf, C. & Liu, S., eds). Williams and Wilkins, Hong Kong: 577–588.

Movin, T., Gad, A. & Reinholt, F.P. (1997) Tendon pathology in long-standing achillodynia. Biopsy findings in 40 patients. *Acta Orthopaedica Scandinavica* **68**, 170–175.

Nelen, G., Martens, M. & Burssens, A. (1989) Surgical treatment of chronic Achilles tendinitis. *American Journal of Sports Medicine* **17**, 754–759.

Orava, S., Osterback, L. & Hurme, M. (1986) Surgical treatment of patellar tendon pain in athletes. *British Journal of Sports Medicine* **20**, 167–169.

Paavola, M., Kannus, P., Jarvinen, T.A., Khan, K., Jozsa, L. & Jarvinen, M. (2002) Achilles tendinopathy. *Journal of Bone and Joint Surgery. American volume* **84**, 2062–2076.

Paavola, M., Kannus, P. & Paakkala, T. (2000a) Long-term prognosis of patients with Achilles tendinopathy. *American Journal of Sports Medicine* **28**, 634–642.

Paavola, M., Orava, S. & Leppilahti, J. (2000b) Chronic Achilles tendon overuse injury: complications after surgical

treatment. An analysis of 432 consecutive patients. *American Journal of Sports Medicine* **28**, 77–82.

Phillips, B.B. (1992) Traumatic disorders of tendon. In: *Campbell's Operative Orthopaedics* (Crenshaw, A.H., ed.) Mosby-Year Book, St. Louis: 1921–1922.

Pierce, G.F., Tarpley, J.E., Tseng, J., *et al.* (1995) Detection of platelet-derived growth factor (PDGF)-AA in actively healing human wounds treated with recombinant PDGF-BB and absence of PDGF in chronic nonhealing wounds. *Journal of Clinical Investigations* **96**, 1336–1350.

Pintore, E., Barra, V., Pintore, R. & Maffulli, N. (2001) Peroneus brevis tendon transfer in neglected tears of the Achilles tendon. *Journal of Trauma* **50**, 71–78.

Puddu, G. & Cipolla, M. (1993) Tendinitis. In: *The Patellofemoral Joint* (Fox, J.M. & Del Pizzo, W., eds). McGraw-Hill, New York.

Raatikainen, T., Karpakka, J., Puranen, J. & Orava, S. (1994) Operative treatment of partial rupture of the patellar ligament. A study of 138 cases. *International Journal of Sports Medicine* **15**, 46–49.

Reddy, G.K., Stehno-Bittel, L. & Enwemeka, C.S. (1999) Matrix remodeling in healing rabbit Achilles tendon. *Wound Repair and Regeneration* **7**, 518–527.

Rolf, C. & Movin, T. (1997) Etiology, histopathology, and outcome of surgery in achillodynia. *Foot and Ankle International* **18**, 565–569.

Romeo, A.A. & Larson, R.V. (1999) Arthroscopic treatment of infrapatellar tendonitis. *Arthroscopy* **15**, 341–345.

Sandemeier, R. & Renstrom, P. (1997) Diagnosis and treatment of chronic tendon disorders in sports. *Scandinavian*

Journal of Medicine and Science in Sports **7**, 55–61.

Schepsis, A.A. & Leach, R.E. (1987) Surgical management of Achilles tendinitis. *American Journal of Sports Medicine* **15**, 308–315.

Sharma, P. & Maffulli, N. (2005) Tendon injury and tendinopathy: healing and repair. *Journal of Bone Joint Surgery. American volume* **87**, 187–202.

Subotnick, S. & Sisney, P. (1986) Treatment of Achilles tendinopathy in the athlete. *Journal of the American Podiatric Medical Association* **76**, 552–557.

Tallon, C., Coleman, B.D. & Khan, K.M. (2001) Outcome of surgery for chronic Achilles tendinopathy: a critical review. *American Journal of Sports Medicine* **29**, 315–320.

Testa, V., Maffulli, N., Capasso, G. & Bifulco, G. (1996) Percutaneous longitudinal tenotomy in chronic Achilles tendonitis. *Bulletin of the Hospital for Joint Diseases* **54**, 241–244.

Testa, V., Capasso, G., Maffulli, N. & Bifulco, G. (1999) Ultrasound guided percutaneous longitudinal tenotomy for the management of patellar tendinopathy. *Medicine and Science in Sports and Exercise* 1509–1515.

van Dijk, C.N. & Kort, N. (1998) Tendoscopy of the peroneal tendons. *Arthroscopy* **14**, 471–478.

van Dijk, C.N., Kort, N. & Scholten, P.E. (1997) Tendoscopy of the posterior tibial tendon. *Arthroscopy* **13**, 692–698.

Wang, E.D. (1998) Tendon repair. *Journal of Hand Therapy* **11**, 105–110.

Yodlowski, M.L., Scheller, A.D. Jr & Minos, L. (2002) Surgical treatment of Achilles tendinitis by decompression of the retrocalcaneal bursa and the superior calcaneal tuberosity. *American Journal of Sports Medicine* **30**, 318–321.

Index